The

Broken

Mirror

The
Broken
Mirror

UNDERSTANDING AND TREATING BODY
DYSMORPHIC DISORDER

Katharine A. Phillips, M.D.

*Butler Hospital and
Brown University
School of Medicine*

OXFORD
UNIVERSITY PRESS

For Ralph

and

for my patients,

whose courage and trust made this book possible

***

OXFORD
UNIVERSITY PRESS

Oxford   New York

Athens   Auckland   Bangkok   Bogotá   Buenos Aires   Calcutta
Cape Town   Chennai   Dar es Salaam   Delhi   Florence   Hong Kong   Istanbul
Karachi   Kuala Lumpur   Madrid   Melbourne   Mexico City   Mumbai
Nairobi   Paris   São Paulo   Singapore   Taipei   Tokyo   Toronto   Warsaw

and associated companies in

Berlin   Ibadan

First published by Oxford University Press, Inc., 1986

First issued as an Oxford University Press paperback, 1998

Oxford is a registered trademark of Oxford University Press

Library of Congress Cataloging-in-Publication Data
Phillips, Katharine A., M.D.
The broken mirror: understanding and treating body dysmorphic disorder /
Katharine A. Phillips, M.D.
p. cm. Includes index.
ISBN 0-19-508317-2
ISBN 0-19-512126-0 (pbk.)
1. Body dysmorphic disorder. I. Title.
RC569.5.B64P48   1997
616.89—ds20   96-4976

7 9 10 8 6

Printed in the United States of America
on acid-free paper

CONTENTS

ACKNOWLEDGMENTS

I want to thank many people and organizations for their role in this book.

I thank my many researcher colleagues for their collaboration on the research discussed in this book, most notably Dr. Susan L. McElroy of the University of Cincinnati School of Medicine, who provided invaluable guidance in starting my research and who continues to be a valued collaborator. Other researcher colleagues deserving thanks are Drs. Harrison Pope, James Hudson, Katherine Atala, William Carter, and Gopinath Mallya of McLean Hospital and Harvard Medical School; Dr. Ralph Albertini of Butler Hospital and Dartmouth and Brown Medical Schools; Dr. Paul Keck of the University of Cincinnati School of Medicine; Dr. Eric Hollander and his colleagues of Mount Sinai School of Medicine; Drs. Jane Eisen, Steven Rasmussen, Mark Zimmerman, Jill Mattia, Doug Beer, Susan Diaz, Joseph Penn, and Caron Zlotnick of Brown University School of Medicine; Drs. Andrew Nierenberg, Maurizio Fava, Jonathan Alpert, Michael Jenike, Lee Baer, Jennifer Soriano, and Richard O'Sullivan of Massachusetts General Hospital and Harvard Medical School; Craig Gunderson and Catherine Carter of Harvard Medical School; Drs. Bruce Lydiard, Olga Brawman-Mintzer, and their colleagues of the Medical University of South Carolina; Dr. Gail Steketee of Boston University School of Social Work; Sarah Taub of McLean Hospital; and Leslie Shapiro and Eyal Muscal of Butler Hospital.

I also give special thanks to my mentors over the years, who have provided invaluable support of my work: Drs. Steven Rasmussen and Martin Keller of Butler Hospital and Brown University School of Medicine; and

Drs. Harrison Pope, James Hudson, and John Gunderson of McLean Hospital and Harvard Medical School.

Without the support of the following organizations, my research and this book would not have been possible: The National Alliance for Research on Schizophrenia and Depression (NARSAD), Butler Hospital and Brown University School of Medicine, McLean Hospital and Harvard Medical School, and The National Institute of Mental Health.

Finally, thank you to those who read through portions of an earlier draft of the book: Dr. Ralph Albertini, Dr. Robert Spitzer, Harry Phillips, Carol Ewin, Barbara Phillips, Suzanne Gluck, Leslie Shapiro, Eyal Muscal, Barbara van Noppen, Chris Saville, Dr. Michele Pato, Dr. Henrietta Leonard, Dr. Fugen Neziroglu, Dr. Robin Goldstein, and my editor Joan Bossert. I am also grateful to Dr. David Veale for his significant contribution to the section on cognitive therapy.

The
Broken
Mirror

To protect confidentiality, all patient names in this book are fictional, and certain details of their stories have been changed. In addition, the longer case descriptions are composites of several cases.

·· *one* ··

Why BDD Matters

Millions of Americans have a secret obsession. They're obsessed with how they look, with a perceived flaw in their appearance. They worry that their nose is too big, their breasts are too small, their skin is blemished, their hair is thinning, their body build is too small—any body part can be the focus of this obsession. It's easy for us to discount these concerns. How can she worry so much about her looks when she's so pretty? Why is he so upset about his hair—it looks fine! But people with these body obsessions suffer greatly, some are severely tormented, some are suicidal.

Most of us care about how we look—we think about our appearance and try to improve it. A recent survey of 30,000 people in fact found that 93% of women and 82% of men care about their appearance and work to improve it. And other surveys have shown that many of us are *dissatisfied* with some aspect of how we look. We're not pretty enough or sufficiently handsome. Who wouldn't like smoother skin, more attractive eyes, a flatter stomach? If we could look better, most of us would. Indeed, most of us try. We wear makeup, buy flattering clothes, check our reflection in mirrors, carefully shave, and curl or straighten our hair, hoping to look okay. But when do normal concerns become an obsession?

While the concerns of body dysmorphic disorder (BDD) echo these normal concerns, they're more extreme. People who have BDD not only dislike some aspect of how they look, they're *preoccupied* with it. They worry too much. They'd like to worry less, but they can't. Many say they're obsessed.

They also suffer. Their worries about their looks cause them significant emotional pain and can interfere with their life. Some BDD sufferers function well despite their distress—no one would ever know how unhappy they are. Carrie, who worried about slight facial blemishes and her "small" breasts, was sometimes late for work because she got stuck in the mirror checking her face. And she missed parties because she thought she looked so bad she didn't want people to see her. Yet she had many friends and did her job well. Because of his supposedly thinning hair, David found it hard to concentrate on his school work and missed the prom, but he still got good grades.

But when BDD is severe, friendships, intimate relationships, and work disintegrate. Jane was so tormented by her "huge" nose, "crooked" lip, "big" jaw, "fat and round" buttocks, and "tiny" breasts that she dropped out of school and couldn't keep a job. She stopped dating and seeing her friends. Because she thought she looked so monstrously ugly, she locked herself up in her house for five years, finally even trying to kill herself.

What's so intriguing about BDD is that people who have it focus on defects that others don't see or consider minimal. Ironically, Jane was actually an attractive woman who had none of the defects she abhorred. David's hair looked fine, and Carrie's breasts were somewhat small, but not noticeably so. But to the BDD sufferer, the problem looks hideous and repulsive, magnified by the mind's eye.

BDD concerns don't make sense to others. How can she worry so much about her hair when it's so nice? How could he be so upset about a few pimples? He should just stop thinking about it. "I'm always telling my wife she looks fine," a high school teacher told me. "Why can't she just stop worrying? Wrinkles aren't that important! I tell her this all the time, but it doesn't seem to help." BDD is a problem because these people *can't stop worrying;* reassurance doesn't put an end to their concern.

Of the many patients I've worked with over the years, those with BDD have been among the most tormented. As a 21-year-old man said to me, "This obsession is the perfect torture. I'd rather be blind or have my arms cut off. I'd be happy to have cancer, because it wouldn't isolate me the way this does, and people would believe that something was wrong with me. They wouldn't trivialize it. I could talk to people about it, and they'd understand."

Since treating Carrie, David, and Jane, I've met and treated many people with BDD. They have all suffered. Families and friends, girlfriends and boyfriends suffer as well. They worry about their loved ones and may endlessly reassure them, hold mirrors, or apply hair tonics—to no avail. They may care for them, pay for surgery, try to find help—for a problem that makes little sense to them. Sometimes they don't even know what the problem is. They know that their loved one is depressed or won't go out, but they don't know why. People with BDD may be too embarrassed to reveal their concern, even to their closest friend or spouse.

After hearing about Carrie's, David's, and Jane's concerns, I decided to learn more about this fascinating and little-known disorder. I hadn't even heard of it during medical school or in the lectures of my psychiatric training. I hadn't noticed any articles about it in scientific journals. I did, however, remember seeing BDD in the psychiatric profession's diagnostic manual. The description there was brief but enough to make me think that Carrie, David, and Jane had this mysterious disorder. I started my search to learn more about it.

I am a physician, a psychiatrist, a clinician, and a researcher. I've been studying and exploring BDD and working with people who have this disorder for the past six years. BDD sufferers have come out of hiding; I haven't had to search for them. They've thought that their face is too wide, their stomach is too fat, or their eyes look ugly. Or that their facial muscles are sagging, their skin has marks or scars, their penis is too small, that . . . . The list goes on. Some search endlessly for an elusive physical cure for what actually is a psychiatric disorder. Many go to doctor after doctor—dermatologists, surgeons, and others—without obtaining relief. Some have surgery after surgery without ever being satisfied with how they look.

Many suffer in silence. People with BDD often feel as though they're harboring a burdensome secret no one will ever understand. Many haven't ever told *a single soul* about their appearance concerns—not even relatives, spouses, or close friends. They feel too embarrassed and ashamed. "I feel foolish talking about my concern," one man told me. "The usual reaction is 'What?!' " Or they fear others will think they're vain. And when they finally divulge their secret, and the people they tell can't see the "defects" or consider them minimal, they feel miserable, isolated, and misunderstood.

One woman had never told her husband about her appearance concerns, even though they'd been married 50 years. "It's a barrier between us," she told me. "It's something I think about a lot, and that I get upset about, but I've never been able to share it with my husband. Even though he's a very understanding person, I'm afraid he wouldn't understand. This is my one secret."

As Cassandra said, "If only I could tell someone what this is about!" Her words reflected what so many people with BDD feel: "I feel so incredibly ridiculous and vain! I also have a feeling of humiliation and shame. I'm miserable, but I can't explain it. It's such a secret. It's as painful as cancer, but I can't tell anyone and get support."

BDD isn't rare. Secrecy and shame are part of the reason BDD is underrecognized and underdiagnosed. Preliminary estimates suggest that it may affect as many as 2% of the U.S. population, which translates into more than 5 million people in this country alone. It affects people of all socioeconomic strata and from all walks of life. BDD also occurs around the world—in Japan, South America, Europe, and other countries.

When I started my research, BDD was virtually unknown, even though it's been described for over 100 years. I myself knew very little about it until some of my patients were courageous enough to reveal their concerns. To learn more about BDD, I've conducted lengthy interviews with approximately 200 people with the disorder, the largest study of this kind. I've also treated many of them. With other researchers, I've done additional studies of BDD, which provide the basis for much of the information here.

I wrote this book because BDD causes so much suffering, it isn't rare, and yet it's virtually unknown. We all need to know that it exists, how to identify it, and what treatments seem to work. Many of my patients have struggled for years with their obsession, having no idea that it's a known disorder with a name and available treatment. Many are relieved to learn they have an identifiable disorder and that they aren't alone in their suffering. And many have significantly benefited from the treatments I'll describe—medications known as serotonin-reuptake inhibitors and a type of therapy known as cognitive-behavioral therapy. With these treatments, some improve partially; others describe their response as miraculous.

This is a new frontier: we still have much to learn about BDD. I considered waiting to write this book until more is known, but although our knowledge is incomplete, there's a great deal we already do know. I decided it was time to let people know that this disorder exists, and to respond to the many people who have asked if a book about it is available. The suffering of my patients convinced me that now was the time to write about this little-known disorder—to get the word out, to have their voices heard.

In the pages that follow, I'll describe what's known about BDD—what patients experience, what I and other researchers have learned about it, and what treatments seem helpful. I will also grapple with some complex questions that have no clear answers but which patients often ask. What causes it? Is it related to other psychiatric disorders? How does it compare to the "normal" appearance concerns most of us have? I hope I convey what my patients would want you to know.

I also hope that BDD sufferers and their family members will use this book to identify and understand their symptoms and seek effective treatment, for there *is* hope for BDD sufferers. As Jane said to me, "I can't imagine any suffering greater than this. If I had a choice, I'd rather have cancer. You need to tell people about BDD. Tell them this is a serious disorder. It's too important to wait."

·· *two* ··

Patients Speak

"I'm surprised to hear other people have this problem. I thought I was the only one."
Alex

Jennifer's Story

*T*his is incredibly embarrassing," Jennifer began. "It's really hard for me to talk about this. I don't want to be here." She fidgeted anxiously in her chair and looked at the floor. Her hands shook, and she seemed close to tears. Jennifer had in fact canceled her first two appointments with me, and she'd finally agreed to come in only at her mother's insistence. I had spoken briefly with her mother on the phone, who said she was feeling desperate— her daughter had a serious problem that neither of them could cope with any longer.

I asked Jennifer if she could explain what was so embarrassing. "I don't like talking about my problem," she said. "You'll probably think I'm silly or vain. But I'm not," she said with tears in her eyes. "This is a very serious problem. I can't even tell you how bad it is." She sat silently for a minute, looking down anxiously, as if trying to decide what to say and how to express it. "Well, I guess I should tell you what it is. I think I'm really ugly. In fact, I think I'm one of the ugliest people in the whole world."

Jennifer was by anyone's standards attractive. She was a 22-year-old woman with long strawberry-blond hair, large green eyes, and a beautiful complexion. She reminded me of the captain of my high school cheerleading squad, a pretty and vivacious young woman. How could Jennifer think she was ugly? What could she possibly believe was wrong with how she looked? I wondered what it could be. I couldn't see any flaws anywhere.

At first, Jennifer was reluctant to discuss the details. "Well, I just think I'm not pretty," she said. "I've felt this way for a long time, and I can't seem to convince myself I'm wrong. I know what you're going to say. You're probably going to tell me I look fine—everyone does—but I know it's not true. I look terrible!"

"What is it about your appearance that upsets you so much?" I asked. "My skin," she replied, after some hesitation. "See all these pimples and scars and marks?" I really couldn't see what she was describing. From where I was sitting, her skin looked clear. Jennifer stood up and walked over toward me. "See these marks?" she asked again, pointing at her cheek and nose. In some of the places she pointed to I could discern some small whiteheads, but I had to be within a foot of her to see them. Even then I had to look closely.

Jennifer sat down again and went on to describe how since her early teenage years she'd been preoccupied with the "acne" and "marks" she'd just pointed out. She also thought her skin was too pale. "I look like a ghost. Everyone else looks really good; I stick out like a sore thumb. I'm the one who looks ugly," she said.

"When did the problem start?" I asked her. "When I was around 11," she replied. "It started with my nose. One of my nostrils stuck out more than the other. I remember catching a view of myself in the mirror one day and panicking. I thought, 'Is that what you look like? You look terrible, like a freak!'

"My nostrils don't really bother me anymore. My skin took over for them. Now all I think about is how bad my skin looks. I think about it for most of the day. People can see it from 50 feet away!" Jennifer cried as she said this—she truly believed that she was ugly and that her ugliness was visible to the entire world.

At this point Jennifer wasn't sure she wanted to continue. It was too upsetting to talk about her problem. But, with encouragement, she managed to go on. "I try not to think about it, but I have to," she said. "I think about it for most of the day. It's the first thing I think of when I wake up in the morning. I rush to the mirror, wondering 'How does it look?' How my skin looks in the morning totally determines how my day goes. Unfortunately, 80% of the time it looks horrible."

In high school Jennifer thought so much about her supposed ugliness that she couldn't concentrate in class. Her preoccupations crowded her mind and sapped her energy. "I dressed up a lot, I got really tan, wore blue eye shadow, and did a lot of things with my hair to distract people from my skin. But it didn't work. I couldn't concentrate on my school work, and I didn't want to be seen. It was too hard for me to stay in school," she said. "I started calling my mother in the middle of the day to pick me up. She didn't want to get me because I was supposed to be in class, but I was so upset and cried so much she'd come and take me home."

While doing her homework, Jennifer spent so much time examining her face in a mirror she kept on her desk that she couldn't complete her assignments. When she started reading, she felt compelled to check the mirror. "I had to see how my skin looked," she explained. "I had to see if it was any worse. Sometimes I'd get stuck there for hours, examining it for imperfections.

"I'd pick at it, too" she added, "which just made it worse. Sometimes I'd pick and pick with pins dipped in alcohol trying to get rid of the pimples and get the pus out. I'd pick at all kinds of things—little bumps, blackheads, any mark or imperfection. Sometimes I'd be up doing this at 1:00 or 2:00 in the morning, and then I'd fall asleep in class the next day, if I even went. Sometimes it would even bleed. I always felt terrible afterward. I'd make such a mess of my skin that I'd get totally hysterical."

As a result of her skin concerns, Jennifer's grades slipped from As and Bs to Ds, and she was put in a class for students with academic difficulties, even though she was bright. After missing many days of school, she dropped out of the ninth grade, even though she'd wanted to go to college. "I really tried to stay in school," she said. "But I couldn't do it. It was too much."

Jennifer also missed parties because, as she explained it, "No one would want to hang out with me because I'm so ugly." When her friends encouraged her to go, telling her how pretty she was, Jennifer didn't believe them. "They were just feeling sorry for me and trying to be nice. How could I go when I looked so horrendous?"

She did date one boy after she'd dropped out of school but saw him largely in her own house. "I hardly ever went out with him because I didn't want anyone to see my skin. I'd have him come over to my house. When he came over, I pulled all the shades down and turned down the lights so he couldn't see how bad my skin looked. But I stopped seeing him because I figured he'd just leave me anyway when he found out how bad I looked."

After dropping out of high school Jennifer tried waitressing three different times, but each time she quit or was fired because she missed so much work. "I wouldn't go if I had even one pimple. Sometimes I left in the middle of the day because I thought the customers were making fun of my skin behind my back." A job as a filing clerk was more tolerable, since she didn't have to be around other people as much, but she had trouble with that job, too. She thought about her skin for most of the day and secretly checked it in a pocket mirror over and over. "I tried not to," she explained, "because it took me away from my work. But I couldn't resist. *I couldn't stop thinking about my face, and I had to check it.* I *had* to make sure I looked okay, but I usually thought it looked bad. When I looked in the mirror I felt totally panicked seeing all those pimples and marks. Sometimes I even had to leave work and go to bed for the rest of the day. It was just like when I was in school."

When Jennifer had to work in a room with several other people and sit under fluorescent lights, she quit her job. "Sitting that close to other people was really hard because they could see how bad my skin was," she explained. "And the fluorescent lights were the last straw. I remember the day I quit. I was doing some filing, and all I could think of was that those awful lights showed up all the marks and pimples and holes in my face. I looked like a monster. I couldn't stop thinking that everyone in the room was looking at me! I tried to calm myself down and focus on what I was doing, but I couldn't. I had a panic attack. I ran out of that room and never went back."

Jennifer went on disability because she was unable to work, and continued to live with her parents even though she wanted to live on her own. Her parents bought her most of what she needed, and she rarely went out. "I do go out sometimes, but mostly at night when no one can see me," she said. "Sometimes I go to a 24-hour grocery store at midnight, when I know no one else will be there. For a long time I've bought most of my clothes through catalogs. I'm too scared to go out—everyone will see how ugly I am," she explained. When she did venture out she first spent at least two hours putting on makeup. "I look as though I'm wearing a mask, but at least I sort of cover up the pimples and scars," she said. She also painstakingly covered herself from head to toe with a bronzer to make her skin less white and to look "less like a ghost." She couldn't go out if there was any chance of rain because her bronzer would streak and run.

"It's getting worse," she said. "Last week, I got up my courage and decided to go out in the daylight, which I hardly ever do. I started driving to the store, and, just my luck, I got stuck in a major traffic jam. I was sitting there, in four lanes of traffic, waiting for the traffic to move, but it wasn't moving, and these people in the other cars were looking at me. All I could think was that they were looking at my face, thinking 'That poor girl; look how ugly she is. How can she go out in public when her skin looks so bad?' I tried to convince myself that it wasn't true, but my heart started racing, and I was sweating and shaking. I couldn't stop thinking that they were laughing at me. I got so panicked I had to leave. So I left my car in the middle of the traffic jam, and I ran until I found a phone booth. I called my mother and I stayed there hiding until she got me. That's how bad it got—I left my car sitting in the middle of the highway!"

Jennifer thought her problem was physical, not psychiatric, so she'd seen at least 15 different dermatologists. Some gave her antibiotics and other medications, but most said she didn't need treatment. "I'm every dermatologist's nightmare," Jennifer said. "I keep going back to see them, asking them over and over if my skin looks okay. I didn't believe them when they said my skin was fine. I wouldn't go away. I asked and asked them about my skin, and I begged them for treatment. A lot of them refused to see me anymore. They're probably all seeing therapists because of me!"

One of the dermatologists had in fact called to refer Jennifer to me for treatment. He told me that Jennifer had beautiful skin but was so obsessed with it that she might benefit from seeing a psychiatrist. But, at that time, Jennifer preferred to continue seeing dermatologists.

She finally did see a dermatologist whom she convinced to do a dermabrasion, a painful face peel usually reserved for treating severe acne. "The dermatologist really didn't want to do it," Jennifer said, "but I was so desperate that she gave in." After the dermabrasion Jennifer felt better about her skin for several months, even though her friends asked her what had happened to it. "They all thought it looked worse because it was red for a while," she said. "But I was thrilled. I didn't care if it was red because at least the pimples and marks went away." But within several months Jennifer's preoccupation returned and was even worse. She then had another dermabrasion, even though her parents implored her not to and the dermatologist was reluctant to repeat it. But Jennifer felt so desperate that it was done. That procedure didn't help her feel any better either. She was so depressed over this, over the fact that her "last hope" didn't help, that she thought about suicide.

When she first saw me, Jennifer still believed her problem was physical, not psychiatric, and she really wanted to see another dermatologist, not a psychiatrist. But her mother had insisted. "All my daughter does is ask me if she looks okay, over and over again, all day long," she told me. "She looks through magazines, asking me if her skin looks as good as the models'. No matter what I say, she can't be reassured. She's a pretty girl—I don't know what to do!" She had even told Jennifer that she'd have to move out of the house if she didn't stop her questioning, but Jennifer couldn't stop. "I have to ask her," Jennifer said. "I ask her at least a hundred times a day. I try not to, but I can't stop."

Jennifer also insisted that her mother hold magnifying glasses and shine light on her face from different angles when she inspected herself in the mirror so she could get a better look at her skin. Her mother reluctantly did it because Jennifer was so upset if she refused, but this took more than an hour a day and never really helped. "If it helped I might be willing to keep doing it," her mother said, "but she just keeps asking me if her skin looks okay and if she has scars, and she just keeps looking in the mirror. It might be hard for you to believe this, Doctor, but this problem is ruining our family—the constant questioning, the constant tears. She won't go out. We've tried to be patient, but nothing we do seems to help. We love our daughter and want to help her, but we can't take it anymore!"

Jennifer's story is not unusual. Although her body dysmorphic disorder was severe, her long struggle is typical of what many people experience. Body dysmorphic disorder, or BDD, is a painful yet virtually unknown psychiatric disorder—one in which normal-looking or even attractive people are preoccupied with a defect or flaw in their appearance. What's unusual about the defect is that it isn't visible—or is hardly visible—to others. People with this disorder may, for example, think that their hair is too curly, too straight, or too thin. Or that they have "veins" on their cheeks, scars on their nose, or skin that's too red or too pale. Or that their nose is too big, their lips too thin, their hips too big, or their breasts too small. Any body part can be the focus of concern. In reality they look fine. Often they have no defect at all. If they do have a flaw, it's generally minimal—something other people don't particularly notice. When I meet someone with BDD, I can almost never figure out what the supposed defect is by looking at them. Other people usually can't either. The "defects" are more in their minds than their bodies.

People with BDD not only focus on a defect that others don't notice—they think about it excessively. They worry. They obsess. It causes them pain. And it often interferes with their life.

BDD is a fascinating disorder. How can a person with no perceptible flaw, or only a minimal flaw, in his or her appearance focus so excessively on something others don't notice? How can an attractive young woman like Jennifer think she looks monstrously ugly—that she's "one of the ugliest people in the whole world"?

I've found BDD particularly intriguing because it's largely undiscovered and unknown. Many people with this disorder have gone from doctor to doctor—dermatologists, plastic surgeons, ophthalmologists, psychiatrists—

without finding out what their problem is. Until very recently, many professionals and laypersons alike had never heard of BDD. Even though this is beginning to change, BDD is still an underrecognized disorder. And even though there's much that we know about BDD, much about it remains mysterious.

Chris's, Keith's, and Andrew's Stories

One of my first patients with BDD was a shy, articulate young man named Chris, who made an appointment with me to be evaluated for depression. When I first met with him, he told me that depression was his problem—that he'd been feeling down, unmotivated, uninterested in things he usually enjoyed. He was having trouble sleeping, and found it difficult to concentrate on his job. His girlfriend had recently left him.

Chris indeed sounded depressed, and it seemed as though he had a fairly straightforward case of depression. But when I asked him if he was bothered by anything else, Chris seemed unusually hesitant and uncomfortable. He was silent for several minutes and seemed to be struggling to decide whether to tell me something. "There *is* something else bothering me. I wasn't sure I'd be able to tell you about it, but I should because it's why I'm here. It's my main problem. I'm depressed because of my hair."

Chris struggled to explain. "This is really embarrassing for me to talk about, but I'm devastated over my hair. I think it's falling out and that I look terrible. I realize I'm probably distorting—that I really don't look so bad—but I can't stop worrying about it." Chris had recently joined a hair club and had tried many hair tonics, which cost him $300 a month—a significant financial burden. But none of these remedies had diminished his preoccupation. Now he was considering getting a hair weave and was saving his money to pay for it.

Chris also worried about his nose—that it didn't look right. He was also reluctant to describe this concern, but explained that he thought his nose was too wide and too long. "I'm so worried about my nose, and especially my hair, that I can't concentrate at work. I had a big assignment last month, and I had a hard time getting it done because I thought my hair looked especially bad. I thought more was falling out than usual. This probably sounds ridiculous to you, but I was so distracted by these thoughts and by the fear that I was going to be bald that I was a week late with the assignment. That was a big blow for me because I'm a perfectionist. I do a good job at work, and I pride myself on getting my assignments done on time.

What was really hard was that my boss called me in to talk about my lateness and to ask me what the problem was. Of course I couldn't tell him what it was. I'd be totally mortified. I made up an excuse about a close friend being sick, even though I hate to lie." Chris worked as an accountant and had deadlines to meet. "It probably sounds ridiculous that I can't meet my deadlines because of my hair. It really shouldn't matter what my hair looks like. But I can't help it!"

Chris was also very nervous going out to parties and bars with his girlfriend. "Before my hair problem began, I didn't have much trouble talking to people when I went out. I was never the life of the party, but I'd go out. I liked to see people, and I never avoided social events that I wanted to go to. But it's really hard for me now because of how I look. When I do go out, it's hard for me to talk with people—I can't concentrate on the conversation. All I can think about is whether my hair looks okay and whether they're noticing how thin it is. I constantly check out their hair and compare it to mine. Then I usually feel worse because I think their hair looks better. That's why my girlfriend left me. She likes to go out and said she can't stay with me if I stay home or leave parties early because of my hair. She thinks I look fine, and she can't understand why I can't just forget about it.

"The final straw for her came last month," he continued. "Last month was a really bad time for me—I'm not sure why. I was supposed to be in her brother's wedding. I went to the dress rehearsal, but on the morning of the wedding I panicked. I looked in the mirror and I thought 'Where's your hair?' I thought I looked balder than ever. I spent about an hour frantically putting gel in it, combing it, and blow drying it, trying to make it look fuller. I even had my girlfriend help me with it, even though she was really frustrated and angry with me. But no matter what we did to it, it didn't look right. I kept trying to convince myself that it really didn't matter— that people would be looking at the bride and groom, not at my hair. But I just couldn't go. I felt so demoralized and desperate."

Chris's problems intrigued me. How was it possible that his hair and nose had caused him such difficulties? His hair was a little thin, but not so thin that I'd noticed it when I met him. And his nose looked fine. Why was he so worried? How could these worries interfere with his job when he'd always been such a high achiever? Why couldn't he go out to parties? How had it gotten so bad that he'd missed the wedding and his girlfriend had left him?

Soon after I saw Chris, another patient, Keith, called me. He said he was calling about something important, and sounded very anxious and agitated over the phone. "Dr. Phillips," he began, "I'm calling about something that's making me feel really panicked. It's been a problem for a while, but I haven't been able to tell you about it." I asked him what it was. "Well, I couldn't tell you about it in person because it's too embarrassing. But maybe I can over the phone. . . . I'm . . . I'm upset about my hair." I was puzzled. Why would he be so upset over his hair? His hair had always seemed fine. And two men with hair problems in the same month? This seemed like an unusual coincidence.

Keith went on to explain that he was very worried that his hair was too thin. "I keep worrying about it, even though it's probably not true," he explained. "I try to stop thinking about it, but I can't." I wondered whether Keith might actually be losing his hair for some reason—perhaps he had an undiagnosed medical illness that can cause hair loss. But I was wrong. Keith continued to explain. "It's actually not my overall hair—it's my bangs. My bangs aren't right. They're too thin and the shape is wrong. I don't think my hair is falling out. I just think my bangs look *really bad.*"

Keith was extremely embarrassed about this. "I'm afraid you're thinking I'm silly to be worried so much about my hair, but I can't help it. I think I look like a dork!" Keith was concerned I wouldn't take him seriously. At that point I thought about my recent meeting with Chris and wondered whether Keith, too, might have BDD. He did.

When I next met with Keith I was surprised to learn that he had many worries about his appearance. He thought that his ears were "too pointy—like Mr. Spock's," that he had "lines" on his face, and that his eyes were "small and beady." His most embarrassing concern was that certain parts of his body—his chest and buttocks—were "shaped like a woman's." I'd known Keith for more than two years and had worked closely with him during that time. He'd told me about many of his problems and had gotten fairly comfortable talking about subjects he found shameful. But this problem had been too embarrassing for him to discuss. In fact, it had taken him more than two years to tell me about it! And he could initially raise it only over the phone, not in person. I commented that he'd seemed comfortable talking about other personal matters—what made this one so hard to discuss? He replied that it was somehow much easier to talk about his depression or his mania—even his sexual problems. For reasons he found difficult to articulate, he was particularly ashamed of his appearance concerns. He was afraid I'd think he was superficial and vain. He also feared that by talking about his "ugly" body parts, I'd notice them even more than he thought I already did. He finally summed it up: "I just didn't have the guts to tell you. It's almost taboo to discuss it. I can't believe I brought it up."

Andrew was another of the first patients I saw with BDD. Like Chris, he came in to be evaluated for depression, not BDD, because he was too embarrassed to divulge his BDD. I may never have found out about Andrew's BDD if I hadn't asked him if he had any ideas about why he was depressed. His answer: "I've had five nose and chin operations, and I don't look any better."

Andrew had BDD for more than 20 years. It started after he had minor nose surgery for a deviated septum, during which he thought the surgeon changed the shape of his nose. In desperation, Andrew had five more operations to improve its appearance. But with each operation, he believed his deformities worsened. In addition, at the time of the second operation the surgeon suggested that Andrew also have a chin implant, which triggered a new obsession that his chin was too small. "My life stopped every year or so to have another operation," Andrew said. He dropped out of college and quit jobs to have the procedures. "Each time, right after the surgery I was ecstatic, because I thought this time I'd finally look right. But when the bandages were removed I was heartbroken. I thought I looked even worse, and I became more deeply depressed."

His family and friends tried to talk Andrew out of the operations, reassuring him that he was a good-looking man with no observable defects. The surgeons also didn't want to operate. "You might wonder why they kept doing more operations," Andrew said. "But they couldn't turn me down because I was so miserable. I *had* to have more surgery. I kept hoping that the operations would help—that I'd look better and that people would like me more and accept me more if I looked better." But with each procedure Andrew became more withdrawn, to the point where he rarely went out and never dated. "A few years ago I got very close to suicide," he said. "I gave my things away and made out a will. I had it all planned—the day, the time, the place—but I chickened out. Sometimes I think I should have gone through with it."

BDD from the Past and Around the World

My search through the professional literature on BBD uncovered few research studies but many case reports—descriptions of a single case or a few cases—of BDD. The reports came from a surprisingly wide variety of countries—England, Italy, France, Germany, Russia, Japan, the former Czechoslovakia, and others. I read about a young man from Germany who thought his cheeks were too "rosy and round" and who, in an attempt to make them thinner, severely starved himself. I read about a young woman from England who worried that her breasts were too small and had been refused breast augmentation surgery. Another young woman from England was so concerned about "lines" under her eyes that she wanted to kill herself. "I am constantly thinking about them, about my face and how I have changed," the author wrote of her preoccupation. "Makeup is just a waste of time. Life is not worth living."

A report from Japan described several cases similar to those I've seen. One was a 25-year-old man who was preoccupied with his "flaccid" nose and who thought his eyebrows had "declined." Another was a 28-year-old woman who was also preoccupied with a supposed nose deformity, which she attributed to having been hit in the nose with a brush. Six nose operations didn't diminish her concern. The third patient, a 25-year-old woman, complained that her eyelid was drooping, her nose was deformed, and the whites of her eyes were yellow. Four surgical procedures hadn't helped, and she in fact believed that one of the operations had given her a snoring problem.

I found descriptions of BDD from more than 100 years ago. I was struck by how such descriptions so accurately described the patients I was seeing. William Stekel, an early twentieth-century author, wrote in 1949 about "the peculiar group of compulsive ideas which concern the body. There are people," he wrote, "who occupy themselves continuously with a specific part of the body. In one case it is the nose; in another it is the bald head; in a third case the ear, the eyes, or (in women) the bosom, the genitalia, etc. These obsessive thoughts are very tormenting."

One of psychiatry's most famous patients—known by the pseudonym "the Wolf Man"—probably had BDD. The legendary Sigmund Freud, the Wolf Man's first psychoanalyst, didn't even mention BDD symptoms in his description of his patient, even though it was a significant problem. Why not? Had the Wolf Man mentioned it to Freud, or had he kept it a secret? Was he too embarrassed to bring it up? Perhaps he wasn't yet worried about his appearance, although BDD usually begins during adolescence. Ruth Brunswick, the Wolf Man's second psychoanalyst, did write about her patient's preoccupation. In 1928 she noted that "(he) neglected his daily life and work because he was engrossed, to the exclusion of all else, in the state of his nose" (its supposed scars, holes, and swelling). "His life was centered on the little mirror in his pocket, and his fate depended on what it revealed or was about to reveal."

This quote describes many of the patients I've seen. Jennifer, too, neglected her daily life and work because she was so engrossed with supposed defects in her appearance. And her life was also centered on the little mirror in her pocket. Without realizing it, when Jennifer repeatedly checked her pocket mirror at work, she was doing what the Wolf Man had done more than half a century before.

Body dysmorphic disorder is a relatively new name for this disorder, having been used only since 1987, when it first entered psychiatry's classification manual of psychiatric disorders. For the previous 100 years, BDD was more commonly known as *dysmorphophobia*, a term coined in the 1880s by Enrique Morselli, a brilliant and prolific Italian psychiatrist, who saw many patients with BDD. Dysmorphophobia comes from *dysmorfia*, a Greek word meaning ugliness, specifically of the face, which first appeared in the Histories of Herodotus. It refers to the myth of the "ugliest girl in Sparta," who, upon being stroked by the hand of a goddess, became the "fairest of all Spartan ladies" and later married the Spartan king. Herodotus writes, "Thither the Nurse would bear the child every day to the Shrine and set her by the Statue and pray the Goddess to deliver her from her ill looks."

In the late 1800s, Morselli saw 78 patients with BDD, which he described as an "idea of deformity." "The dysmorphophobic patient," he wrote, "is really miserable; in the middle of his daily routines, talks, while reading, during meals, everywhere and at any time, he is caught by the doubt of deformity." Subsequently, BDD was described by some of Europe's most prominent turn-of-the-century psychiatrists, such as Emil Kraepelin and Pierre Janet. Janet considered BDD to be relatively common. In 1903, he described a 27-year-old woman he called Nadia, the gifted and intelligent daughter of a distinguished French family. Nadia worried about many aspects of her appearance, including her red and spotted skin, her feet and supposed tallness, and her "long and ridiculous" hands. Nadia worried that no one would ever love her because she feared she was "ugly and ridiculous," and for five years she confined herself to a tiny apartment that she rarely left. "If they saw me in plain light, people would be disgusted," Janet wrote of Nadia's concern.

"Beauty hypochondria" (*"Schönheitshypochondrie,"* in German) and "one who is worried about being ugly" (*"Hässlichkeitskümmerer,"* in German) are other colorful labels used in the 1930s to describe a BDD-like preoccupation with imagined ugliness. "Dermatologic hypochondriasis" depicted a BDD-like syndrome that focused on supposed defects of the skin and hair.

The vivid case descriptions written during the past century bear testimony to BDD's long history and to the fact that people from a variety of cultures have suffered from it. Indeed, BDD is well known and recognized in certain countries—Japan, for example—but has escaped adequate recognition in many others, including the United States.

While it's not entirely clear why BDD has been largely unknown in the

United States and certain other countries, one likely reason is that it's often kept secret. Keith wasn't my only patient to take several years to tell me about his concerns. Some people, like Jennifer, tell family members and friends about their worries and may even describe them to doctor after doctor, but many others keep them secret.

Some have finally gotten up the courage to mention their concern to someone they trust, but when they're reassured that they look fine, they feel misunderstood. They may interpret reassurance to mean that the person they've told doesn't take them seriously and doesn't understand their suffering. As a result, they may never mention it again.

Others don't realize their problem is psychiatric. They go to surgeon after surgeon, dermatologist after dermatologist, hair club after hair club seeking a nonpsychiatric cure for a psychiatric problem. This, too, has contributed to BDD's underrecognition. If people with BDD do see a psychiatrist, they may be too ashamed to bring it up. They may muster up only enough courage to talk about the depression and anxiety that people with BDD often experience, thus keeping their suffering a secret even from those who can help them.

"No One Takes Me Seriously": Letters from BDD Sufferers and Their Families

BDD is not a rare disorder. While only preliminary data on its prevalence are available, they suggest that it's far more common than is recognized. Preliminary data from a number of researchers suggest that BDD may affect:

- 1–2% of the general population

- 4 to 5% of people seeking medical treatment in an outpatient setting

- 8% of people with depression

- Up to 12% of people seeking psychiatric treatment in an outpatient setting

---

These numbers translate into many millions of people in the United States alone. While these findings need to be confirmed in large-scale studies, I and my fellow researchers have been surprised by the relatively high rates of BDD we've found in patient groups we've studied. When stories about BDD have run in newspapers and magazines, I've been deluged with calls and letters. I hear from people who wonder if they have BDD and want treatment, from family members who think a loved one may be suffering from the disorder, from professionals asking for information, for consultations on their patients, and sometimes for help for their own family members. One woman, who read about BDD in her local newspaper, wrote the following:

> I am 45 years old—and I don't ever remember not feeling this way. It is very difficult to discuss with anyone, as no one seems to take me seriously or can relate to the amount of pain I feel. Therapy has helped me work on many of my other issues, but I seemed to skirt around this more serious problem, which didn't get addressed. . . . The hardest part for me in this is that no one takes me seriously and so I never feel heard. It is very distressing and has affected many areas of my life.

The sense of isolation and aloneness implied in this letter is more directly conveyed in the following letter, which a woman wrote to me after seeing a story about BDD on *Dateline NBC* in 1993:

> I am 29 and never knew that there was anyone else out there who thought the same way I do about themselves.

Another woman wrote me about her brother's long struggle with severe BDD:

> My 49-year-old brother has suffered from body dysmorphic disorder his entire adult life. He has been hospitalized, had shock treatment, taken drugs, and received psychotherapy on and off for years as he imagines people are making fun of his looks. Nothing has helped him. Now, thank God, this disorder is finally being recognized and hopefully can be successfully treated.

The following letter conveys that this disorder can indeed be treated successfully. The young woman who wrote it had responded to psychiatric treatment after several years of suffering:

> My history of BDD is relatively short, but very painful! I had what would probably be a mild case of it years ago in regards to my eyelids. I chose to have cosmetic surgery done and instead of remedying the situation, I became obsessed—I was sure that my eyelids looked even worse and terribly abnormal. It consumed me. I consulted six more cosmetic surgeons, mirrors began to be a terrible problem, I became reclusive, and I thought about it from the minute I woke up until I fell asleep. It was a nightmare. I'm sure you're familiar with the story. Anyhow, this went on for two years before I got help....I'd have to say I'm about 85% recovered from the BDD and that is a *big* relief!

In contrast to this hopeful letter, I received an extremely sad one sent to me by a woman whose son had been preoccupied with the shape of his head. She had just read about BDD in her local paper and realized that this was the disorder from which he had suffered for so long. She started her letter with the following:

"I read the enclosed article nearly a month after my dear son hanged himself in sheer desperation. Until we read the reporter's words, none of us had any perception of my son's suffering and feeling that no one could help him. . . . My son had been telling us for many years how he felt and that he wanted to die.

The last letter shocked and haunted me for a long time. I spoke with the woman, who told me of her family's and her son's suffering and of her long and unsuccessful quest for a diagnosis and effective treatment. No one could tell her what his problem was. And she felt that no one had truly understood the depth of his suffering. She blamed herself for this. She felt she should have understood. In retrospect, her son's suffering and hopelessness couldn't have been clearer, but at the time it *had* been hard to understand—he was a handsome young man whose head looked completely normal. Her self-blame made his death all the more painful.

The tragedy of this young man's death and other stories I heard spurred my resolve to learn more about this serious and underrecognized disorder—to understand who gets it, how to identify it, and how to treat it.

Hope for BDD Sufferers

In many ways, we're only beginning to understand BDD, and much more research is needed. At this time, there are more questions than answers. What causes BDD? Is it rooted in a person's biology, life experience, or societal expectations? Is it a disorder of the brain, the mind, or society? Why do some people get it but others don't? Is it related to eating disorders, like bulimia and anorexia nervosa—disorders that also involve distorted body image? Or is it related to obsessive compulsive disorder, a disorder characterized by obsessive thoughts—for example, about contamination or harm—and compulsive behaviors that, like those of BDD, often involve checking and reassurance seeking?

How is BDD related to koro, a disorder in which men fear that their penis is disappearing into their abdomen and will kill them? And where exactly should we draw the line between BDD and the normal concern with appearance that so many people have? Is BDD simply an exaggerated version of this normal, common concern—a more intense, problematic variant of it? Or is it something different?

While continued research is essential, we aren't totally in the dark. There's much that we *do* know—what people with BDD experience, what other problems and disorders commonly accompany it, how it affects peoples' lives. Promising preliminary evidence suggests that this disorder often responds to psychiatric treatment. The suffering of many people with BDD—including Jennifer, Chris, and Keith—has been significantly alleviated by treatment. Some are completely free of their tormenting concern.

Jennifer's symptoms were alleviated by clomipramine (Anafranil), a certain type of antidepressant medication known as a serotonin-reuptake inhibitor. After several months on this medication, she began to notice that she thought about her skin much less often—only an hour a day instead of most of the day. It became much easier to stay away from mirrors. Her preoccupation no longer tormented her. She also felt somewhat better about how she looked. She still thought that she had "some pimples," but she realized they weren't particularly noticeable. They were no longer devastating. As she explained, "This is more of a normal dislike—it isn't taking over my life anymore. I've put this problem in perspective. I don't love my skin, but I can accept it. It no longer ruins me." She stopped asking her mother about her appearance, and she's been able to leave her house, go into stores to shop, and look for a job.

Keith responded to a combination of a serotonin-reuptake inhibitor known as fluoxetine (Prozac) and a type of therapy known as cognitive-behavioral therapy. He stopped worrying about his appearance almost entirely. Like Jennifer, he now finds it much easier to go out in public because he no longer thinks that everyone is staring at him. The serotonin-reuptake inhibitors, antidepressant medications with antiobsessional properties, are particularly promising for BDD. Those currently marketed in the United States are fluoxetine (Prozac), fluvoxamine (Luvox), clomipramine (Anafranil), paroxetine (Paxil), and sertraline (Zoloft). Another promising treatment is cognitive-behavioral treatment, in which patients are helped to stop their compulsive behaviors and face the situations they fear.

The field of psychiatry is rapidly advancing; some of the things we now know about the workings of the brain were barely imaginable even a decade ago. Many advances—such as those in brain imaging—will be applied to this disorder and are likely to exponentially increase our knowledge. A statement made by a neuroscientist about his area of research struck me as particularly applicable to BDD: "We are at the foothills of an enormous mountain range."

·· *three* ··

What Is Body Dysmorphic Disorder?

"One day I saw my face in a certain light, and I panicked. I thought, 'Is this what you've looked like all along? How awful! How can you live with this?'"
                                                                          Lauren

"My Problem Isn't Very Severe": Do I Even Have Body Dysmorphic Disorder?

Sarah, a 24-year-old medical student, called me after she'd seen *Dateline NBC's* 1993 piece on BDD. "My problem isn't very severe; I'm not sure I have body dysmorphic disorder," she told me over the phone. "My concern with my appearance isn't that extreme, but it probably *is* excessive. It's a problem for me."

I looked forward to meeting with Sarah. At this point I'd seen many people with severe BDD—people like Jennifer and Andrew—but fewer people with mild BDD, and I was interested in what she'd have to say. Did she have mild BDD? Did she even have BDD? I also hoped I could be helpful. She *had* said her concern was a problem.

When I first saw Sarah I had no idea of what her concern could be. She was very appealing—quiet yet also animated—with a lovely smile. She did have a few small pimples on her chin, but only a few, and to my eye they were barely noticeable. Nonetheless, this is a concern of many people with BDD—perhaps it was hers.

But it wasn't. We started off talking about medical school and the hospital rotation she was on. She was sleep deprived but loved her work and what she was learning. She was trying to decide what her specialty would be—perhaps pediatrics. "My work is going well," she said. "But I'm having problems with my social life. It's hard for me to get into relationships. I isolate myself because of my appearance worries."

Sarah went on to describe what bothered her. "I don't like my thighs," she said. "They're flabby. They have this rippling look, and the skin isn't taut. I also worry a lot about varicose veins on my legs and ankles. I think they look *really* bad. They're dark purple, and some of them bulge out of my legs. They bother me a lot. I get very upset when I think about these things—very nervous and anxious. It causes me a lot of emotional turmoil. It's worse on some days than on other days; some days aren't so bad, but it can be very upsetting."

I asked her if there was anything else that bothered her. "Well, my hair too," she replied. "It's just not right. Sometimes it's too flat; sometimes it looks asymmetric. I can spend a lot of time combing it. And I've never been very happy with my weight. I'm always on a diet. In fact, I've gained a few pounds in the past month because there's always candy on the ward where I'm working now. But my weight doesn't stop me from doing things the way my other concerns do. I don't like it, and I'm trying to change it, but I don't really consider it a big problem."

"Do your other concerns cause you problems?" I asked. "Yes, they do," she answered. "I avoid the beach even though I love it. If I go, I worry about my thighs and my veins the entire time, and I can't have fun. And I wear pants even on really hot summer days—even if it's 90 degrees out. It's pretty uncomfortable, and it probably looks pretty strange. It also makes my feel phony—why can't I just be myself? Why do I care so much about how I look? I don't have an answer to that question, which is very frustrating. I try to talk myself out of my concerns, but I can't, and that adds to my frustration.

"I've seriously considered moving to a colder climate," she added. "I probably will when I begin my residency. The summers in New England aren't that long, but they're much too long for me! In a colder climate I won't seem so strange wearing pants all the time, and I won't have to turn down invitations to the beach. I think I'll feel less self-conscious.

"But the bigger problem is that I've avoided dating because of these things. I finally got up the courage to go out with someone I'm seeing now. I like him a lot, and I want the relationship to continue. But my appearance is interfering. It sounds stupid, but I'm afraid he'll reject me when he sees my veins and my thighs! This worry is a burden and a hindrance. I'm afraid I'll never be able to get married because of it."

Sarah stopped at that point, and she looked upset. "I'd really like to get married sometime," she said. "I don't want this to get in the way. The big problem right now is that I haven't told my boyfriend about these things. It's hard to be intimate. I try to hide my legs, but that's pretty hard to do when you spend a lot of time with someone and are romantically involved with them."

I asked Sarah if there were factors other than her appearance that might be contributing to her relationship problems. She responded by saying that she had often asked herself this question. "I've always been somewhat shy and reserved," she said. "But I've always wanted to go out with men, and I've always strongly felt that I wanted to get married someday. But maybe there *are* other reasons for my intimacy problems. My parents didn't have a good marriage, so maybe I'm unconsciously afraid of getting seriously involved with someone. I've always been somewhat sensitive to rejection, so I do think I hold back to some degree before getting involved with men. But at the same time, I'm also pretty trusting. I really don't know how to answer your question. Perhaps the best I can do is say that my appearance concerns are a *big part* of my relationship problems. I think if I didn't worry about how I look, I'd risk more in relationships.

"People tell me I'm attractive and that men find me attractive, but I find it hard to believe them. I can't be reassured. Actually, *overall* I think I look fine. But the things I told you about are very upsetting. My sister has seen my thighs and thinks they look fine. She keeps asking me to go to the beach with her because she loves to go too. But I rarely go. I feel much too self-conscious."

It did sound as though Sarah had BDD. She was very distressed over her concerns, and her relationships had suffered because of them. I wondered how bad the defects that she described really were. Were they slight or nonexistent, or were they as grotesquely unsightly as she thought? I couldn't see her legs because she was wearing pants, but presumably the defects were less severe than she believed—her sister, at any rate, thought she looked fine.

I also wondered about her hair. She had mentioned that this was a problem. I couldn't see anything wrong with it. It was a beautiful deep auburn and was cut fashionably short. I asked her to tell me about it. "Yes, my hair's a problem, too," she said. "It really bugs me because it never looks right. First it's too flat, then one side sticks out more than the other." She pointed to demonstrate. "But it's more than a bad hair day. It's upsetting."

Sarah went on to describe how she sometimes got stuck in the mirror trying to get her hair right. "I comb it and recomb it, style it and restyle it. I apply mousse, then hair spray, then I use a curling iron. When it doesn't look right, I wet it and start all over again. Sometimes I do this literally for hours."

I wondered how she managed to function as a third-year medical student. These students spend their time on the wards with patients and usually are very busy. How could she be doing her work if she was spending hours a day in the mirror? "Has this gotten in the way of your work at all?" I asked her. "Well I try really hard not to let it," Sarah replied. She seemed anxious, and her voice was starting to quaver. "I try not to ever look in the mirror when I'm at work, because when I do I can get stuck there. If my hair looks bad, I can't resist fiddling with it and then the whole routine can start. Once I start, I have to complete it. I've actually been late for rounds and lectures because I got stuck. My friends have even come looking for me in the bathroom when I've been late for rounds and the whole team was waiting for me. That was really embarrassing! I know I told you at first it wasn't really a problem at work. But I guess sometimes it is a little bit because sometimes I'm late."

Many people with BDD don't like to admit the difficulty their symptoms cause them. Many try to ignore them and go on with their job, with raising children, with their lives. Some make a valiant effort to keep a stiff upper lip. But it's usually a struggle, even when the BDD is relatively mild.

"A big problem is that the patients' rooms have mirrors in them. If I can prevent myself from glancing in them when I enter their rooms I do much better. My preoccupation stays under better control, and I don't get stuck there. The mirror acts like a switch. When I look in, the obsession turns on, and it can get pretty out of control."

Despite her useful strategy of avoiding mirrors, Sarah still encountered a problem when she got up each morning. "I need to look in the mirror to get myself ready for the day," she explained. "And that's a problem because I can get stuck there, and I've been late for work." A few months earlier, however, she had come up with an idea that worked—getting ready after her shower and before putting in her contact lenses. "Then the mirror's steamed up, and without my contacts in I'm practically blind. So I really can't see myself very well, but that's actually good. I just comb my hair and walk out without really seeing it. It's very anxiety provoking for me to do that because I'm petrified that my hair looks terrible. But I tell myself it probably looks fine and that the anxiety is nothing compared to what I feel when I get caught up in the grooming."

Sarah also avoided shopping malls with lots of mirrors in them and kept her distance from mirrors when buying clothes. "Getting my hair cut is especially hard—I *hate* getting it done," she said. "I keep my eyes glued to a newspaper or magazine the whole time so I don't get too upset. I *want* to look in the mirror, but I don't."

Like Sarah, most people with BDD have a special and torturous relationship with mirrors. Most check excessively, and some get stuck there for hours each day, caught between a desire to flee the unattractive image they see and a compelling desire to fix it. But fixing it isn't simple and often is unattainable. Because looking in mirrors can generate such intolerable anxiety, people who've found ways to avoid them usually say they're better off.

"But it's not easy to avoid mirrors," Sarah added. "I feel I'm almost physically pulled to them when I go near them—as if there's a magnet in them. It takes a lot of willpower not to look in." To help with this, she had left only one mirror hanging in her apartment and had even hidden a few reflecting items she sometimes felt compelled to check herself in. "I keep my toaster hidden away in a cupboard rather than keeping it on the counter," she said. "It has a very shiny surface, and sometimes I checked myself in it, which could be a problem. That strategy may sound silly, but it helps."

Sarah returned to talking about how her symptoms affected her work. "My legs cause less of a problem at work because I can cover them, and I don't see them in mirrors. But they still bother me. When I see patients' legs I think of my own and how ugly they are. Sometimes it really upsets me. But I'm very serious about my work, and I just try to get my mind back on what I'm doing. I usually manage."

Sarah was in fact doing very well in school, and her patients liked her a great deal. She was especially commended for her sensitivity to her patients' suffering. "Maybe it's because I myself suffer with this problem," she said. "You may think that sounds really bad—in fact, incredibly insensitive!" she said with a laugh. "How can I compare my appearance problems to the suffering of my patients who have cancer or are amputees? I realize how ludicrous that sounds, and I feel very guilty even saying it. It makes me feel spoiled and vain. But, you know, even though I think I have a pretty mild case of BDD, it still causes me a lot of pain. I try to tell myself that it's silly—that it shouldn't bother me so much—but it still bothers me a lot. I worry that I'll always be alone in life because of this problem."

A Spectrum of Severity

Mild BDD, like Sarah's, can be distressing and can interfere to some extent with living. But it isn't devastating. When BDD is very severe, it can destroy virtually every aspect of one's life. Some people, like Jennifer, stop working and stay in their homes, sometimes for years. Some adolescents drop out of high school or college. Parents may stop caring for their children because they're so preoccupied with their appearance that they can't focus on their children's needs. Some people with BDD think they look so ugly that they never date or marry. Some don't even buy food because they're unable to leave their home. Others, in an attempt to look better, lose dangerous amounts of weight.

Some even get into life-threatening accidents. Jennifer ran through red lights because she couldn't tolerate being looked at while waiting for the light to change. One man was so preoccupied with his reflection while washing windows that he fell off a three-story ladder. Others are so intent on examining their face in the rearview mirror while driving that they get into car accidents. One man *planned* to get into a car accident. He felt so hopeless over his facial "defects" that he planned to crash his car so he could destroy his face and have it completely surgically reconstructed. He explained that the car accident was necessary because 15 surgeons had refused to do the procedures he requested; even if he could find a surgeon willing to operate, his insurance company wouldn't pay for it, so the accident was necessary. Another woman was equally desperate; she was so distressed by the shape of her breasts that she repeatedly slashed them with a knife. Some suffer so intolerably that they attempt suicide. Some succeed.

But most people with BDD don't get into serious accidents or act in self-destructive ways. Like Sarah, those with milder BDD live relatively normal lives. They work, they see friends, they date, they raise families. I treat college students who get good grades and graduate, homemakers who successfully juggle raising children and running a home, accountants who meet their deadlines, and doctors who give their patients superb care. Many people with this disorder are productive; some are very high achievers. All of them suffer, but they manage, sometimes very well.

A psychiatrist colleague of mine wondered if a patient of hers had BDD but thought the diagnosis was unlikely because he was functioning so well. This colleague had treated several other people with BDD whose functioning had been severely impaired by their symptoms, and she consequently thought that *all* people with BDD had severe difficulties with work, socializing, and other aspects of life. But it turned out that the patient in question, who was a college professor, did in fact have BDD. He managed to perform well at work because of the effort he made to keep his symptoms from interfering. The patient, however, viewed his functioning as less than optimal. He hadn't applied for a job he'd wanted because he feared he'd be turned down because of his "awful" appearance. And he'd once refused a promotion that would require more work because his preoccupations were so taxing. "Even though I'm very high functioning and successful," he explained, "I'm not working up to my capacity, although no one would ever know it."

So BDD's severity spans a spectrum, ranging from relatively mild to life-threatening. In this way, BDD is like other medical problems. Severe diabetes can lead to hospitalization and serious medical complications, such as blindness, whereas people with a milder form of the illness can remain active and productive. Heart disease, too, spans a spectrum from severe to mild; it can severely limit one person's ability to work and engage in leisure activities but impose few or no limitations on another person's activities and enjoyment of life.

Psychiatric problems are no different. Depression can be severe and life-threatening: a severely depressed person may be unable to eat, sleep, or get out of bed, and may even commit suicide. But depression can be milder: many depressed people, despite their suffering, manage, with effort, to function fairly normally. No one would ever know they were depressed. One person with a severe phobia may not be able to leave her house; another person with a milder case may go out despite her fear. BDD is similar. When it's severe, it's as crippling as any serious psychiatric or medical illness. At the milder end of the spectrum, it's more manageable and even shades into normality.

Some people I've seen, who had heard or read about a particularly severe case of BDD, have told me they thought they didn't have the disorder because their symptoms "weren't that bad." Others, with severe BDD, thought they might not have the disorder because their symptoms were *so severe* there couldn't possibly be other people who had the same problem, who had suffered as much as they had. But they all had BDD.

BDD varies from person to person in other ways. Some people are preoccupied with their hair, others with their buttocks, others with their legs, testicles, or eyebrows. Any body part can be the focus of concern. Even among people concerned with the same body part, exactly what they dislike can differ. One person might think her hair is too flat, whereas another believes his sticks out too much. One person may think his skin is too red, whereas another feels hers is too white.

One man unfortunately dropped out of a treatment group I ran for people with BDD because he thought his problem was different from everyone else's. He felt he didn't fit in because he was the only one who worried about his hair; other people had other appearance concerns. He also felt different because he thought he was the only one who'd get uglier each week—he would get balder and balder, whereas everyone else would return looking the same. He couldn't tolerate being the only one who would look worse every week.

What he didn't realize is that *although no one with BDD has exactly the same experience as anyone else with BDD, all people with BDD have certain things in common.* The severity may differ, the body areas may differ, the behaviors may differ from person to person, but there are many commonalities. Everyone with BDD is concerned with some aspect of their appearance that they consider ugly, unattractive, or "not right" in some way. Everyone is preoccupied—thinking and worrying about their body excessively. Everyone is distressed or doesn't function as well as they might because of their preoccupation. The details differ from person to person, but these basic themes are shared by all.

How Is BDD Defined?

The basic features of BDD—what *everyone* with the disorder experiences—are described by BDD's diagnostic criteria. These criteria, on the next page, are from DSM-IV (the *Diagnostic and Statistical Manual, Fourth Edition*). DSM-IV is the manual used in the United States and many countries around the world by mental health professionals to make psychiatric diagnoses. Although the criteria may seem skeletal, they are useful because they provide guidelines for identifying who does and does not have BDD.

Criterion 1 is the core definitional criterion that describes the preoccupation occurring in BDD. People with BDD have more than an occasional thought that they don't look right—they're preoccupied. They think excessively about their supposed appearance problem; some people in fact find it difficult *not* to think about it. They say such things as "I think about it a lot," "It's always on my mind," "It's like a second reel that's always going," or "I'm obsessed." People with BDD generally spend at least an hour a day thinking about the supposed defect.

The definition then states that the defect is imagined or slight. Some people with BDD "imagine" their defects, in the sense that they're preoccupied with something that others don't perceive. Other people with BDD actually have a physical defect, such as mild acne, a scar, or slightly thinning

---

Table 1   Definition of Body Dysmorphic Disorder

---

1. Preoccupation with some imagined defect in appearance. If a slight physical anomaly is present, the person's concern is markedly excessive.

2. The preoccupation causes clinically significant distress or impairment in social, occupational, or other important areas of functioning.

3. The preoccupation is not better accounted for by another mental disorder (e.g., dissatisfaction with body shape and size in anorexia nervosa).

---

hair, but by definition the flaw is slight. Nonetheless, they're preoccupied with it and consider it ugly and clearly visible to others. A study from England, which used an objective measure of facial appearance known as morphoanalysis, found that in BDD the focus of dissatisfaction is usually normal.

But the word "imagined" is complicated and can be problematic. While some people with BDD realize that they imagine their defect—that it really looks okay and they're blowing it out of proportion—others are certain their view is correct. They think they *really do* look terrible and balk at the word "imagined." They worry that if they're imagining their defect, they may be labeled as "crazy." Some insist that because they're not imagining the defect, they must not have BDD, even though they really do. One person asked me, "My problem is really there; it's true. Do you deal with true things or only imaginary things?" He thought that if I dealt only with "imaginary things," then I wasn't the doctor he should be seeing.

It isn't known whether people with BDD see what other people see but *interpret* it differently, considering the body part unattractive when others don't. Or do they actually *see* the body part differently? Most likely, one of these two possibilities pertains to BDD. The question isn't so much whether the defect is "real" versus "imagined," but rather why it is that people with BDD perceive their appearance differently from other people.

Yet another knotty issue is how to determine whether a defect, if present, is "slight," which is required by BDD's definition. If the defect is very obvious to others—if it's immediately noticeable—then by definition the person doesn't have BDD. But what if the defect is more subtle? Who's to judge whether it's slight or not? These questions take us into a subjective realm where reality and distortion can't always be clearly differentiated. To some extent, just as beauty is in the eye of the beholder, so is ugliness. If someone with BDD thinks her legs are huge, but I think they're only "slightly" big, who is right? Should a woman who's 5'11" and preoccupied with her height be considered "slightly" tall? In some cases, I don't notice the defect when I meet someone, but when it's pointed out I can see that it's actually there. Is such a defect "slight" or "nonslight"?

It's helpful to consider what *most people* observe. I often have corroboration from others—clinicians, family members, or friends—who agree that the defect is nonexistent or slight. The most common reason people with BDD are turned down for surgery or other medical treatment is that the physician can't perceive the defect or considers it too minimal to treat. One patient was referred to me by a dermatologist who described her as "a woman with beautiful skin." Many of my patients have been brought to me by family members who recognize that their loved one has an inaccurate view of how bad the defect is. I and several dermatologists did a study in which we independently rated the severity of skin defects and found that in general we closely agreed about which defects were slight and which were clearly noticeable, which suggests that such judgments can be made with reasonably good agreement and "objectivity."

Sometimes—although not always—BDD sufferers themselves agree that the defect is really only slight and they have a distorted view of how bad it is. As one young man told me, "My view of my appearance is illogical—I know I really look okay. I'm making a mountain out of a molehill."

If the defect is slight, then BDD's definition requires that the person's concern is "markedly excessive"—that is, they must be preoccupied. In addition, they typically overreact to the minor defect in terms of how it affects their life. Charles, a college student, left his dorm room only once during a two-week period when his mild acne worsened. He missed his classes and avoided all social activities. He even didn't visit a close friend who just learned he had cancer. True, Charles had some pimples, but hardly enough to warrant such extreme avoidance. Charles qualified for BDD because his defect, while present, wasn't particularly noticeable and his reaction was excessive.

What if I can't assess the severity of the defect because of its location? This is another challenge in diagnosing BDD. Many people with an "unassessable" defect have another supposed defect that's visible and can be assessed, which allows the diagnosis to be given. For example, although I didn't evaluate one patient's buttocks, I could see that his concern with his "crooked" eyes was unfounded. In other cases, an "unassessable" defect has been assessed by someone else who thinks it's fine; men with penis concerns often say that spouses and doctors alike have told them the size is normal.

This information also allows a presumptive diagnosis of BDD to be made. Making the diagnosis can also be complicated if noticeable scarring has been caused by skin picking; if it can be ascertained that the acne or scarring was fairly mild before the picking began, the person is a candidate for the BDD diagnosis.

I should emphasize, however, that in my experience the need to make difficult judgment calls is the exception rather than the rule. Of the patients I've seen, only 5% have had an unassessable defect in the absence of others I could assess. Fewer than one-third have had an actual defect, and in only some cases was it difficult to determine whether it was "slight" or clearly present. Most of those I've seen had what I considered a nonexistent defect. In some cases, the body part of concern is actually very attractive. One woman obsessed with her "ugly" hair actually had hair that was widely considered unusually attractive. While she despaired because she thought it was "frizzy and ugly," other women asked her who her hairdresser was so they could have theirs done in a similar style. Another young woman had been asked to work as a model, and as a child she'd been told that she would someday be Miss America; she, however, believed that such requests and statements were motivated by pity for her ugliness.

It's worth considering whether people with more noticeable, "clearly present" defects (who don't qualify for a BDD diagnosis because of the obvious nature of their deformities) might nonetheless have features of BDD. Do people with birth defects, accident victims, or others with very noticeable physical flaws have experiences similar to those of people with BDD? Are they preoccupied with their flaw? Do they suffer as a result? Does it interfere with their functioning? Do they feel very self-conscious in social situations?

I've met some individuals with obvious defects for whom the answers to these questions are "yes." And research findings suggest that, for some individuals, the answers are "yes." Although by definition they don't have BDD because their defect is very obvious, they're preoccupied, distressed, and sometimes impaired by their appearance concerns. It's possible that much of what I'll be describing in this book applies to them as well. And what about people with physical features that, strictly speaking, aren't defects or flaws—for example, tattoos they no longer like? Do some of them have features of BDD? Some appear to. This is another important question that needs to be studied.

To return to BDD's definition, I've already briefly discussed criterion 2 in Table 1 (distress or impairment), noting that degree of distress and impairment varies considerably. This criterion is very helpful; requiring distress or impairment for the diagnosis helps guard against overdiagnosis.

Not everyone who's worried about his or her appearance has BDD. After all, concern with appearance is very common, especially during adolescence. Studies have shown that most people dislike at least some aspect of how they look. And this concern is no doubt amplified by the messages we get from fashion magazines, clothing advertisements, and makeup commercials. Magazines, television, billboards, and movies are filled with beautiful and glamorous people who, intended or not, set a certain standard for how we should look.

So criterion 2 attempts to draw a line between normal and excessive concern and indicates that people with normal appearance concerns shouldn't be considered to have a psychiatric disorder. A problem with this criterion, however, is that it isn't clear exactly where the line should be drawn. What if someone is quite distressed about her appearance but hasn't suffered any impairment as a result; she works and leads a fairly normal social life. Does she have BDD? How much distress is required for the diagnosis? And how much impairment? While this issue of where to distinguish between "normal" and "abnormal" also applies to other psychiatric and medical disorders, it's particularly complicated with regard to BDD because BDD echoes the very common concern so many of us have with how we look. Where normal concern leaves off and BDD begins is sometimes a difficult judgment call. But in cases of moderately severe or severe BDD—like Jennifer's, Chris's, and Andrew's—it's crystal clear that the suffering and impairment are significant and, therefore, the diagnosis applies.

The purpose of criterion 3 (the preoccupation isn't better accounted for by another disorder) is to ascertain that people with anorexia nervosa and certain other psychiatric disorders don't get misdiagnosed with BDD. Anorexia nervosa is a disorder in which people—usually young women—think they're too fat and lose excessive amounts of weight to avoid being fat. Sometimes they become skeletal but still fear they are, or will become, fat. According to DSM-IV definitions, someone whose only concern is that she's too fat and who is significantly (about 15% or more) underweight (and who meets certain other criteria for anorexia) should be diagnosed with anorexia nervosa, not BDD.

But the relationship between BDD and anorexia gets complicated when we consider the following: some researchers suggest that the core disturbance in anorexia nervosa isn't a problem with eating or food, but with body image. Indeed, people with anorexia fulfill criterion 1 for BDD in that they're preoccupied with a defect in their appearance (being fat) that others don't perceive. This view raises the very interesting and even heretical question of whether anorexia might be a form of BDD. If so, we would need to delete BDD's criterion 3. The interesting relationship between eating disorders and BDD is one that I'll return to later. In the meantime, I'll note that a person can receive diagnoses of both anorexia *and* BDD, if, for example, she thinks that she's too fat *and* her nose is too bumpy.

The DSM-IV criteria for BDD provide a useful common language for patients, clinicians, and researchers alike. They help researchers ascertain that they are all studying the same phenomenon. It's important that what I call BDD is what a researcher elsewhere calls BDD; this allows a coherent body of knowledge about the disorder to be developed. The criteria also allow clinicians to make the diagnosis, which, in turn, guides treatment. They can also be helpful to patients. As a man with BDD said to me, "I read DSM to find out what was wrong with me. It was a relief to know what I had. Finally, I'd found the road and a sign on the road telling me where I was."

While the criteria are useful guidelines, they do have the limitations I've discussed. In addition, in no way do they convey the experience of people with BDD. They don't tell us about their lives—the private torment, the fears, the isolation. Nor do they adequately convey what is unique about each person's experience.

Patients' experiences tell us far more than criteria ever could. Jennifer and Sarah had certain things in common with Jane, whose story follows. They all fulfilled the diagnostic criteria for BDD: each was preoccupied with physical defects that were nonexistent or minimal and generally went unnoticed by others, and each was significantly distressed or impaired by her concerns. But their experiences were quite different. Sarah's symptoms were relatively mild, and she functioned well despite them. Jane's symptoms, in contrast, were very severe. She couldn't work and had been hospitalized. She even thought she was so ugly that people stared at her through binoculars, and she believed that drivers were so distracted by her "ugliness" that they got into car crashes when they saw her.

"My Biggest Wish Is to Be Invisible"

I clearly remember meeting Jane. As she rose from her chair in the waiting room I was struck by her long dark hair, soft features, and deep blue eyes. She was in her mid-thirties, fashionably dressed, tall, thin, and stately. She looked kind and earnest—but very timid and anxious. As she entered my office she explained that a friend had driven her to her appointment because she was too afraid to drive alone—which had everything to do with why she had come to see me.

"My biggest wish is to be invisible," she began. Despite her severe anxiety, she had the courage to get straight to the heart of the matter. Many people who see me are far too anxious to talk about their appearance right away. "Why do you want to be invisible?" I asked. "So no one will laugh at me and think I'm ugly," she replied. "That's my biggest fear." On the one hand, Jane's statements were hard to understand. She seemed a lovely woman, both her demeanor and her appearance. At the same time, I thought I understood. By now I had seen scores of people with BDD and knew this was how many of them feel.

"I think I have this disorder you're studying," she continued. "And I'm *totally* paralyzed by it. I think I have a really bad case. I haven't worked in ages. And you may not believe this, but I've hardly left my house in six years. This is one of the few times. That's why I couldn't come alone—I was much too scared." I had heard many people say they couldn't leave their house because they thought they were too ugly—but six years?

Jane wanted to start at the beginning. "My hatred of my appearance began when I was 12," she began. "I became obsessed with my nose; I thought it was too big and shiny. It started when I heard a boy in my class make a comment about Jimmy Durante. I can't even remember what he said, but he was snickering, and I was sure it was a mean comment. I thought he might be making fun of *me*—of *my* nose. I couldn't be sure, but I kept worrying that maybe there *was* something wrong with my nose, even though I'd never worried about it before. After that I started lifting up my lips to raise my nose so it wouldn't look so big. After a while, I couldn't concentrate in school because all I could think of was my nose. I didn't do my final eighth-grade project because I couldn't stand up in front of the class and have people see my nose. I skipped school that day and got an F. All my grades dropped—I went from straight As to Ds and Fs. I got very withdrawn, and I stopped seeing my friends."

"What were you like before then?" I asked. "I really wasn't very concerned with how I looked," she replied. "I was very active, a good student, and I had lots of confidence. But I was always very sensitive. And I wasn't very interested in boys and thought I should have been, so I wondered if something was wrong with me. But basically I was fine. Then the nose problem started, and my life went downhill. I've thought about it every day since.

"When I was 16 things got even worse," she continued. "When I was much younger I'd fallen against a table and got a slight scar on the top of my lip, but it never really bothered me until I was 16, when I got it surgically revised. Now I realize that was a mistake. Obviously, I got the revision to make the scar less noticeable, even though it was pretty faint, but it just made it worse. After the operation, I noticed a funny irregularity in a certain light, and it's been a disaster ever since. I think about it all the time—24 hours a day. I even have dreams about it. In my dreams people ask me things like, 'What's that thing on your lip?' and then they make nasty comments about it."

Jane's concern with her faint scar started at the time she was having problems with her boyfriend. "Maybe it was the stress," she said. "But I don't want you to misunderstand," she added. "Some of my therapists have tried to convince me that my appearance concerns are just a symptom of other problems—that they aren't my real problem. After years and years of trying to figure this out, I've finally come to the conclusion that they're wrong. *My obsessions have a life of their own.* They're a problem in their own right! They're not just a symptom of other problems." Jane started crying as she said this.

"I've been incredibly frustrated when I've been told that this isn't my real problem and that I had to figure out what my real problem is," she said. "*This* is a real problem. I do have other problems. I don't want you to think this is my only one. I've had problems with my parents, and I don't get along with my brother. Our family has had some serious financial problems. But this obsession is the biggest problem in my life. *This* is the problem that's kept me in my house for six years. I don't know if it's related to my childhood. Sometimes it feels *chemical,* totally out of my control, as if there's something biological driving it." Jane had fortunately found a therapist and a psychiatrist who took her concerns seriously and who treated her BDD as a legitimate disorder. That attitude alone had helped her greatly.

Jane returned to her story. But first she pulled her suede jacket up over her chin and mouth so I couldn't see her face from the nose down. She smiled slightly through her tears. "I have to hide my face before I tell you about this one," she said. Then she became completely serious. "It started when I was in my early twenties. I started worrying about my jaw when a surgeon I'd seen for a nose job said my nose was fine but my jaw was too big. I was totally devastated by that comment, and I've been haunted ever since. How could a simple comment like that trigger such a strong obsession that I've had ever since?"

Over the years, Jane had also worried about other things—that her breasts were too small and her buttocks too "big and round." "I tried to go to school to become a fashion designer—I was told I had a lot of talent—but I had to drop out. I couldn't go. I couldn't let people see how bad I looked. So many of my body parts were totally unpresentable. Then I tried working, but I stayed only a few weeks at each place. I felt I was really ugly and really unlikable. I just couldn't let people see me. It got worse and worse. I stopped dating, and then I stopped going out at all. I'm sure I'll never get married because of this. How can I? I never meet anyone. I'm totally isolated.

"My sister and grandmother started buying my clothes and food. I started spending my entire day in my parents' house. Sometimes I watch television, but mostly I walk back and forth between the bedrooms on the third floor, thinking about how ugly I look. When relatives come over, I stay upstairs and don't see them. I don't even see them on holidays like Thanksgiving. I feel overwhelmed and hopeless and out of control. Sometimes I panic and think 'I can't tolerate this. I'm going to die. I have to kill myself. I wish I could be put to sleep.' "

Jane started crying again. Her pain seemed too much to bear. "The hardest part of this is the isolation. I didn't see my own mother for two years, even though she lived in the same house with me. I was so ashamed of my appearance and that I'd dropped out of school and wasn't working that I completely avoided her. My family has no idea that I have this problem. I've kept it a secret. It's immature for me to be so concerned with how I look. I've been too ashamed to tell them."

Jane then described the one time she'd left her house in six years. "I got sick," she explained. "I tried putting off going to the doctor, but the pain got pretty intense. My grandmother convinced me to see him. When I finally went, I covered my face with bandages, so no one could see how I looked."

I thought of someone I'd seen several times in the town where I live. His face was notably disfigured—reddened and deeply scarred—and his nose and lips were misshapen. He looked as though he had birth defects and had suffered third-degree burns. This is what Jane *felt* she looked like—so deformed that when she left her house she covered her entire face with bandages.

"So coming here today was a big event. I haven't been out in so long that I was afraid to drive by myself. Sometimes when I drive I get especially freaked out because I think everyone is looking at me as they drive by and that they're thinking how ugly I am. Sometimes I think my face will frighten them so much that they'll crash their cars."

Jane had received a lot of treatment, both surgical and psychiatric. A nose job didn't help her feel any better about her nose, so she had it redone. The second procedure wasn't helpful either. The revision of the scar on her lip actually triggered a new obsession. She continued to seek surgical treatment but finally stopped after four surgeons refused to do any further procedures.

"Later, when I realized my problem was psychiatric, not physical, it was still really hard for me," Jane said. "The first time I was hospitalized, the doctors and nurses on the psychiatry ward hadn't heard of BDD, so it was hard for them to understand me or take me seriously. I think they tried, but they didn't really get it. No one knew my inner torment. They tried to reassure me and talk me out of my concern, telling me I looked fine. The reassurance just made me feel pathetic. It felt patronizing. If I'd had any other problem, they would never have taken that approach. They would have realized it doesn't work."

Jane had received cognitive-behavioral therapy, a type of therapy that focuses on helping patients resist compulsive behaviors, such as mirror checking, and facing feared situations, such as social situations. She had also been treated with many psychiatric medications, including antipsychotics, lithium, tranquilizers, antidepressants, and others. A type of antidepressant known as a monoamine-oxidase inhibitor had been very helpful for several years but then stopped working. Because she then became so severely depressed over her appearance, Jane received electroconvulsive therapy (ECT), also known as shock therapy. This treatment, which is often extremely effective for severe depression, did temporarily help her depression somewhat but not her BDD. "It's still on my mind all the time," she said, "and I still consider suicide because of it."

Jane had also been in several support groups for people with a variety of psychiatric difficulties such as anxiety and depression. "Everyone else was pretty open about their problems, and I was to a certain extent. I talked about my depression and my family problems. But I couldn't discuss my appearance. I told them there was a big thing I was worried about, but I couldn't tell them what it was, even though I was in the group for four years. It was too humiliating, and I was afraid they wouldn't understand. I was afraid they'd focus on my defects more and notice how horrendous they looked. And I was afraid of their reaction, which I'd hear negatively, no matter what. That's what *always* happens. If someone says I look nice, I think that means I must have looked bad some other time. Or if someone says I have nice eyes, that must mean that something else about me is ugly. Or what if they didn't say something positive about my appearance the next time they saw me? I'd assume that meant I looked terrible! My *biggest* fear was that they'd *validate* my concern. I couldn't take the risk. So my isolation continued."

At the time she saw me, Jane was considering a consultation for a cingulotomy, a type of brain surgery that patients with severe psychiatric disorders sometimes undergo when other treatments haven't worked. Its effectiveness in BDD isn't known because it hasn't been studied. "I really don't want to have brain surgery," she said, "but I can't go on suffering like this."

I didn't treat Jane, but I spoke with her several times after I'd seen her. I'd recommended to her and her doctor that she postpone the surgery consultation and try a new combination of medications. With her new medications (a higher dose of fluoxetine [Prozac] than she'd taken in the past plus a medication called buspirone [Buspar]), she gradually felt better. Four months after I'd seen her she gave me a call. "You won't believe this," she said. "The medications have helped immensely. I can get out of the house, and I'm doing volunteer work as a receptionist." It was hard to believe that she had made such progress—even harder to believe that she was doing something that required her to interact so closely with people. "I still have BDD feelings," she said, "but I can view it more rationally. I can tell myself that people aren't looking at me. It's a real triumph to allow people to get so close to my face."

I heard from Jane again about six months later. Although her BDD wasn't entirely gone, she was still feeling much better, and was still successfully volunteering. But about a year later, she called to tell me that she'd been feeling tired and more depressed. It appeared that her depression had returned. She decided to stop her medications, and her BDD symptoms gradually came back. The last time I spoke with her she was trying other medications and still struggling with her symptoms.

I hope that these stories, and others throughout this book, will convey *both* the common themes of BDD—what all people with this disorder share— *and* the uniqueness of each person's experience. Everyone with the disorder has much in common, yet each person's experience is his or her own. And even though BDD is quite different in some ways from normal appearance concerns, it also echoes them—it is an amplified, exaggerated, and sometimes quite distorted version of what most of us experience.

·· *four* ··

How Do I Know If I Have BDD?

Why BDD Is Underdiagnosed

BDD isn't rare. Dr. Mark Zimmerman and Jill Mattia, of Brown University School of Medicine, and I found that approximately 4% of 316 people seeking medical treatment in an outpatient setting had probable BDD. Of 500 people seeking psychiatric treatment in an outpatient setting, we found that 12% had probable BDD—yet the BDD diagnosis was missed by the patient's clinician in all cases. While preliminary, these numbers translate into many millions of people.

These percentages are surprisingly high—in fact, many mental health professionals might be skeptical of them. If BDD is really this common, why don't they see more patients who have it? The likely explanation is that BDD is underrecognized and underdiagnosed for some of the following reasons.

Secrecy and Shame

BDD is often a secret disorder. The diagnosis isn't made because the symptoms aren't revealed. Many people I've seen have never mentioned their appearance concerns to others. Many who've been in treatment with a mental health professional have never discussed their BDD symptoms, even though they were a significant problem. Courage is usually needed to bring them up and discuss them. *If the concerns aren't asked about, they may not be revealed.*

Reasons for secrecy and shame include the following:

- Worry about seeming superficial, silly, or vain;

- Worry that once the perceived defect is mentioned, others will notice it and focus on it more, resulting in even more embarrassment and shame;

- Fear that disclosure of the worry will be met with reassurance that the BDD sufferer looks fine. Many people with BDD interpret this response, although honest and well-meaning, to mean that they were foolish to have mentioned it, or that their emotional pain isn't being taken seriously or understood. If they get this response, they may not mention it again.

Lack of Familiarity with BDD

Many, including health professionals, aren't aware that BDD is a known psychiatric disorder that often responds to psychiatric treatment. Despite its long history, BDD entered psychiatry's diagnostic manual, DSM, only recently. When I began my research, most of the mental health professionals I queried had never even heard of BDD. Fortunately, this is changing, but BDD is still among the lesser-known psychiatric disorders.

Trivialization

BDD is easily trivialized. Why should he care so much about a few pimples? How could she be so worried about her face when she's so pretty? The fact that BDD sufferers generally look fine, combined with the fact that appearance concerns are so common in the general population, contribute to its trivialization. BDD is easily mistaken for vanity. But anyone who knows someone like Jennifer or Jane is only too aware of how serious—even life-threatening—the disorder can be.

Misdiagnosis

BDD is often accompanied by depression, social anxiety, and other symptoms that are often easier for BDD sufferers to discuss. Thus, they may receive the diagnosis of depression or social phobia, but not BDD. In addition, patients who reveal their BDD symptoms are sometimes told the symptoms aren't their "real problem"—that their real problem is low self-esteem, a relationship problem, or another issue. Although these problems may coexist with BDD, the BDD itself should also be diagnosed and treated if present.

Pursuit of Nonpsychiatric Medical and Surgical Treatment

Many people with BDD see dermatologists, plastic surgeons, and other physicians rather than mental health professionals. They search, usually unsuccessfully, for a cosmetic solution to a body-image problem. Most people are unaware that BDD is a known psychiatric disorder for which psychiatric treatment is often effective.

Screening Questions for BDD

How do you know whether you or someone you know has BDD? For the time being, psychiatric diagnoses—including BDD—are made primarily on the basis of asking questions that ascertain that DSM-IV criteria for the disorder are fulfilled. There are as yet no blood tests, brain-scanning techniques, or other tools sufficient to diagnose psychiatric disorders, although such tools are being worked on.

I've developed several "diagnostic instruments" for BDD, which consist of questions useful in making the diagnosis. The set of questions (the BDDQ) on the next page is in a self-report format; that is, the patient fills out the questionnaire. The other set of questions, which is included in Appendix B (the BDD Diagnostic Module), is asked by a clinician. Both sets mirror the DSM-IV diagnostic criteria for BDD discussed in the last chapter, and they ascertain whether these criteria are fulfilled.

What follows is the BDDQ, or Body Dysmorphic Disorder Questionnaire, which assesses whether BDD may be present.

Body Dysmorphic Disorder Questionnaire (BDDQ)

Name _____

This questionnaire assesses concerns about physical appearance. Please read each question carefully and circle the answer that best describes your experience. Also write in answers where indicated.

1. Are you very concerned about the appearance of some part(s) of your body that you consider especially unattractive?   Yes   No

   If yes: Do these concerns preoccupy you? That is, you think about them a lot and wish you could think about them less?   Yes   No

      If yes: What are they? _____
      _____

      Examples of areas of concern include: your skin (e.g., acne, scars, wrinkles, paleness, redness); hair (e.g., hair loss or thinning); the shape or size of your nose, mouth, jaw, lips, stomach, hips, etc.; or defects of your hands, genitals, breasts, or any other body part.

      If yes: What *specifically* bothers you about the appearance of these body part(s)? (Explain in detail): _____
      _____

(NOTE: If you answered "No" to either of the above questions, you are finished with this questionnaire. Otherwise please continue.)

2. Is your main concern with your appearance that you aren't thin enough or that you might become too fat?   Yes   No

3. What effect has your preoccupation with your appearance had on your life?

   • Has your defect(s) caused you a lot of distress, torment, or pain?   Yes   No

   • Has it significantly interfered with your social life?   Yes   No

   If yes: How? _____
   _____
   _____

   • Has your defect(s) significantly interfered with your school work, your job, or your ability to function in your role (e.g., as a homemaker)?   Yes   No

continued

If yes: How? _____
_____
_____

- Are there things you avoid because of your defect(s)?   Yes   No

  If yes: What are they? _____
  _____

- Have the lives or normal routines of your family
  or friends been affected by your defect(s)?   Yes   No

  If yes: How? _____
  _____
  _____

4. How much time do you spend thinking about your defect(s) per day
   on average? (circle one)

   (a) Less than 1 hour a day
   (b) 1–3 hours a day
   (c) More than 3 hours a day

You're likely to have BDD if you give the following answers on the BDDQ:

- Question 1: Yes to both parts
- Question 3: Yes to any of the questions
- Question 4: Answer b or c

Question 1 establishes whether preoccupation is present, and question 3 establishes whether significant distress or impairment are present. Regarding question 4, while the BDD criteria don't require that the defect be thought about for a specified amount of time a day, it's useful to ask this question. If at least one hour a day is spent thinking about it, I'm more likely to diagnose BDD. In fact, I have significant reservations about diagnosing BDD in anyone who spends less than an hour a day thinking about their defect, because I'd generally consider them insufficiently preoccupied to fulfill criterion 1 for the diagnosis. Everyone I've given the diagnosis to has at some point spent at least this much time focused on their concern.

A note of caution about the BDDQ is that it's intended as a screening instrument, not a diagnostic one. What this means is that the BDDQ can suggest that BDD is present but can't necessarily give a definitive diagnosis. The diagnosis is ideally determined by a trained clinician in a face-to-face interview. There are several reasons for this. First, in general, clinical judgment should be used to confirm that answers on a self-report questionnaire indicate the presence of a disorder; for example, is any distress or impairment that's reported on the questionnaire problematic enough to warrant a psychiatric diagnosis? In addition, for BDD to be diagnosed, it must be ascertained that the physical defect is nonexistent or slight. Finally, as required by DSM-IV criterion 3, a clinician should ascertain that appearance concerns aren't better accounted for by an eating disorder. (A "yes" answer to question 2 raises the question of whether an eating disorder is a more accurate diagnosis.)

Typical, as well as less common, BDD concerns—what people worry about and what body areas they dislike—are described in the next chapter. Although a preoccupation with virtually any body part may qualify for this diagnosis, the question of whether a concern with weight alone qualifies for a diagnosis of BDD is controversial. This is an issue I'll discuss further in Chapter 12.

Additional information about the BDDQ, including its psychometric (measurement) properties, is included in Appendix B. That appendix also includes the clinician-administered counterpart of the BDDQ (the BDD Diagnostic Module), a brief set of questions determining the presence of BDD, along with a clinician-administered instrument that assesses the severity of BDD symptoms (the Yale-Brown Obsessive Compulsive Scale modified for BDD).

Clues: Mirror Checking, Grooming, Skin Picking, and Others

The BDDQ questions ask about the core definitional features of BDD—what's required for the diagnosis. But BDD has some features that, while not necessary for the diagnosis, can provide clues to its presence. These include frequent mirror checking, excessive grooming, face picking, and reassurance seeking.

I've sometimes observed strangers doing things that have made me wonder if they have BDD. I once saw a young man in a parking lot who stood outside his car repeatedly checking his hair in a side-view mirror, frantically combing and recombing it. He wasn't simply taking a quick glance, as many people would—instead he seemed "stuck" there, and appeared extremely agitated and distressed over the state of his hair. I once drove behind a woman on a busy highway for about 20 miles who spent most of the time looking in her rearview mirror fixing her hair, rather than looking at the road. And what about the young woman I saw at a baseball game who seemed to have normal body hair except for that on her arms, which was completely absent? Had she removed it through excessive "grooming," trying to improve "excessively" hairy arms? Did any of these people have BDD? Without talking with them, I couldn't make the diagnosis. But their behaviors were clues to the diagnosis that made me wonder.

Some of the more common clues to BDD are in Table 2.

Table 2   Clues to the Presence of BDD

1. Do you often check your appearance in mirrors or other reflecting surfaces, such as windows? Or do you frequently check your appearance without using a mirror, by looking directly at the disliked body part?

2. Do you avoid mirrors because you dislike how you look?

3. Do you frequently compare yourself to others and often think that you look worse than they do?

4. Do you often ask—or want to ask—others whether you look okay, or whether you look as good as other people?

5. Do you try to convince other people that there's something wrong with how you look, but they consider the problem nonexistent or minimal?

6. Do you spend a lot of time grooming—for example, combing or arranging your hair, tweezing or cutting your hair, applying makeup, or shaving? Do you spend too much time getting ready in the morning, or do you groom yourself frequently during the day? Do others complain that you spend too much time in the bathroom?

7. Do you pick your skin because you're trying to make it look better?

8. Do you try to cover or hide parts of your body with a hat, clothing, makeup, sunglasses, your hair, your hand, or other things? Is it hard to be around other people when you haven't done these things?

9. Do you often change your clothes, trying to find an outfit that covers or improves disliked aspects of your appearance? Do you take a long time selecting your outfit for the day, trying to find one that makes you look better?

10. Do you try to hide certain aspects of your appearance by maintaining a certain body position—for example, turning your face away from others? Do you feel uncomfortable if you can't be in your preferred positions?

11. Do you think that other people take special notice of you in a negative way because of how you look? For example, when you walk down the street, do you think others are noticing what's unattractive about you?

12. Do you think that other people are thinking negative thoughts about you or making fun of you because of how you look? Are you "paranoid" because of this?

13. Is it hard for you to leave your house, or have you actually been housebound, because of how you look?

14. Do you frequently measure parts of your body, hoping to find they're as small as, as large as, or as symmetrical as you'd like?

15. Do you spend a lot of time reading about your appearance problems in the hope that you'll reassure yourself about how you look or find a solution to your problem?

16. Have you wanted to get cosmetic surgery, dermatologic treatment, or other medical treatment to fix your appearance when other people (for example, friends or doctors) have told you such treatment isn't necessary? Have surgeons been reluctant to do cosmetic surgery, saying the defect is too minor or they're afraid you won't be pleased with the results?

17. Have you had cosmetic surgery and been disappointed with the results? Or have you had multiple surgeries, hoping that with the next procedure your appearance problems will finally be fixed?

18. Do you work out excessively to improve your appearance?

19. Do you diet, even though others tell you it isn't necessary?

20. Do you avoid having your picture taken because you think you look so bad?

21. Are you late for things because you worry you don't look okay or because you're trying to fix an appearance problem?

22. Do you get depressed or anxious because of how you look?

23. Have you felt that life wasn't worth living because of your appearance?

24. Do you get very frustrated or angry because of how you look?

25. Does it take you longer to do things because you're distracted by appearance worries or related behaviors such as mirror checking?

26. Do you feel more comfortable going out at night, or sitting in a dark part of a room, because your defects will be less visible?

27. Do you have panic attacks or get very anxious when you look in the mirror because of how you look?

Many of these questions ask about behaviors, such as mirror checking and reassurance seeking, that many people with BDD perform (these are described in Chapter 7). Other questions ask about consequences of BDD—for example, being housebound (these are described in Chapter 8). A "yes" answer to any of the above questions doesn't necessarily indicate that you have BDD. But "yes" answers—especially many "yes" answers—suggest that BDD may very well be present and that further evaluation is warranted to determine whether it is.

Additional Clues: Depression, Social Anxiety, and Other Symptoms

Many people with BDD are depressed. Others have problems with alcohol, drugs, or anxiety. Some have panic attacks. Indeed, BDD often coexists with other psychiatric symptoms and disorders, which can provide additional clues to its presence.

I have carefully assessed the frequency of other psychiatric disorders (e.g., depression) in people with BDD. Conversely, I and other researchers have studied the frequency of BDD in patients with other psychiatric disorders. These findings are shown in greater detail in Appendix C. What these study results suggest is that major depression is very common in people with BDD. Major depression is characterized by depressed mood, decreased interest and pleasure, and other symptoms, such as sleep and appetite disturbance. (See Appendix A for a further description of this and other psychiatric disorders.) While major depression is fairly common, affecting 10 to 20% of the general population at some point in their lifetime, the lifetime rate of depression in people with BDD is strikingly higher than this—over 80%. In addition, the depression is often quite severe.

In a study I did with Drs. Andrew Nierenberg, Maurizio Fava, and their colleagues of Harvard Medical School, we found, conversely, that BDD is also surprisingly common among people with major depression. In fact, we discovered that among nearly 250 depressed patients, BDD was more common than obsessive compulsive disorder, which affects 2% to 3% of the general population. This result is striking because, as a little-known disorder, BDD generally isn't looked for in people with depression. In addition, we found that depressed people who also had BDD had onset of depression at a relatively young age and that their depression was unusually persistent. These findings suggest that depressed people—especially those with long-standing depression—should be asked whether they have BDD.

Certain other disorders also commonly co-occur with BDD and may provide clues to its presence. One of these is social phobia, an excessive fear of social or performance situations due to a fear of doing something embarrassing or humiliating. Another is obsessive compulsive disorder, characterized by obsessions (intrusive, recurrent, unwanted thoughts that are difficult to dismiss despite their disturbing nature) and compulsions (repetitive behaviors that are intended to reduce the anxiety caused by obsessions). People with these disorders, too, should be asked whether they have symptoms of BDD. It's important to inquire, because BDD sufferers may be too embarrassed and ashamed to volunteer their symptoms. In the depression study I described, not a single person revealed his or her BDD symptoms until specifically asked about them, reflecting the often secretive nature of BDD.

BDD Can Be Misdiagnosed

In addition to being *under*diagnosed, BDD can easily be *mis*diagnosed as another psychiatric disorder. This occurs because BDD can produce symptoms that mimic another disorder, such as social phobia. Some of the disorders BDD can easily be confused with are the following.

- **Social phobia** *(an excessive fear of social or performance situations due to a fear of doing something embarrassing or humiliating):* BDD often causes social anxiety and withdrawal. The social anxiety may be quite noticeable, but the BDD symptoms may be kept secret. This can lead to a misdiagnosis of social phobia. If social phobia symptoms are largely due to BDD, BDD rather than social phobia should be diagnosed. Some people have *both* BDD and social phobia, in which case both diagnoses should be given.

- **Agoraphobia** *(anxiety about being in places or situations from which escape might be difficult or embarrassing, or in which help might not be available, in the event of having a panic attack or panic-like symptoms):* Because people with BDD may think they're too ugly to leave their house, or because they fear that others are taking special notice of their defect, they may feel anxious in and avoid a variety of situations. Thus, BDD can be misdiagnosed as agoraphobia. People with features of agoraphobia should be asked whether they're anxious in and avoid situations because of how they look.

While most people with a diagnosis of agoraphobia don't have BDD, some of them do, and the BDD can easily be missed.

- **Panic disorder** *(recurrent panic attacks that come out of the blue followed by concern about having more attacks, worry about the consequences of the attacks, or a significant change in behavior related to the attacks):* Some people with BDD have panic attacks as a result of their BDD. They feel intensely uncomfortable and fearful—and experience physical symptoms, such as a pounding heart, sweating, or trouble breathing—because they're so upset by how they look. These attacks of extreme anxiety can be triggered by the mirror or by thinking that someone is staring at or making fun of the perceived defect.

    Panic attacks that are caused by BDD shouldn't be diagnosed as panic disorder. To receive a diagnosis of panic disorder, the panic attacks must come "out of the blue," rather than triggered by a particular situation or by symptoms of another disorder. It's important to ask people with panic attacks whether anything consistently triggers them. Sometimes BDD is the cause and should be diagnosed. Panic attacks may be the initial clue that leads to the diagnosis of BDD.

- **Trichotillomania** *(recurrent pulling out of one's hair, resulting in noticeable hair loss):* Some people with BDD pull out their hair to improve their appearance. They may, for example, pull out eyebrow hair to improve the "hideous shape" of their brows, or pull out head hair to make it look "acceptable." Hair pulling in response to a perceived defect in appearance should be diagnosed as BDD, not trichotillomania.

- **Obsessive compulsive disorder** *(obsessions [intrusive, recurrent, unwanted thoughts that are difficult to dismiss despite their disturbing nature] and compulsions [repetitive behaviors intended to reduce the anxiety caused by obsessions]):* Many people with BDD are misdiagnosed as having obsessive compulsive disorder because of the obsessional nature of BDD concerns and the repetitive nature of many BDD behaviors. Although BDD and obsessive compulsive disorder have much in common (as I'll discuss further in Chapter 12), BDD should be diagnosed if the thoughts focus on appearance.

BDD is usually easy to recognize if the reasons for misdiagnosis and underdiagnosis, as well as the clues in this chapter, are kept in mind.

But what's most important is taking your own concerns or those of someone else seriously. Reassurance may be taken to mean that the problem isn't really being listened to or understood. Asking about and listening to the concerns—and taking them seriously—is the best approach to take.

·· *five* ··

BDD Comes in Many Forms

"I'm the ugliest thing in the world. I hate my skin and my hair, and my hips are too fat. I hate how I look. I feel repulsive. It's the first thing I think of in the morning: how am I going to look today?"

Janice

Overview of Body Parts and Behaviors

Every time I meet someone with BDD and listen to their experience, I hear familiar themes. In some ways, their experience is similar to that of others with BDD (although they may find this hard to believe). But each person's story is also in some ways unique.

This is illustrated by Table 3 on the following pages, where I've listed 20 examples of body areas of concern, along with accompanying behaviors and consequences of the concern. Sufferers can dislike any part of their body and can engage in an unlimited variety of behaviors to cope with their concern. But although each person's experience is unique, certain patterns and themes are also evident.

The first description in the table refers to Carol, a young woman who thought that her thighs were too flabby and her nose misshapen. In reality, her thighs were taut; on close inspection, her nose was slightly misshapen,

Table 3   Examples of Preoccupations and Associated Behaviors*

Appearance Concerns	Associated Behaviors
1. Thighs too flabby Nose misshapen	1. Believes others take special notice Avoids mirrors Avoids swimming and social activities Had nose surgery
2. Thinning hair	2. Problems with girlfriend Social avoidance Consulted a dermatologist
3. Hair "never right" Body shape abnormal (hips too wide, shoulders too narrow, waist too high and wide)	3. Checks mirrors and windows excessively Buys excessive hair products Gets excessive haircuts and perms Questions others about appearance Wears baggy clothing Avoids fashion magazines, gym class, swimming, and social activities
4. Beard growth asymmetric Eyes too small	4. Believes others take special notice Checks mirrors excessively Compares self with others Shaves excessively Wears tinted glasses to hide eyes Grew long hair to cover face Avoids magazines, social activities, dating Housebound
5. Lines around mouth Hair loss Chin too prominent and asymmetric Teeth crooked, curved, and too large Cheeks sunken Nose too large	5. Believes others take special notice Excessively checks and avoids mirrors Compares self with others Questions others Avoids social activities and dating

continued

Table 3   *(continued)*

Appearance Concerns	Associated Behaviors
	Difficulty working Had braces several times
6. Facial skin and muscle tone flabby Hair too curly Dark circles under eyes	6. Checks mirrors and other reflecting surfaces excessively Frequent hair perms and straightening Frequent makeup application Compares self with others Avoids shopping, school, social situations, dating, and sex
7. Nose bumpy and too small at tip after surgery Facial and body hair excessive and dark One tooth longer than another	7. Believes others take special notice Excessively checks and avoids mirrors Avoids dating Had teeth filed Saw an endocrinologist to evaluate body hair Had electrolysis
8. Thinning hair Shrunken and sagging facial muscles Facial skin too loose Lips too thin Cheekbones asymmetric Penis too small Body build too small	8. Avoids mirrors Repeatedly touches doorknobs to tighten skin Excessively lifts weights Wears a hat Stuffs shorts and wears shirts down to knees to cover crotch Grew a beard to cover face Missed school Avoids shopping and social activities Leaves the house only at night Uses numerous hair tonics
9. Ugly face	9. Checks mirrors, car bumpers, and windows excessively Late for school

continued

Table 3　Examples of Preoccupations and Associated Behaviors *(continued)*

Appearance Concerns	*Associated Behaviors*
	Difficulty interviewing for jobs
10. Penis too small 　　Wrists and body build too 　　　small 　　Pot belly	10. Believes others take special 　　　notice 　　Checks mirrors excessively 　　Compares self with others 　　Avoids showers in gym class 　　Covers crotch with long 　　　clothes and wears bulky 　　　clothes 　　Lifts weights excessively 　　Avoids dating and sex 　　Consulted a urologist for 　　　penis surgery
11. Nose too large 　　Hair too curly 　　Forehead too high 　　Face too long and thin 　　Breasts too small	11. Believes others take special 　　　notice 　　Checks nose, brushes hair, 　　　and applies makeup 　　　excessively 　　Asks others for reassurance 　　Wears padded bras 　　Holds head in certain 　　　positions so nose looks 　　　smaller 　　Covers forehead with bangs 　　Spends large sums of money 　　　on hair products 　　Unable to go to school, 　　　work, swim, or socialize
12. Waist fat 　　Nose too wide 　　Chest hair asymmetric 　　Pubic, underarm, and leg hair 　　　ugly	12. Believes others take special 　　　notice 　　Checks mirrors and store 　　　and car windows 　　Changes clothes frequently 　　Sits and stands only in 　　　certain positions so waist 　　　isn't visible under clothing 　　Shaves body hair 　　Avoids commercials and ads 　　　with "gorgeous people"

continued

Table 3 *(continued)*

Appearance Concerns	Associated Behaviors
	Avoids dating, sex, swimming, shopping, and public transportation
	Had several nose jobs and liposuction
13. Circles and puffiness under eyes Lines on face Legs too thin and long Stomach too fat Buttocks misshapen	13. Believes others take special notice Checks mirrors and other reflecting surfaces excessively Questions others Compares self with others Avoids salty foods Takes diuretics (water pills) Camouflages with makeup Avoids swimming Had liposuction
14. Thinning hair Hips too slim Acne scarring Large pores on face Shoulders too broad	14. Believes others take special notice Compares self to others Avoids haircuts Got a hair weave Picks skin
15. Nose unattractive Chin and neck too large and wide Facial rash and acne Body too fat	15. Believes others take special notice Avoids mirrors Worries nose will break or otherwise be damaged Compares with others Covers face with hands Seeks reassurance Sleeps and uses alcohol to avoid thinking about appearance Avoids restaurants, other public places, and dating Housebound
16. Acne Eyes dull Breasts too small	16. Believes others take special notice Checks mirrors excessively

continued

**Table 3   Examples of Preoccupations and
Associated Behaviors** (continued)

Appearance Concerns	Associated Behaviors
	Camouflages with makeup
	Combs eyelashes excessively
	Stopped working; avoids dating and other social activities
	Housebound
17. Eyes "harsh, tired, and heavy" Face too wide Nose too large Body too fat	17. Believes others take special notice Checks mirrors and car rearview mirror excessively Wears bulky clothing Drinks excessive alcohol to decrease preoccupation Avoids beaches, parties, and vacations
18. Acne Hair sticks up and looks "bizarre" Skin "blotchy" (different colors and freckles) Nose too bumpy and long Too short and thin	18. Checks mirrors and store windows excessively; also avoids mirrors Compares with others Arranges and combs hair excessively Applies makeup excessively Picks skin Avoids haircuts because can't look at self in the mirror Questions others, asking for reassurance Lifts weights excessively Avoids direct eye contact Avoids shopping, dating, and other socializing (including weddings and other important events)
19. Hair "not right" (too flat, frizzy, and bangs too short or too long) Chin too small Eyes not big and bright enough and the wrong color	19. Believes others take special notice Checks mirrors excessively Combs hair and applies makeup excessively Questions others

continued

Table 3   *(continued)*

Appearance Concerns	Associated Behaviors
Hips too wide	Cuts hair impulsively Touches hair frequently to make sure it's "all right" Buys excessive number of hair products Avoids vacations to humid places, going outside on windy days, and swimming to avoid messing up hair Avoids shopping and public transportation
20. One buttock too fat (asymmetric) Stomach too fat	20. Exercises excessively Diets excessively Questions others Sleeps excessively and uses drugs to forget appearance concerns

*The descriptions are examples of what people with BDD experience; they don't provide a comprehensive list of all BDD concerns.

but not noticeably so. She nonetheless believed these defects were clearly visible to other people and that others even took special notice of them. Because she was so upset by her reflection, she avoided mirrors. She also avoided swimming, which she greatly enjoyed, many social events, and dating.

Which Body Parts Are Disliked?

It's interesting that William Stekel's observation from many decades ago—in which he commented on concerns with the nose, balding, ears, eyes, breasts, and genitals—are supported by recent research findings. My data, as well as that of several other researchers, suggest that people with BDD are usually concerned with specific parts of the body and that this concern can involve almost any body part but often focuses on the face. I've found that BDD preoccupations most often involve the skin, hair, or nose.

Table 4 illustrates that BDD can strike virtually anywhere. On average,

Table 4   Location of Perceived Defects in BDD

Body Part	Percent (%) of Patients with Concern*
Skin	65
Hair	50
Nose	38
Eyes	20
Legs/knees	18
Chin/jaw	13
Breasts/chest/nipples	12
Stomach/waist	11
Lips	11
Body build/bone structure	11
Face size/shape	10
Penis	9
Weight	9
Cheeks/cheekbones	8
Teeth	7
Ears	7
Head size/shape	6
Fingers/toes	5
Arms/wrists	5
Forehead	4
Hips	4
Height	4
Hands	3
Buttocks	3
Ugly face (general)	3
Feet	3
Facial muscles	2
Shoulders	2
Neck	2
Eyebrows	2

*The percentages add up to more than 100% because people are usually concerned with more than one aspect of their appearance.

people are concerned with three to four body parts over the course of the disorder. It's likely that worries about certain body areas—for example, the breasts and genitals—are underreported because of embarrassment, and that their true percentages are higher than those listed here.

Some people with BDD also have "subclinical" concerns with certain aspects of their appearance; that is, in addition to the body parts they're preoccupied with, they dislike other aspects of how they look, but not to the point where they're preoccupied with them or experience distress or impairment as a result. Heather, for example, was preoccupied with her "wide" nose and her weight, but her weight wasn't a significant concern and didn't preoccupy her. "It's much less severe than my nose," she said. "I don't like it, but it's not really a problem." In my research, I've made an effort to identify the body parts that are the focus of preoccupation, and have listed only excessive and problematic concerns in Table 4. If I had identified all the body parts which people had any dissatisfaction with whatsoever, the percentages for each body area would be much higher.

Some people with BDD think they sometimes look okay. As one woman said, "When my hair looks okay, I think I look attractive. But when it's bad, which it often is, I think I'm really ugly." People who are worried about minor acne may think they look fine when their skin is better—but when it's "broken out," it's a disaster.

I've found that skin concerns, especially concerns with facial acne or scarring, are most frequent. BDD sufferers use a variety of terms for such imperfections—not only acne or pimples, but also "bumps," "marks," "small black dots," "white spots," or "ugly things." But virtually any aspect of the skin can be disliked—facial pores that are considered unusually large, veins, capillaries, red marks, white marks, or other skin flaws. Some people think their skin is the wrong color—typically too red or too white. Others are preoccupied with wrinkles, lines, sagging, shriveling, or stretch marks, which they may consider a sign of aging.

Like Jennifer, who was preoccupied with pimples, scars, and facial marks, as well as her "ghost-like" skin color, some people have multiple skin concerns. Ellen was excessively preoccupied with supposed facial acne, scars, and veins, which were barely discernible to other people. Like Jennifer, she excessively checked mirrors and repeatedly asked her mother for reassurance—for example, "Do you think this pimple will go away? Will I have a scar?" To improve her skin, Ellen spent lots of time applying makeup and picking, sometimes using pins. She also compulsively washed her hands to avoid causing pimples while she picked. Dermatologic treatment temporarily diminished Ellen's preoccupation, but, as she described it, she became "more sensitive to smaller imperfections," resulting in no overall improvement in her concern.

Hair concerns—often that the hair is thinning or the hairline receding—are also very common. James, a teacher, thought his hair "never looked right." He feared that it was thinning and that other people laughed at him because he was going bald. Each day he applied hair potions that cost him hundreds of dollars a month. Although his friends said his hair looked fine, he was so upset over it that he bought a thousand-dollar hairpiece. But this didn't help. As he stated, "I was never satisfied; I still battled myself and wanted to get rid of it." In fact, James was so unhappy with his hairpiece that he destroyed it in a fit of rage.

While men are more likely than women to worry about thinning hair, women have this concern as well. One woman stated that her mother had very thin hair, and that she feared she would eventually look even worse than her mother, becoming completely bald. This patient found it difficult to come in to see me because she feared she became "balder and balder" with each visit.

Getting a haircut is usually a very distressing—even traumatic—event for people with hair concerns. "I'm terrified of getting my hair cut," Jon told me. "Getting the right haircut is *crucial*. There's very little stability in my life because of the BDD. How I feel and function depends on how I happen to look and the quality of my haircut."

Hair concerns may also involve other body hair. Men may be preoccupied with supposedly uneven, light, or heavy beard growth. Men or women may think they have too much or too little body hair. Marie, an attractive 24-year-old nursing student, worried that she had "excessive" and "dark" hair on her nose and arms. She thought about her hair nearly "all day every day," and she repeatedly looked at her arms, tweezed her hair at work, and, using special lights, checked her facial hair in mirrors for an hour a day. She tried to hide her hair with makeup, had electrolysis, wore long sleeves in the summer, and covered her face with her hands. Marie described her preoccupation as "severely upsetting," saying that she felt "masculine" and "like a freak" whom no one would ever love.

Nose concerns are also very common. People with BDD often worry that their nose is too large, bumpy, or misshapen. Less commonly—sometimes after nose surgery—they think it's too small. One woman thought her nose was "bumpy and swollen"; a middle-aged man thought his was "puffy." People with nose concerns are especially likely to have surgery—often repeated surgeries. One woman I treated first thought her nose was too large, and then, after surgery, felt it was too small. A college student first believed his nose was too long, but then, after surgery, thought his nostrils were too wide.

Several years ago I had an interesting conversation with a psychiatrist from Japan who was familiar with BDD. He was surprised to learn that I'd found that nose concerns are usually that the nose is too large; in his experience, the concern is often that the nose is too small. In addition, concerns with hair loss are uncommon in Japan. These observations raise the interesting question of whether cultural factors shape the specific content of the belief.

Larger bodily areas may also be involved. I've seen many men who are preoccupied with their overall body build or bone structure, thinking they look too small. Some of them wear many layers of clothing to enhance their size, and some excessively lift weights. Others—often women—are concerned that they're too large or are overweight. Although only 9% of the people I've seen were excessively concerned with their weight, another researcher has found that this is a common concern of people with BDD.

While people with BDD are concerned with, on average, three to four different body parts over time, some are preoccupied with as many as ten or more. Sometimes concerns with different body areas are present simultaneously, and sometimes they're present sequentially. I've identified three common patterns over time:

1. 40% are concerned with one body part—or one set of body parts—over the course of the disorder. One man was concerned with his receding chin and never developed another concern. Another became concerned simultaneously with his "sunken" eyes and "swollen" nipples; he remained concerned only with these two things, without developing new concerns.
2. An approximately equal percentage (37%) are concerned with one body part and then add new parts over time, with continuation of their previous concerns. For example, at the age of 13, Ted worried that his ears stuck out, then at 18 became additionally concerned with his crooked lip, and then at the age of 25 started to worry about a scar on his neck. At age 25, he had all three concerns.
3. The third pattern is more complex. It's also less common, occurring in 21% of the people I've seen. Over time, concerns with one or more body parts disappear and other concerns emerge. Jane, whom I described in chapter 3, fit this pattern. She first worried about her nose and then a scar on her lip. Later, she became preoccupied with her jaw, breasts, and buttocks, but, over time, she stopped worrying about her buttocks. One concern can begin when another ends. One man stated after nose surgery that his nose looked more acceptable, but his "stomach took over for (his) nose."

While some people with BDD want to be unusually attractive or look "perfect," in my experience many people don't—they simply want to look normal. They might not *mind* looking like Elvis Presley or Marilyn Monroe, but this isn't what they're obsessed with. What they're obsessed with is getting rid of the defect and looking normal. They want to no longer look like the Elephant Man; they want to no longer stand out in a crowd. They say things like, "I don't want to look tanned like George Hamilton; I just want to look *not pale*." "Being average looking is okay. My goal is to be acceptable." As one man said, "I don't care whether I'm attractive. I just want to look normal. I wouldn't mind looking like Beetle Bailey; I just don't want things on my face."

"My Face Is Falling"

People with BDD use various terms to describe their perceived appearance problem. They may say that the defect, or their appearance more generally, is ugly or unattractive. Or they may say that it looks defective, flawed, wrong, odd, not right, or off. Some people use words like "monstrous" or "hideous" to describe the perceived flaw. One man said he looked like a cartoon character, and a woman said that she resembled a distorted figure from a Salvador Dali painting.

For simplicity's sake, I'll generally use the term "defect" or "flaw" to refer to these various appearance concerns. I'll also use this term to refer to more than one concern and to more general concerns with appearance not so easily pinpointed or confined to a specific body part or parts.

While people with BDD usually describe the flaw in quite specific and understandable terms—for example, "My ears are pointed," "I have a scar right here on my neck," "My hairline is receding," or "My waist is too wide"—they sometimes express it in ways that are vague and hard to understand. One man, for example, was preoccupied with his "inadequately firm eyes." A woman described in a published case report complained of "a funny and crinkly nose," and another stated, "the skin under my eyes joins my nose in a funny way." A woman I interviewed was extremely distressed because her face was falling. I tried very hard to understand what she meant. After much discussion, it seemed that she thought that her facial muscles were wasting away and that her facial skin was sagging. But she thought "my face is falling" best described her concern.

Instead of describing a specific concern with a particular body part, some people say that their general appearance, or their entire face, is ugly. In some cases the concern really is somewhat vague and can't be described more specifically than "There's something wrong with how I look" or "I think my face is ugly." In other cases, a vague description like this is given because of embarrassment over discussing the specifics, or because of a fear that describing the problem more specifically will draw more attention to it. After all, it's much easier to say, "There's something wrong with how I look" than "I think my penis is too small." As one woman said, "I told my doctor about my aging fears, but not about the wrinkles or hair. It's easier to talk in generalities."

The first two times I saw Larry, he told me, "I just don't like my face; I don't like how it looks. It feels different from everyone else's." "Is there anything in particular that you don't like?" I asked him. "No, nothing specific—I just don't like it," he replied. It wasn't until the third time I saw him that he felt comfortable enough to reveal the specifics: that his nose was too wide, his forehead too small, and his eyes too beady. "I was much too embarrassed to tell you these things before," he said. "I feel ashamed."

"I Look Like a Gorilla"

Some people find it easier and more accurate to describe their appearance concerns in terms of animals, other people, or even food. One of the first people with BDD whom I saw had many appearance concerns, one of which was his "egg-shaped head." Another person said he looked like a chicken. This was, in his view, the best description of his appearance and was as important as his specific concerns—wrinkles on his face, a large nose, a thin face, and sunken cheekbones. In a published report a person complained of "chipmunk cheeks." A woman who was concerned about excessive facial hair described herself as a gorilla. Such unflattering descriptions reflect how the person *thinks* he or she looks. They help us see how people with BDD see themselves and how they think others see them.

Other people with BDD compare themselves to other people, stating that they look like a burn victim, the Hunchback of Notre Dame, Gomer Pyle, or the Elephant Man. One man who disliked his hair said he looked like Kramer on the TV show *Seinfeld*. His hair actually looks nothing like Kramer's.

Some people with BDD associate their perceived defect with a family member or relative. "My looks remind me of my father, who I dislike," a 40-year-old woman told me. "He was ugly emotionally and physically." Some men who are concerned with thinning hair express a concern that they look like a bald uncle or will end up looking like their bald father. Others say that they've always been told that they look like a particular relative, and their worry focuses on what they consider a prominent and unattractive aspect of that relative's appearance.

"I'm Not Feminine Enough"

Some people with BDD associate their perceived defect with other characteristics that they consider negative, such as aging or a lack of masculinity or femininity. In the same breath, they may, for example, mention their worry about wrinkles and aging. While they're concerned with the perceived ugliness of the wrinkles per se, they're also upset because they consider them a sign that they're getting old. One woman I saw had been hospitalized because she was so desperate over the belief that her appearance had changed, and that new lines on her face made her look 10 years older than she actually was.

Lack of femininity is a concern described by some women. Often, they're worried that their breasts are too small. Or they may be concerned with excessive facial hair, which they think makes them look masculine. The concern that they're not feminine enough can be as distressing as the perceived defect itself. One young woman who worried that her breasts were too small said that she felt she "really wasn't a woman, because breasts symbolize femininity." Even though she was frequently asked out on dates and was often reassured that she was quite feminine, she nonetheless had this view of herself.

Marie, the nursing student preoccupied with supposedly excessive facial hair, told me, "The hair makes me masculine looking. When I was young, I had short hair, and people sometimes mistook me for a boy. Maybe that has something to do with it. The hair makes me feel masculine and like a freak."

Similarly, men who are concerned that their penis is too small often say that they feel unmasculine and that women don't find them desirable. "It makes me feel unmanly, like I'm not masculine enough," one young man told me. "It's embarrassing and something I feel I need to hide. What I obsess about is I'm half of a man." Another said, "My penis doesn't look ugly, but it looks unattractive and unmanly. All of my concerns are related to maleness. I have shame about being a man."

A quiet, intelligent young man told me, "It's not so much that I'm ugly but that I look nerdy. I've always done very well in school, but I'm not good in sports. When I was younger I was skinny and I wore thick glasses. I want my nose to look more masculine—I look like a little nerd with my long nose."

Fear of the Future: "Soon I'll Be Totally Bald!"

A prominent theme for some people with BDD is fear of the future. They worry that their perceived defect will become worse and uglier with time. "I always fear the future," a pretty young woman told me. "I fear my skin will get worse and worse."

"I get very depressed over my appearance because I truly believe it will get worse as I get older," Carmella said. "I don't think I can live with myself if my hair keeps getting thinner and my wrinkles get worse. How can I go on? My problems that won't get worse—like my teeth—don't cause me such horrible panic and unmanageable distress." Olivia feared that she wouldn't be able to work in the future because she'd look worse as she aged. "No one will want to hire me when I'm older and even uglier," she said. Eric feared that his hair would get thinner and thinner and that he would soon be completely bald. "Bald guys are total rejects," he told me. "My life will be over when I lose all my hair."

Fear of the future sometimes focuses on a belief that the person used to look fine but now their looks have been ruined and will continue to deteriorate. "Sometimes when I look in the mirror I get an image of how I used to look," Ed said. "It only lasts for a minute. Then I see how I look now, and I worry about next week and next year. Will I get even uglier?"

"My Face Is Asymmetrical"

Symmetry concerns are relatively common: of those I've seen, one third had this concern about at least one aspect of their appearance. They're worried that one side of their body doesn't perfectly match the other, or that certain features are uneven or off balance. One woman was preoccupied with having more freckles on one side of her face than the other. A 25-year-old man worried that one side of his face was different from the other—that his bone structure was asymmetrical. Another man obsessed about the supposed asymmetry of his eyebrows—that one was a little higher. A teenager I saw was concerned that one eyelid hung over one of his eyes more than the other one.

Some people are concerned that the length of their hair is uneven and may spend hours a day cutting it to make it perfectly even. A college student told me, "I'm obsessed with having my hair an even length. It *has* to be even. I compulsively cut it to even it up. I cut it every morning, and then I carry scissors with me and cut it throughout the day. I try to resist—I've thrown away a lot of scissors—but I can't. I've even hit my hands with a hammer and slammed them in a car door so I'd stop cutting. But that didn't work either. I *have* to make my hair even so it will look better!"

"I'm Not Big Enough"

A variation on the BDD theme that affects men is the fear that their body build is too small and not muscular enough. Mark, a muscular man in his twenties, was preoccupied with the belief that his upper body was too thin and that he wasn't big, strong, and masculine enough. To build himself up, he drank protein drinks every day and lifted weights for hours daily, which he called an "obsession." He also frequently asked his father, "Do I look okay? Am I getting bigger?"

Mark always wore long-sleeved shirts to hide his "skinny" arms and avoided going to the beach, where his body would be more exposed. He also avoided being around other people because he was so embarrassed by his supposed smallness. When I met Mark, he was wearing five layers of T-shirts and sweatshirts to look bigger.

"Reverse anorexia" is a term coined by Drs. James Hudson and Harrison Pope of Harvard Medical School to refer to the syndrome that Mark had. It resembles the eating disorder anorexia nervosa (see page 319 for a description), except that the symptoms are reversed, with sufferers thinking they're too small rather than too large. Reverse anorexia meets criteria for BDD and has many features in common with more classic BDD. It also raises important questions about the relationship between BDD and anorexia nervosa, which I'll discuss in Chapter 12.

"I Look Depressed"

Jacob's and Max's experiences were another variation on the BDD theme. "I look depressed," Jacob told me. "I feel my mouth is unattractive and that I'm not likable because I look depressed. Looking depressed equals looking like something people don't want to see, which is distasteful." Jacob thought he looked depressed because his mouth was turned down, and he'd considered surgery to straighten it.

In addition to thinking his mouth was too small, Max felt he didn't have the right expression on his face. "I keep trying to get the right expression on my mouth, like the popular kids," he said. "I get caught up in the mirror thinking 'Which way does my mouth look the best? Most natural, most attractive?' My mouth feels ugly and wrong. I'm afraid of offending other people with my appearance."

Both Jacob and Max were concerned about looking unattractive, but they also expressed their concerns in a less typical way, by focusing on their facial expression, which they thought would be offensive or distasteful to others. Such concerns differ somewhat from classic BDD concerns and illustrate that human experience doesn't always neatly fit into our diagnostic categories.

"My Fingers Are Getting Shorter"

"Sometimes my hand gets fat, and all of my fingers get shorter," Jim told me. "I actually *see* them change—it's a process I perceive. They aren't fat and short all the time. It happens two or three times a day. It can happen when I'm around other people, especially good-looking people, or when I'm feeling nervous. Some of my doctors thought maybe I had a seizure disorder or another neurological problem, but I don't. I know it's impossible for this to happen, but it's what I see."

Occasional people with BDD have an experience like Jim's—their body parts sometimes change shape or size and become unattractive in the process. Jim also saw his eyes come closer together at times, and his cheeks changed from thin to fat and back to thin again. "My cheeks look bad when they're fatter," he said, "and my eyes look strange when they're closer together."

While reports of body parts frequently changing size or shape in such a dramatic way are uncommon, and raise the question of whether a neurological disorder is present, they echo what many people with BDD say—that they sometimes look worse than at other times, or that their perception of the defect can change. For example, facial scars can look worse, and moles can look bigger, at some times than at others. Reports such as these raise the interesting question of whether people with BDD actually see something different from other people, whether they experience a visual illusion.

"I'm Afraid My Nose Will Break!"

There are still other bodily concerns. About 10% with BDD think that the unattractive body part—for example, their nose—is fragile and in danger of breaking, or that the body part doesn't work correctly. They believe, for example, that their legs are too skinny *and* that they can't walk correctly. Or that their lip is misshapen *and* their speech is slurred. Or that their nose is crooked *and* they make whistling noises when they breathe. And some believe that they have an underlying illness, such as cancer, that's responsible for their appearance problem.

Julie had one of these variations on the BDD theme. "I have a nose problem; I hope you're an expert on noses," she began when I first met her. I assumed that she, like most of the people I'd seen, was concerned with how it looked. Indeed, in the past Julie had worried that her nose was too big and bumpy. But now her concern was different. "This is very humiliating because it sounds so silly. My concern is irrational, and I'm afraid you'll think I'm crazy," she told me. "No one understands my problem. The problem is I'm totally obsessed that my nose is fragile and is going to break. It's tormenting me!

"I worry all day long that I've damaged it. Whenever I bump it or brush against something, I panic. I think I've ruined it. If I blow my nose and see blood, I think I've damaged it. Sometimes I even think that I've hurt it by crinkling it up or letting cigarette smoke get near it! I constantly look in the mirror for evidence of damage. If I see any little problem—a spot or a pimple or a tiny vein—I think it's evidence I've ruined my nose. It can be anything. Sometimes it's a blackhead or a broken blood vessel. Other times it's a pore. Sometimes I feel tingling and aching in my nose, which means I must have broken it. I try to talk myself out of it, saying things like 'You'd have to hit it with a sledge hammer to damage it.' But that doesn't really help."

Julie also developed what she called a "sniffing obsession." "When I was wondering if I'd hurt my nose, my nose felt funny when I sniffed, so I had to keep sniffing to see if it was OK. It was a way to check on whether I'd damaged it."

The problem had started when Julie had had nose surgery 20 years earlier to remove a small bump. After surgery, the surgeon commented, "I worked really hard on your nose, so take care of it and don't damage it." Julie interpreted this to mean that her nose was fragile, and it triggered her obsession. For the next eight years, she secretly visited her surgeon as often as twice a week. "I never told anyone I was doing this, not even my husband. I was much too ashamed. I kept going to the surgeon to ask about my nose—I wanted reassurance that it wasn't broken. It was a compulsion to run for reassurance. I even dragged my three kids with me, and sometimes I'd wait for two hours. The office staff thought I was crazy, and they tried to keep me from the doctor. When he reassured me, I felt a little better, but only for a few minutes."

When she first saw me, Julie was more worried about her nose than usual, because she'd just seen a television show on "botched" nose jobs. "I've been so preoccupied that I haven't been able to keep up the house or keep a job," she said. "And it's hard for me to enjoy social activities. I don't even bother going a lot of the time. I'm so focused on my nose that I can't think of anything else. I don't plan social events because I'm afraid my nose problem will flare up and I won't be able to go.

"It's a huge problem in my marriage, too," she added. "My first husband left me because of it. I drove him nuts! I asked him all day long about my nose and whether I'd damaged it, and I'd have him hold magnifying glasses and special lights to check it for damage."

During childbirth, Julie was so fearful that her nose would be damaged that she hadn't even felt labor pains. When having dental work done, she was so afraid the dentist would damage her nose by bumping it while she was anesthetized, and that she'd be unaware of the damage, that she didn't use Novocain. She preferred the intense physical pain of unanesthetized dental work to the emotional pain of unrecognized nose damage.

"The Walking Concept Was Erased"

Some people with BDD worry that their supposedly unattractive body part doesn't work correctly. Ben was concerned not only that his legs "looked funny" but also that he couldn't walk normally. As a teenager he'd been preoccupied with his supposedly thin upper lip, but several years later, as he put it, "my legs replaced my lip." His problem began with pain in his right foot, for which he consulted a physician, who diagnosed a fallen arch. This diagnosis frightened Ben, and he incorrectly assumed that he'd never be able to walk again. He then worried about his walking "all day long," wondering whether his walking would become abnormal.

Eventually, Ben began to think that he couldn't walk normally. "The walking concept was erased," he said. "It was as if I'd had a lobotomy." He also started worrying that the muscles in his legs "were becoming thin like toothpicks and disappearing." Although several doctors tried to reassure him that his walking, as well as his legs' appearance, were normal, Ben couldn't be reassured. "I felt crippled," he said. "The damage was already done."

Concerns such as these—as well as those involving bodily fragility—resemble typical BDD beliefs in that they are distressing preoccupations about one's body. But they differ from typical BDD concerns in that they don't focus on appearance per se. The patients I've seen with such concerns have usually also had a more typical BDD concern that involved the same body part; that is, they worried that the fragile or malfunctioning body part was also unattractive or deformed. Whether less typical concerns such as these should be considered to constitute BDD, or a separate disorder such as hypochondriasis or obsessive compulsive disorder (see Appendix A for definitions), is unclear, although the similarities between them and BDD concerns are striking.

"I'm Shrinking Because I Have Cancer"

A few patients I've seen have attributed the perceived defect in their appearance to an underlying medical illness. A woman who believed that her shoulders and upper body were shrinking attributed this supposed change to cancer. Because she feared she was "shriveling up," she'd seen countless physicians and had had numerous tests, all of which were normal. Ben, the young man I just described who worried that his legs were becoming thin and atrophied, also worried that these changes were attributable to multiple sclerosis.

Robert attributed his appearance problems to hypothyroidism. He had initially worried that his hair was falling out, for which he'd seen several dermatologists. Most of them reassured him that his hair was normal, but one prescribed a steroid, later discontinued by another physician. He then saw a nutritionist, who prescribed vitamins and iodine. As a result of excessive iodine intake, Robert developed hyperthyroidism, and the iodine was discontinued. Even though his thyroid tests normalized, Robert became convinced that he was now hypothyroid. He became preoccupied with the thought that his eyes were sunken and that his skin had "lost its firmness and tone," which he attributed to the supposed hypothyroidism. Eventually, he became immersed in the concern that his "whole appearance had changed," thinking about it all day long and berating himself because he believed that he had ruined his appearance by making himself hypothyroid.

In addition to BDD, all three of these people received a diagnosis of hypochondriasis—a preoccupation with the idea that one has a serious disease. It's interesting that in the International Classification of Diseases (ICD-10), the international counterpart of DSM–IV, BDD is considered a type of hypochondriasis, although, as I'll discuss in chapter 12, BDD and hypochondriasis do seem to have some important differences and are probably distinct rather than the same disorder. Only a few of the hundreds of people with BDD I've seen have attributed their appearance concerns to a bodily illness.

BDD By Proxy

I once got a call from a woman who was very upset about her daughter's nose. "I worry that it doesn't look right, that it's crooked," she told me, "even though everyone else says it looks fine. *She* doesn't worry about it, but *I* do! I know I'm too upset about it, and it's causing my daughter problems. I keep pushing on it to make it straight, and I'm afraid I'm ruining her self-esteem."

Like this woman, some people don't worry about their *own* appearance—they worry about the appearance of someone else. They obsess that their son's ears are sticking out or their boyfriend's hair looks wrong, when in fact these body areas look okay. They may insist that their loved one get surgery, even when it isn't necessary. I call this phenomenon "BDD by proxy"—that is, excessive worry about someone else's appearance, which may or may not cause the person to worry about it themselves. This is another variation on the BDD theme.

"I Feel More Air Where My Hair Used to Be"

Subtle tactile sensations in the area of the perceived defect are fairly common in BDD. About 30% of people with BDD experience sensations such as itching in the area of perceived blood vessel markings, tightness in the area of perceived acne, "gritting where fat rubs together," or "too much air" in the area of perceived hair loss. Usually, these sensations are fairly mild and not problematic.

But in some instances, the sensations are troubling because they're a reminder of the defect's presence or because they're painful. Some people with concerns about the appearance of their lips, for example, feel they're dry and cracked, which can be irritating and unpleasant. The woman who thought her shoulders and upper body were shrinking as a result of cancer also had prominent and constant shoulder pain. The pain was in and of itself a troubling problem.

"All I Really Care About Is My Skin"

People with BDD generally think that other aspects of their appearance look okay. But they're so focused on the perceived defect that they consider these other aspects less important. They believe the defect is the most obvi-ous and important part of how they look. They tend to view themselves not as an attractive person with a small bump on their nose, but as one whose most obvious and prominent feature is a grotesque nose. Thus, many consider themselves to be unattractive overall.

Some people with BDD are so intensely and exclusively preoccupied with the supposed defect that they're oblivious to other aspects of their appear-ance. Matthew had been so focused on his mild acne, it was all he could "see." He told me, "Before I got better with the medication, I was just one big pimple, without any feet or even any toes!"

Ellen, too, was so intensely and exclusively focused on her skin that she had little sense of how the rest of her body looked. Nor did she really care. In fact, when she gained 25 pounds, she didn't notice it until her friends pointed it out. Even then, she didn't really care. "All I really care about is my skin," she stated. "When my skin looks good, I'll be happy with how I look."

Like Ellen, some people with BDD don't seem to notice or be bothered by aspects of their appearance that would probably concern most people. Instead, they're preoccupied with a defect that others consider nonexistent or slight. Jeremy, who was in his early thirties, was nearly bald. But this didn't bother him. What troubled him were tiny bumps on his nose that were barely visible. He explained that he wasn't concerned about his hair because hair loss was natural, whereas his acne should have resolved 10 years ago.

Similarly, a woman I saw had large, deep, red ulcers on her legs as a result of a medical illness. But they didn't particularly bother her, and she often wore shorts, even on cool days. Instead, she was preoccupied with her supposedly wide nose and her "sunken and dull" eyes, which other people considered attractive. Another woman concerned with her breasts told me, "My husband tells me that if I'm going to be upset about my appearance, I should worry about my stretch marks. But I can't do anything about them, so why should I care?"

These observations raise some fascinating questions about BDD, which I'll speculate about later. Why do some people with BDD focus on one area whereas others focus on others; in other words, how does the body part get "selected"? What do people with BDD actually see? Do they see what other people see, or do they see something different? And how can some people with BDD become so intensely focused on a defect that others can't see, or consider minimal, while ignoring aspects of their appearance, such as leg ulcers, that are obvious to others?

·· six ··

Painful Obsessions

"It's constantly on my mind. And it's unbelievably painful. People don't understand. If you told someone, they'd think you were off the wall."　　**Matt**

"I Can't Get It Out of My Mind"

"*I*'m obsessed about my appearance," a 50-year-old secretary told me. "I think about it all the time. It's a crazy way of thinking. It's torturing me. . . . It's always in the back of my mind. I can't push it away. It's like a clock ticking. It's always there, taunting and haunting me." Another woman said of her preoccupation: "It feels like a magnet. I can't get my mind away from it. I constantly fight with it."

Most people with BDD actively think about their appearance problem for at least an hour a day. Of those I've seen, about a quarter think about it for 1 to 3 hours a day, and another quarter for 3 to 8 hours a day; most (about 35%) think about it for more than 8 hours a day. The remaining 10% think about the defect for less than an hour a day, but for a substantial period in the past they'd thought about it for at least an hour a day.

Some people think about their perceived defect "all day, every day"—it's always on their mind, making it difficult to focus on anything else. One

woman said, "My BDD is a shadow—it's always with me. I can't get rid of it." Others say that they "actively" think about it for only part of the day, but they're always "aware" of their concern; it's always in the back of their mind. Some say they always have "two reels going." With one reel, they focus on the matter at hand; with the other, they're thinking about how they look.

One man described his preoccupation with his "small" head as follows: "It's constantly there. I can't get it out of my mind. It's like a monkey on my back. I never stop thinking about it, not even for a day or an hour. I even obsess in my sleep." Another said, "It's always there. Even if I'm focusing on other things, it's still there. It's like a radio that's *always on.* You may not hear it for a while, but if you stop and think about it, you know it's there." Ray told me, "I was very preoccupied. It was all I could think of. My mind would go back and forth from the hair to the chest and from the chest to the hair, back and forth like a yo-yo."

Susan described her thoughts about her facial freckles as "invasive." "They force themselves into my mind." Other people, however, experience their thoughts not as invasive but as something that's "always there," to the point where they seem a part of themselves.

Most people with BDD realize that they spend too much time thinking about their appearance. But others don't. The thoughts are so much a part of their life that they don't realize they worry too much. They think that everyone worries about their appearance for hours a day.

What do the thoughts consist of? They vary, but they're usually quite negative—for example: "There's a pimple on your face; everyone's going to see it and think you're ugly" or "I'm disfigured. It's ugly. I deviate." One person thought, "You stick out in a crowd; you look ridiculous. People are looking at you funny because of your ears." Jane told me, "I have two tapes playing in my head at all times: one of them says not to worry and another says I'm ugly."

Some people's thoughts focus on what they consider a bad outcome with surgery. "I *constantly* think about the operation I had on my nose," Greg said, "and I think, 'It's not me. Now it's too short and too thin. It looks like a woman's nose, not a man's nose.' And I obsess about how angry I am at the doctor and how I shouldn't have had the surgery. I also think a lot about what all the different surgeons have told me. Things like 'You could have something done, but it's not a good idea,' or 'Don't do anything to it; it could get worse.' "

Some people have nightmares about their concerns—they're haunted, even while they're sleeping. In their dreams, their worst fears come true. One woman described the following dream: "I have nightmares of getting my hair cut. All of my hair is getting cut off the front. I wake up in a panic." Another woman told me, "I dreamt I was walking down the street and suddenly I had a lot of hair on my face. People were pointing at me and laughing at the gobs of hair on my face." A woman who disliked her hair described this dream: "I dreamt a friend of mine with beautiful long hair was getting married. All of the bridesmaids except me also had beautiful hair. The bride told me I couldn't be in the wedding unless I wore a wig. I couldn't even be in the church because of my hair, and I had to leave."

One reason these preoccupations take up so much time is that they're difficult to resist and control. Many people do try to resist them by pushing them aside and trying to focus on something else. But many find their preoccupations so powerful that they don't even make an effort to divert their attention away from them. I've found that 10% of people with BDD always attempt to resist the preoccupations, 21% usually try to resist them, and 30% make some effort to resist them. But 23% rarely try to resist them, and 17% make no effort whatsoever to resist them—they simply let them enter their mind. Degree of resistance can fluctuate, however, with more of an effort made to resist the thoughts at some times than at others.

Control over the thoughts is usually limited. Almost no one with BDD says they have complete control over them. Most people (46%) report having little control, and 18% report having no control. Inability to resist and control the preoccupations is a particularly difficult aspect of BDD. "I try to ignore them, but I can't," one man told me. "They won't leave me alone. It's like trying to will away a headache; you can't just make them stop." The woman who was concerned about her supposedly shrunken shoulders said, "My concern about this takes over—it's controlling me. It's very scary. I can't stop it." Another woman stated, "One of the hardest things about this disorder is that I can't control my own thoughts! They have a life of their own. I feel powerless over them. I try to resist them and distract myself from them. Sometimes I can, even though it's difficult. But often I can't. It seems so silly—I should be able to stop thinking them. But I usually can't."

Sometimes people with BDD are told to just stop worrying about how they look. If only it were this simple! Lack of control over the preoccupation and thinking about it too much are the core features of BDD. People with BDD would love their problem to disappear and simply forget about it; after all, they, more than anyone else, would like to end their suffering. But they can't—*this is what BDD is all about.*

Cassandra had little control over her preoccupation. "I'm so agonized by my body dysmorphic symptoms," she said. "I feel a complete lack of freedom, like I'm a caged animal. It cuts you off from the freedoms of life. I can't get out of it. I can't escape from the thoughts. I wish there was a way of reaching greater freedom."

"It's Like an Arrow Through My Heart"

When I met Bill, a 40-year-old landscaper, he was so profoundly distressed over his appearance that he couldn't put his pain into words. I first met him in a darkened room in the hospital. He was wearing a baseball cap that was pulled down over his forehead and partially covered his eyes. His head was down in his knees.

While looking down at the floor, he started to tell me about his problems. He was anxious and very hesitant to discuss them. He had no friends, and he'd just been fired from his job. He felt that life wasn't worth living. When I asked him what he thought the cause of his difficulties was, he replied, "It's really hard to talk about this, Doctor. I don't know if I can. It's too embarrassing, and it hurts too much."

Eventually, Bill told me what had happened and why he was in the hospital. He was worried about his nose, which he thought was covered with huge pockmarks and pores. Except for the pores, he thought he looked fine. But he believed the pores made him grotesque and ugly, like the Elephant Man. He'd thought about them for hours a day for the past 15 years. He wore the hat to hide them. And he'd insisted on meeting with me in a dark room so I couldn't see them.

"I can't begin to describe this to you," he said. "It's humiliating and very embarrassing. Who am I to complain, when so many people are worse off than me? To lose control over your life because of marks on your face—it's embarrassing, and it seems ridiculous! But every morning when I get up, I want to die. I rush to the mirror and see the marks. I can't face it anymore. Every day, the holes look like they're getting bigger. I go back and forth between the mirror and my bed, feeling hopeless. I feel a pain and terror. I think 'How can I face this? How can I go on living if I look like this?' " He tried to conceive of other equally painful experiences. "Maybe it's how a woman feels after she's been raped. Maybe it's how cancer victims feel. It's like an arrow through my heart.

"It ruined my life. I got very depressed. I stopped seeing people. I was so obsessed I couldn't work and I got fired. It crushed me. Before I came into the hospital, I went to a hotel room to kill myself. I kept looking at myself in the mirror, thinking I couldn't live with the marks. I was scared, because I wanted to die, and I hated myself. I paced around the room, arguing with myself, telling myself it was stupid to be so worried about the marks. But everyone could see them—I couldn't hide them! I decided I couldn't go on living like this, and I tried to suffocate myself."

Many people with BDD describe their pain in similar ways. A young man told me, "The pain is unbearable, unremitting. My life is a devastation. It's so painful it's hard to put it into words. Every day is hell."

Descriptions such as these may sound extreme, even melodramatic. But these people weren't being melodramatic. Many of them understated rather than overstated their suffering. Most were very embarrassed and hesitant to describe their emotional pain and even apologized for it, thinking they were selfish or silly for suffering as much as they did.

But their pain is very real and profound. Of all the patients with various psychiatric problems whom I've worked with over the years, some of my patients with BDD have been the most severely distressed and tormented.

The distress and emotional pain some people with BDD experience are less severe than Bill's—the pain spans a spectrum of severity. I've found that 8% report that their preoccupations cause mild distress; 33%, moderate distress; 40%, severe distress; and 18%, extreme and disabling distress. At the less severe end of the spectrum, people are distressed by their appearance concerns, but they don't find them devastating. They aren't in despair over them, and don't consider killing themselves because of them. Their distress is manageable and tolerable. Nonetheless, they suffer.

I've tried to understand the reasons for the pain. One is that the thoughts are so often present and difficult to control. It's unpleasant to spend so much time thinking unbidden thoughts that interfere with focusing on other things and take time away from enjoyable or important activities. In addition, the content of the thoughts—believing that you're unattractive, defective, ugly, or disfigured—is very distressing. One man tried to explain: "Think about how you'd feel if someone cut your nose off. That's how I feel about how I look."

In fact, many people with BDD wish they were worried about some other body part instead, because they think it would be less painful. A young woman who thought she was losing her hair said, "I wish I worried about something else, like my skin. At least I could cover it with makeup. But I can't change my hair." But a young woman who disliked her skin said, "I wish I worried about something else, like my hair because I could wear a wig. But I can't change my skin. The scars are there forever."

Another woman similarly said, "I'd rather worry about a big nose because you could just get a nose job—and your nose is supposed to be there anyway. Scars aren't supposed to be there, so it's worse." The source of this pain is a belief that another body part could be more easily covered or fixed, whereas the disliked body part is unchangeable. This creates feelings of helplessness and despair.

Another source of the pain is that people with BDD think other people view them as disfigured, even repulsive. Furthermore, they believe that they can't easily hide their flaw from others. People who worry about their facial features—the most common location of BDD concerns—point out that a facial flaw is particularly painful because it's on their face, which is where other people generally focus and fix their gaze, so hiding it is very difficult.

In addition, BDD symptoms are often accompanied by feelings of low self-esteem, inadequacy, embarrassment, humiliation, and shame. Although not universal, these feelings are very common. Many people with BDD feel badly about who they are. They feel rejected by others, and assume that others will judge them negatively.

"I've always disliked myself so much I can't imagine people liking me or how I look," Sonya told me. "My appearance concerns are all tied up in feelings of inferiority. They make sense to me, because they're related to low self-esteem, feeling like damaged goods." A man with BDD said, "When I go into a store I feel like the lowest thing in the store. Maybe people and women would like me more and accept me more if I looked better." "My face is the source of all the pain in my life," a 35-year-old artist said. "I feel hopeless about it. It's a feeling I'll never belong anywhere or be happy. It's a feeling that I'm unacceptable. I feel the outside world sees me as unlovable, rejected, unacceptable, ugly."

The importance of low self-esteem in BDD reflects what is known about the link between appearance and self-esteem in the general population. Research has found that judgments about appearance are closely linked to self-esteem, with negative views of one's own appearance associated with low self-esteem.

It's my impression that shame is so common in BDD, it may even be intrinsic to the disorder. Pierre Janet, one of the greatest psychopathologists of all time, underscored the importance of shame in BDD. In fact, he referred to BDD as an obsession with shame of the body. In his 1903 description of Nadia, a 27-year-old woman, he noted her embarrassment and shame over many aspects of her "ugly body," including her skin, hands, legs, and feet, and a fear that no one would ever love her because of her "ugliness."

A close relationship between BDD and shame makes sense because the preoccupation itself involves strongly negative feelings about oneself— thoughts of being unappealing and defective. This view of the supposedly defective body part often extends to the person more generally. One woman said, "Whenever I see myself, I see something very inadequate. The one word I associate with my body is shame." A high school teacher said, "Shame is central to my appearance concerns. BDD equals ridicule." Men may be ashamed because they consider it unmasculine to worry so much about how they look.

Another source of suffering is feeling selfish and vain for being so preoccupied with such "trivial" concerns. Like Sarah, some people with BDD feel it's wrong—even immoral—to be so focused on how they look. This is what I call the "double whammy" of BDD: not only do BDD sufferers have painful thoughts they can't stop thinking, they also berate themselves for having those thoughts. Many feel guilty and consider themselves morally weak and defective because they're so preoccupied with something they feel is so trivial. They feel ashamed of being ashamed.

As one woman told me, "I shouldn't be so worried about this. I get down on myself because I am. It's hard for me to talk about it, because appearance shouldn't matter. I don't want to be the kind of person who cares so much about something so superficial. I can't even talk about my problem because I'm so ashamed of it. I refer to it as 'you know what.' " Another woman had similar feelings, "It sounds very superficial, but it isn't. I feel ridiculous thinking about it. I feel spoiled and shallow. I feel guilty because I could be blind or crippled. I *try* not to think about it, but I can't."

Some people with BDD don't consider their appearance concerns trivial, pointing out that attractiveness is important and highly valued in our society. Thus, their concerns seem justified. But more common are feelings like the following: "I feel like a horrible, terrible person because I'm so concerned with my breasts. How could I be so vain, so concerned with my appearance? It shouldn't be that important to me." This woman berated herself even more when she learned that her best friend had breast cancer. "I felt even more strongly that I was a bad person—here I was obsessing about how big my breasts were when my best friend had breast cancer and had to have a mastectomy. I feel like this is a very selfish disease that I can't control. I'm the one who deserved the mastectomy!"

Rather than a problem of excessive vanity, BDD should be viewed as an illness like depression or anorexia nervosa or heart disease. It has a life of its own and doesn't reflect moral weakness. If people could stop thinking about their preoccupation, they would. If they could put an end to their suffering by simply willing their symptoms away, they would. The self-blame only adds to their pain.

Others feel guilty because they think they should be able to fix the problem—for example, by dieting or working out enough. Still others are self-critical because they feel responsible for creating the defect; they believe that something they did ruined their appearance—something that might have been prevented. "I look in the mirror, and I say 'What did I do!?' " Tina said. "I get really down on myself because I destroyed my looks by picking at my skin."

Tom believed that he ruined his appearance by using Accutane, a medication for severe acne. The Accutane did get rid of the few pimples he had, but it also made Tom's skin slightly dry, which, in his view, was catastrophic. He blamed his dermatologist but mostly blamed himself. "I ruined my skin," he told me. "I ruined my looks. I can't believe I did this to myself!" Tom's guilt and self-blame became obsessional and extreme and greatly increased his suffering.

Isolation from others is one of the more emotionally painful aspects of BDD. Such feelings often stem from the belief that others consider the BDD sufferer defective and unlikable. A college student didn't go home for the holidays because she thought her family would be repulsed by her skin and wouldn't love her. As she said, "I fear being an outcast." Another student said, "I'm afraid I won't be able to lead a normal life—date, have sex, have friends. I feel like a freak because I have a defect. No one could ever love me."

A young man told me, "Maybe people, especially women, would like me more and accept me more if I were better looking. I often ruminate about my ugliness and think I can't survive because people choose their friends and partners on the basis of looks. I'm disgusting and repulsive. I'm overwhelmingly lonely."

Contributing to the isolation is the feeling that other people don't seem to understand or take their concerns seriously. After all, people with BDD look fine to others, who are usually incredulous or reassuring. "I feel foolish talking about my concern," one man said. "The usual reaction is 'What?!' " When someone has a medical problem, they usually have observable and "understandable" symptoms, like a rash, or test results, like an X–ray, that confirm that the illness is "real" and justify the person's distress and limitations. The same is true for many psychiatric disorders. An adult with anorexia nervosa who weighs only 70 pounds is clearly ill. A panic attack, too, is observable and obviously not under the person's control; the physiologic arousal of the attack—for example, rapid breathing or sweating—is dramatically obvious and "real" to anyone who might witness it. Even though others may not fully understand the symptoms, they know that something is wrong and that the person is suffering and needs treatment.

But BDD is different. Because the BDD sufferer looks fine, it's hard for others to understand the preoccupation and the pain it causes. How can someone be so obsessed with something that, in the eyes of others, doesn't exist? Or if a slight defect is present, how can it interfere so much with their life? Why can't they just forget about it? It generally makes little sense to others. As a result, people with BDD often feel misunderstood, set apart, and alone.

"I've been very isolated with my concern because people thought I was crazy," one man told me. "They didn't understand, so I've kept it largely to myself. It's an extremely private inner turmoil. I feel alone." "The pain is as bad as when my dog who I'd had for 15 years was put to sleep," a college student told me, "but that was easier because people can understand your grieving. People can't understand BDD."

"A Neon Sign Is Pointing at My Face!"

One reason BDD is so painful and embarrassing for many BDD sufferers is they think others take special notice of—and even mock—their defect. If someone glances in their direction, they assume they're being looked at in horror—that the glance reflects the fact that their defect is repulsive and cannot go unnoticed. One man concerned about a minimal scar on his neck said, "I know people are smirking at me when they see me. When I cross at a crosswalk I think people in cars are thinking, 'I wonder what happened to him. Look how ugly he is.' " Another man worried about mild acne said, "When I go out, I think everyone's noticing it. I think they're thinking 'What's that ugly thing on his face?' It would be like if you painted big red marks all over your face and then walked down the street. Everywhere I go I feel like a neon sign is pointing at my face!"

People with BDD usually think that others can *see* the defect, but what I'm describing here goes beyond this. The phenomenon I'm depicting—known in psychiatric terms as *referential thinking*—is that others take *special notice* of the defect. Benign events in the environment unrelated to the person—or events that are related to them but have nothing to do with the supposed defect—are interpreted as referring to the flaw in a negative way. Sixty-five percent of the people I've seen have such experiences—for example, thinking that others are staring at, talking about, or making fun of how they look. About half of them think that other people probably are taking special notice of them, and about half are completely convinced of this. Some use the term "paranoia" to describe their experience.

This was a serious problem for Jennifer, who left her car in the middle of a traffic jam because she thought other people were noticing the imperfections on her skin. When she walked down the street, she believed that people stared at her skin and thought, "That poor girl—look at her skin. It looks terrible!" When she entered a restaurant she believed the acne and marks distracted people from their meals, and she could eat out only if she hid in a booth in the restaurant's darkest corner. Even then, she had to look down at the menu while ordering her food so the waitress couldn't see her face. At work she thought her co-workers and the customers were laughing at her behind her back. It was because of these experiences that she often left work in the middle of the day and eventually quit her job.

Conversations may be erroneously interpreted to refer to the person with BDD. "Whenever people talk about shaving or beards, I think they might be referring to *my* beard," Bart told me. "They're really mean." Some BDD sufferers think that others can see the defect from impossibly long distances. One man thought that other people could see his minimal acne from 20 feet away, and Jennifer believed hers was visible from 50 feet. A man who sang in a choir thought the entire audience could see a small scar on his neck.

Experiences such as these are similar in some ways to what we all experience. We've all had the feeling of noticing that someone has been looking at us and we may wonder why. Do we remind them of someone they know? Are they interested in the book we were reading? Were they noticing our glasses because they were considering buying a similar pair? It's possible that they were observing our appearance—perhaps something negative. But it's also possible that they were noticing something positive about how we look. Were they even noticing us at all? Perhaps they were looking over or behind us. Or they were looking in our direction but thinking about something else, like the report they had to give at work that day or what they needed to buy at the supermarket. The possible explanations are varied and endless.

But people with BDD generally don't seriously consider, or even think about, these various possibilities. They assume that the person was looking at and thinking about *their appearance.* In particular, they assume the other person was scrutinizing the *defect* and thinking about it in a *negative way.*

This way of thinking isn't limited to people with BDD. Some people with very obvious and noticeable physical deformities think in a similar way, assuming the behavior of others is a negative reaction to their physical deformity, even when it isn't. And studies by social psychologists show that physically normal individuals may also think in this way. In a very interesting experiment by Robert Kleck and A. Christopher Strenta, normal-appearing young adults were told that a noticeable and authentic-looking facial scar was being applied to their face with cosmetics, but it was then removed without their knowledge. These study subjects subsequently believed that the "scar" had a strongly negative impact on how other people behaved toward them and that others rejected them because of it. In other words, the subjects erroneously found plenty of "evidence" that others were reacting negatively to their "physical defect" (which they didn't actually have). This misattribution is surprisingly similar to that of people with BDD. Importantly, the researchers noted that misattributing social outcomes to one's supposed physical deformity can lead to low self-esteem and social withdrawal, which may in turn negatively influence interactions with others.

I've tried to present other possible explanations to patients. Perhaps the other person wasn't actually looking at you. Perhaps they were thinking about something else. Perhaps they were looking at you but not in terms of your appearance. Perhaps they thought you seemed to have an appealing personality. But most people with BDD find it hard—if not impossible—to believe such explanations. They *see themselves* in terms of their imperfect appearance and assume that others must be doing the same. Often, it's only after they respond to psychiatric treatment that they can consider other explanations and actually believe them.

One handsome young man was convinced that people on the subway were distracted from conversations and reading the newspaper by his hair, and that they thought things like "That poor man! He's practically bald! How can he leave his house looking like that? He'd be pretty handsome if it weren't for his hair." Only after he'd responded to psychiatric treatment could he recognize that others didn't take special notice of his hair and when they did notice him, it was often in a positive way that had nothing to do with his hair.

Sometimes the referential thinking experienced by people with BDD is more unusual. Jane thought that other people stared at her nose through binoculars. Another thought that people said "She's ugly," or muttered "Dog!" under their breath as she walked by them. Quite understandably, she was very reluctant to be around others. When Alex was a child, he thought his mother left the table during meals because he was so ugly. "This happened more often as I got older and uglier," he said.

Steven's experience was a particularly poignant example of referential thinking. He was often pursued by women who found him very attractive, but was convinced that he was ugly—in particular, that his facial structure "wasn't sophisticated or full enough." When he was around others, especially young women, he thought that they took special notice of him—but in a negative, not a positive, way. He was sure they were snickering and laughing at the shape of his face, and he felt mortified, deeply shamed, and sometimes angry. I would guess that, most of the time, any laughing Steven observed had nothing to do with him. But I wouldn't be surprised if other people, especially young women, sometimes *did* notice Steven—in a positive way.

Some BDD sufferers have described a no-win variation on this theme. "If people look at me I think it's because I'm ugly," one woman told me. "If they *don't* look at me, it's because I must be ugly. And if they look at me and then look away, they must be thinking that I'm not worth looking at. I feel shut out and rejected."

These types of experiences reflect important aspects of BDD. One is that many, if not most, people with BDD erroneously believe that other people view them negatively no matter what. This is in keeping with their generally low self-esteem. Second, people with BDD generally experience interactions with other people in terms of their appearance. They look at the world through "appearance-tinted glasses," viewing themselves through this lens and assuming the rest of the world does as well. They find it hard to believe that others don't focus on appearance as much as they do. Furthermore, people with BDD find it difficult to believe that other people generally don't focus on the defect that the BDD sufferer perceives.

One aspect of treatment is to help patients understand that although appearance may in fact be important, most people value many different aspects of the people they know and love, such as their warmth and personality. And when others do notice the BDD sufferer's appearance, they're unlikely to focus on the perceived defect.

Experiences such as these can be as problematic and painful as the core BDD preoccupation itself. Feelings of being mocked and rejected contribute to feelings of shame, defectiveness, and isolation. "People always stare at me," Joyce said. "I feel transparent. Whenever I hear people whispering I think they're saying mean things about me and how I look. It's very painful, and I avoid people because of it."

"Foggy Glasses on the Brain"

Stephanie realized her view of her appearance wasn't accurate. "I have X-ray vision," she said. "No one else would see the marks on my face. My mind is playing tricks on me. *It magnifies every crazy little thing!* I look in the mirror, and a mark *jumps out* at me. I see it a mile away, but I know that's stupid."

Hal also realized that he had an inaccurate view of how his skin looked. Sometimes the acne was actually there, but it was slight and not anything other people noticed unless he pointed it out. But, in his mind, it would grow to hideous proportions so it was all he saw when he looked at his face. "My imagination goes haywire," Hal said. "In my mind, this little pimple becomes a massive ugly thing that everyone is staring at. It's as if you drew huge red circles around any tiny imperfection on your face. That's how it seems to me, but I know I'm distorting how bad it is." "I think one of my testicles is longer than the other," Louis said, "although logically I can't see it. It doesn't make any sense, yet my concern won't ever go away." Another man similarly said, "This is irrational. It's a very small detail that no one else would notice. I'm like an anorexic. I'm distorting but I can't stop thinking about it."

In psychiatric terms, these patients had good insight—they recognized that their view of their appearance was inaccurate. Even though they couldn't stop thinking about it, they realized that they really weren't terribly ugly. As one man said, "I have a foggy pair of glasses on my brain."

But many people with BDD don't recognize that their view is different from that of others. They think it's *probably* accurate. Others with BDD think their view is *definitely* accurate; they're *completely convinced* that it's right and undistorted. Those who think the defect *probably* is as bad as they think it is, but who can acknowledge that their view might be distorted, in psychiatric terms have *overvalued ideation;* that is, their insight is poor. They say things like, "It's *probably* as bad as I think it is. I don't *think* I'm distorting, but it's a possibility." Or "I'm *pretty* sure my skin looks as bad as I think it does, but I'm not convinced. My concerns make sense to me and seem realistic, but deep down I know I'm probably exaggerating my deformities and blowing them out of proportion." There's an element of doubt. Often, they're not sure what to believe. "I think I look atrocious," one person said, "but maybe I don't. I probably do, but there's a question mark in my head. Your mind doesn't know how to tell the truth from the nontruth."

Anita had overvalued ideas. "I've always been called beautiful," she said, "but *I've* always thought I looked odd and ugly. And I think other people think I look ugly, like a freak." Anita was fairly convinced that her view was accurate, but she also questioned it: "Sometimes I think maybe other people are right and I'm looking at my nose too closely. Maybe it looks okay, and the bump isn't so bad. Maybe my teeth actually are pretty even. If so many people ask me to be a model, maybe I don't look that bad. How could all those people be wrong?" Yet Anita still doubted what everyone told her.

Some people with BDD don't have good insight or overvalued ideation. Instead, they're completely convinced that their view of the defect is accurate and undistorted. They can't be persuaded by others that it's inaccurate. There is no element of doubt. They say things like, "I'm 100% convinced that I'm right. I'm not exaggerating how bad it is. Everyone else is wrong. No one can talk me out of this. There's no question mark." Or "If you said you didn't see it, I wouldn't believe you, because *I* see it." Or "I see it in pictures. I know what I see." One man said, "I'm as certain of what I see in the mirror as you are that the box on this table is rectangular, not round."

Frustrated friends and family members often bear testament to the tenacity and fixity of the beliefs, which they've vainly tried to argue the person out of. In psychiatric terms, such thinking is considered *delusional*; that is, the individual firmly holds on to a belief that others don't share. People with absent insight (delusional thinking) may try to convince others of how terrible the defect looks. Some show photographs to document supposed changes in their appearance, or present evidence that they're right—for example, hair on a towel or in the drain may be considered evidence that hair loss is excessive.

One possible explanation for this view is that they actually *see* something different from other people; that is, they have a different perceptual experience. Another possible explanation is that they see what we see but consider it very unattractive, perhaps because they have high standards. Yet another possibility involves excessive focusing on a minimal defect, which might lead to a distorted view of the importance, or even the appearance, of the supposed defect. I'll discuss these possible explanations further in Chapter 11.

Thus, insight in BDD ranges from good, to poor (or overvalued ideation), to absent (or delusional thinking). Three percent of the people I've seen currently had excellent insight, 9% had good insight, 28% had fair insight, 18% had poor insight, and 41% had absent insight (delusional thinking). Fifty-two percent had been delusional at some point for at least several weeks.

One way to conceptualize the relationship among these degrees of insight is to use the model of a spectrum, also known as a dimensional model. This model is illustrated below.

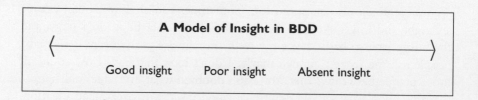

A Model of Insight in BDD

Good insight   Poor insight   Absent insight

According to this model, one type of insight isn't clearly differentiated from other types but instead shades imperceptibly into another. The different types of insight vary only by degree rather than constituting discrete categories. One reason to think this model is accurate is that sometimes it's difficult to definitively classify a person's insight as clearly belonging in one category instead of another. Sometimes it seems to fall right on the boundary. In addition, insight can move between the different types rather than always remaining the same. A sales clerk told me, "Some days I think my skin's not so bad, but other days I'm convinced." Marie often had fairly good insight that her facial hair wasn't excessive, stating "Most of the time I know it's not real or that bad; my view is very distorted." But at other times she thought her concerns made some sense—that "maybe it's really there."

Bill, too, had changing insight—sometimes it was poor, sometimes it was absent. "Sometimes I sort of believe people when they say the pores look normal. I think maybe I *am* distorting and that they're not so bad—maybe they're just normal looking. But most of the time I'm totally, 100% convinced. I think they're huge and ugly, and I know that people laugh at them. Then no one can talk me out of it—when they try to, I think they just feel sorry for me and they're trying to make me feel better."

Sometimes insight varies according to the situation. Some people who think that they may not look so bad become convinced that they look terrible when they look in the mirror. They lose the insight they had. Cassandra recognized that she had a distorted view of her freckles. "Yes, they're there. But they're not so bad. I know that no one else thinks they're hideous, and I know I'm blowing them out of proportion. But sometimes, they seem really bad. I look in the mirror and I panic. I think, 'They really *are* that bad!' " Julie, who worried about damaging her nose, had a similar experience. "Most of the time, I know my worries are ridiculous. But sometimes I'm looking in the mirror and I see a mark—evidence of damage. I try to tell myself it's not really so bad, but when I see it in front of me, I sometimes think this time the damage is real!"

Sometimes insight gets poorer when the BDD sufferer is around other people. One man told me, "Sometimes I distort, and sometimes I don't. When I don't go out, I think I imagine the acne. I know I'm making a mountain out of a molehill. But when I go out, I can become 100% certain that it's awful and hideous. I think other people definitely see it. I can change between these points of view within an hour." Sometimes, other kinds of stressors, and anxiety, also seem to temporarily decrease insight. And insight may improve with psychiatric treatment. Hannah, who had been concerned with acne and red and white facial discoloration, realized after treatment with fluvoxamine (Luvox, a serotonin-reuptake inhibitor) that her view had been distorted. She now recognized that her skin looked fine. She was so certain of this that she even went swimming, without makeup—something she'd never done before.

The insight issue is important for several reasons. One is that in DSM-III-R (the version of DSM used from 1987 to 1993), people with absent insight (delusional thinking) were considered to have a disorder different from those with good or poor insight (nondelusional thinking): those with the delusional form of BDD were diagnosed with delusional disorder (see page 320 in Appendix A for a definition), whereas those with the nondelusional form were diagnosed with BDD. But my and my colleagues' data suggest that these two supposedly separate disorders probably constitute a single disorder characterized by a range of insight, as illustrated by the dimensional model I've discussed. That is, the single disorder (BDD) appears to span the entire spectrum of insight, including delusional and nondelusional thinking, with the delusional form being more severe.* The possibility that the delusional and nondelusional forms of BDD are in fact the same disorder, with a range of insight, is acknowledged in DSM-IV, the current version of DSM.†

This issue is important for another reason. My research findings—although preliminary—suggest that people with the delusional and nondelusional forms of BDD respond to the same medication—the serotonin-reuptake inhibitors (antidepressant medications with antiobsessional properties). What's surprising about this finding is that this class of medications

* We found that patients with the delusional form were similar to those with the nondelusional form in nearly all ways (such as gender, course of illness, and treatment response), although those with delusional thinking appear to have more severe BDD—they're more preoccupied, distressed, and impaired by their symptoms.

† According to DSM-IV, patients with delusional BDD may receive a diagnosis of *both* delusional disorder *and* BDD. This isn't an ideal solution, because people in reality have one disorder, not two. But it's nonetheless useful because it acknowledges that the two disorders may in fact be the same. It doesn't make sense to consider the same person to have one disorder at one time of the day and another disorder at another, or to have one disorder when alone and another disorder when with other people, or to have one disorder when symptomatic and another when improved with treatment.

The insight/delusionality issue is complicated. Insight isn't easy to measure, and there aren't yet any widely used, clinician-administered instruments (questionnaires) that measure delusional thinking in a reliable and valid way. Another complicating factor is that people with BDD sometimes *feel* differently than they *think*. They may *feel* as though their appearance is unacceptable, but, when they think about it rationally, they realize they look fine and that their view of their appearance is distorted. Which is more important, and which should be measured—the thinking or the feeling view? When I assess insight, I assess the thinking point of view. But both are important and need to be taken into account during treatment.

isn't typically thought to effectively treat people with delusional thinking. Even more surprising, it appears that medications commonly used to treat delusional thinking may not be effective, when used by themselves, for delusional BDD. While preliminary, these findings are intriguing.

My and my colleagues' research finding that people with delusional BDD have more severe BDD than those with some insight fits with my clinical impression that some of the most severely distressed people I've worked with are those who don't realize that they *might* look okay, who derive no comfort from the *possibility* that they might look fine, who are imprisoned by their absolute certainty that the perceived defect is ugly.

Some of them wish they had a physical illness instead, because they think they'd suffer less and that other people would take their worry seriously. "This BDD experience is horrible," said Drew, a 40-year-old teacher who was completely convinced that he had "stuck-out" ears and was balding. "It's much worse than physical pain or disease. It's caused me so much pain and mental anguish for the past 30 years. . . . If I was told today I had a brain tumor I'd be *very* upset. But the reason I'd be upset is because I'd have to shave my head and have my ears seen! And I'd need a toupee to cover my bald head. That would be my major concern, not the cancer."

·· *seven* ··

Mirror Checking, Grooming, Camouflaging, Dieting, and Other BDD Behaviors

"His life was centered on the little mirror in his pocket, and his fate depended on what it revealed or was about to reveal."

Ruth Brunswick, 1928

"I Have This Ritual Every Morning . . ."

Amanda had grown up in a family where appearance didn't really matter. "So I don't know why I worry so much about it," she said "It's ridiculous—I shouldn't really care. But I do." Amanda thought that overall she looked acceptable, but disliked her hair, which she thought stuck out and "looked bizarre." She was also overly concerned about a faint scar on her face and thought her neck was too large.

To look better, Amanda spent hours a day arranging and combing her hair. "I don't do it all at once," she said, "but if I added up all the time I spend, it would be a lot. I have this ritual every morning where I take a shower, and then I take at least an hour in front of the mirror getting ready to go to work. I stay in the bathroom looking in the mirror, combing and recombing my hair. I blow dry it and put gel on it, and then I comb it again. I try arranging it in different ways so it doesn't stick out in the wrong places. I go through the whole process at least five to ten times so I can look decent enough to leave the house. I try to make it look better, but it never really works."

During her morning ritual, Amanda also applied and reapplied makeup to cover her slight scar. Sometimes, she picked at it. She also checked mirrors at work. "When I'm at work, I go into the bathroom to see if I look okay and to check my makeup and my hair. I'm drawn to the mirror. Sometimes I get stuck there, combing my hair. It's a problem because it makes it hard for me to do my job. I'm supposed to be waiting on people, but I'm in the mirror instead."

Amanda worked as a sales clerk in a clothing store and sometimes kept her customers waiting too long. "My boss isn't exactly pleased with my job performance because sometimes I'm not waiting on people, and he's wondering where I am," she said. "I think he knows I'm in the bathroom, which is kind of embarrassing. I'm surprised he hasn't fired me yet. I'm actually thinking of leaving, because it's not the right job for me. I meet new people all day long, and they all get too close to my face. I'm wondering what they're thinking about my hair and the scar—I'm sure they're thinking I look bad. I feel nervous all day, and I can't look people straight in the eye because I feel so self-conscious about how I look."

Amanda considered moving to a colder climate so she could more often cover her neck with a turtleneck. "I don't know whether I'll go that far, but it's a little ridiculous to be wearing a turtleneck when it's 60 or 70 degrees out, which is what I do sometimes. My neck looks huge, and I need to cover it," she explained. "In a colder climate, I wouldn't look so strange wearing turtlenecks all the time. And working in a clothing store, I'm supposed to dress well. During the summer I can look pretty weird."

Amanda performed several behaviors characteristic of BDD: mirror checking, excessive grooming, skin picking, and camouflaging. Jennifer, Jane, and Sarah also did some of these things, as do most BDD sufferers. These behaviors are done to examine, hide, or improve the supposed defect, or to be reassured that it doesn't look so bad. Most people check their perceived defect in mirrors or other reflecting surfaces. Others compulsively pick at their skin. Most BDD sufferers frequently and secretly compare themselves with others. Others question family members or friends, sometimes over and over again: Do I look okay? Can other people see the problem? Sometimes they try to convince others that the defect looks really bad, asking such questions as "Can't you see this on my face?"

Camouflaging the perceived defect with clothes or a hat is also common, as is seeking plastic surgery, dermatologic treatment, or other medical treatment. People with BDD may go to doctor after doctor, asking for blood tests, medications, or surgical procedures. Sometimes they have treatment after treatment, without finding the cure they're hoping for.

The table on the next page summarizes the more common behaviors associated with BDD and their frequency as reported by the people I've seen. Nearly everyone with BDD (close to 100%) engages in at least one of these behaviors. The average number performed is four, and some people do as many as seven.

Although the behaviors in Table 5 are particularly common, there are others, such as repeatedly measuring the "defective" body part (e.g., one's waist), reading about the problem area (e.g., books on hair growth), and excessive weight lifting. These behaviors, too, are generally intended to obtain reassurance, fix the defect, or hide it from others.

Some behaviors are more unusual and creative. Rob, a 30-year-old factory worker, was preoccupied with his supposedly loose facial skin, receding hairline, and small penis. To tighten his skin, he did something unusual: repeatedly touching doorknobs. While he realized that this behavior didn't really make sense—touching a doorknob wouldn't actually tighten his skin—Rob nonetheless did it, *hoping* he might look better. For his hair, he used a fairly conventional camouflaging technique—wearing a hat. But for his worries about his penis size, he tried a more unusual approach: sewing an extra pocket in his underwear so he could stuff it and enhance his apparent penis size. A teenage boy kept candy balls or wads of paper in the side of his mouth to widen his supposedly thin face. This, too, was a less typical form of camouflaging.

Questioning and reassurance seeking can also take unusual forms. While most reassurance seekers ask family members or friends, one woman questioned total strangers, in the ladies' room and even in elevators in busy public buildings. "I asked them, 'Would you tell me—do I look okay?' I knew I looked bad," she told me, "but I couldn't face it, so I tried to get people to tell me I looked okay."

A man tied up his calves with rope while he slept to try to make them smaller. A teenage boy who thought his facial features were asymmetric tried to "straighten them out" by tying socks around his head, sometimes so tightly that he hurt himself. He reasoned that this technique might stretch his skin and somehow fix his problem. These were their ingenious— yet ineffective—attempts to cope with their painful preoccupation.

Some behaviors are more avoidant than compulsive; they involve *not doing* rather than excessive doing. Some people avoid having their picture

Table 5   Common BDD Behaviors

Behavior	Percent (%) of People with Behavior
Comparing body part with others/scrutinizing the appearance of others	91
Checking appearance in mirrors and other reflecting surfaces	84
Camouflaging	84
• with clothing	48
• with posture	44
• with makeup	35
• with hand	23
• with hat	16
Seeking surgery, dermatologic, or other medical treatment	72
Questioning: seeking reassurance or attempting to convince others that the supposed defect is unattractive	42
Excessive grooming (combing hair, applying makeup, shaving, removing hair, etc.)	35
Mirror avoidance*	35
Touching the defect	33
Skin picking	27
Other repetitive behaviors	27

*Avoidance of all mirrors for at least several days in a row.

taken—they're missing from their family photo albums and high school yearbook, or they destroy all photos ever taken of them. One man avoided doing chores around the house because he feared any activity would make his calves larger. Some people avoid showering or washing or brushing their hair because they fear more hair will fall out. A teenage boy refused to eat foods like ice cream, which would wet his supposedly red lips and make them redder and more noticeable. The strategies that people devise to decrease their discomfort with their appearance are limited only by their imagination.

Compulsive Behaviors: "I Can't Resist"

Most BDD behaviors have certain things in common. They're generally time consuming and difficult to resist or control. They sometimes decrease but may also increase emotional distress. And they can interfere with day-to-day functioning. In all these ways, BDD-related behaviors resemble BDD-related thoughts.

Typically, behaviors are performed over and over again. The repetitiveness seems related to doubt or dissatisfaction about what was seen or done. Did my nose *really* look okay? Maybe I didn't get a good enough look. . . . My hair *still* isn't right! I can't go out until it is! . . . I don't *really* believe that I look okay; she just said that to be nice. I have to ask again!

People with BDD can spend hours a day doing things—such as grooming—that many people without BDD do in minutes. Or they frequently do things, like seeking reassurance, that most people without BDD do rarely or even at all. In more extreme cases, people spend up to 10 hours a day in front of the mirror, or 12 hours a day picking their skin. Table 6 on the next page shows the amount of time people with BDD report spending each day on their BDD-related behaviors.

BDD behaviors are sometimes described as compulsive—there's a strong drive to perform them and they're difficult to resist or control. Some people try to resist, but others don't—they "give in," or simply do them "automatically." As Jennifer said of her mirror checking: "I couldn't resist: I *had* to check my face. I *had* to make sure I looked okay." This is one reason behaviors may be done over and over or for long periods of time. As one woman said, "My rituals are like an itch that I have to scratch."

How much control do people with BDD have over their behaviors? When they try to resist doing them, how successful are they? The most common response to this question is little control, with 36% giving this response. Very few report having complete control.

The degree of resistance or control experienced may vary depending on the activity. Many people with BDD resist asking for reassurance. They may feel a very strong urge to ask, but they anticipate that others will think they're vain or consider their question strange, and they successfully resist the urge. In contrast, people with BDD typically don't resist camouflaging. They simply do it. They put on their hat or their baggy clothes, without trying to stop the behavior. This may be because camouflaging doesn't necessarily take much time—it's often done just once at the beginning of the day, so resistance is less necessary. Or it may be that people don't usually feel worse after covering up, so there's less reason to resist it. People often

---

Table 6   BDD Behaviors: Time Spent, Resistance, Control, Anxiety, and Interference*

TIME SPENT ON BEHAVIORS
- None   6%
- Less than 1 hour a day   20%
- 1 to 3 hours a day   38%
- More than 3 and up to 8 hours a day   30%
- More than 8 hours a day   6%

ATTEMPT TO RESIST BEHAVIORS
- Always try to resist   8%
- Try to resist most of the time   13%
- Try to resist some of the time   26%
- Rarely try to resist   21%
- Never try to resist   33%

CONTROL OVER BEHAVIORS
- Complete control   7%
- Much control   8%
- Moderate control   27%
- Little control   36%
- No control   23%

ANXIETY EXPERIENCED IF BEHAVIOR ISN'T PERFORMED
- No distress   13%
- Mild distress   13%
- Moderate distress   25%
- Severe distress   25%
- Extreme and disabling distress   26%

INTERFERENCE IN FUNCTIONING DUE TO BEHAVIORS
- None   26%
- Mild   16%
- Moderate   30%
- Severe   22%
- Extreme and disabling   6%

---

*From the Yale-Brown Obsessive-Compulsive Scale for BDD (BDD-YBOCS), which rates severity of BDD thoughts and behaviors. See Appendix B for a more detailed description of this scale.

feel worse after mirror checking or skin picking, which may contribute to a desire to resist and control these behaviors.

The behaviors are usually preceded by an upsetting thought, such as "How does it look?" "Do I look okay?" Or "I know I look terrible and I have to fix it!" Associated feelings of worry, anxiety, and tension drive people to perform their behaviors. In response to the question, "How anxious do you think you'd get if you *didn't* perform your behavior?," 26% report that they would experience extreme and disabling distress (see Table 6). Twenty-five percent would experience severe distress, and 25% moderate distress. Only 13% said they would experience mild distress, and 13% no distress.

Thus, many people perform their behaviors before their anxiety becomes unmanageable, to ward off and avoid an even more painful emotional state. The anxiety they avoid by doing the activity is often interpersonal in nature. They fear that others will see how bad they look and will ridicule or reject them.

Are the behaviors successful in diminishing tension and anxiety? Perhaps. A common response to the question "Do you feel less anxious after checking the mirror?" is "Some of the time." Many people *sometimes* feel less anxious after mirror checking, if they think they look a little better than usual, or at least not as bad as they feared. They may also feel less anxious if they checked themselves in a "good" mirror, in "good" light, or on a "good" day. But they sometimes feel *more* anxious—if they think they look as bad as, or worse than, they feared.

Many people with BDD *usually* feel worse after mirror checking—more anxious, tense, and worried. They check to reassure themselves that they look okay, but often their worst fear is confirmed: they think they look as bad as or even worse than they feared. The distress can become so unbearable that it fuels hopelessness and thoughts of suicide.

Why would someone who usually feels *more* anxious after mirror checking keep checking? The usual explanation is that they *sometimes* feel less anxious after checking, and they hope this will be one of those times. One man told me, "I check in the *hope* that I'll look better this time—that *this* will be one of the times that my fear and anxiety decrease. There's a small chance, a hope."

Not uncommonly, anxiety and distress diminish temporarily after the behavior is done, but then, after some time has passed, the unpleasant feelings return. People who pick their skin, for example, may feel better immediately after picking, but then, several hours later or the next morning, they feel much worse, after they've surveyed the damage they've caused. Similarly, reassurance seekers may feel better temporarily—for a few minutes or hours—after being told they look fine, but, with the passage of time, their anxiety returns as they begin to doubt the veracity of what they were told. The temporary decrease in anxiety and distress may actually reinforce the behavior, impelling the BDD sufferer to perform the behavior once again.

For some people, the behaviors are minimal enough so they don't inter-fere with functioning or quality of life. But, for many, the behaviors are unmanageable and a major problem in and of themselves. Fifty-eight per-cent reported that their behaviors interfered with their functioning to a moderate, severe, or extreme extent.

A homemaker who spends two hours a day checking mirrors doesn't have as much time for her children and running the household. A teenager may spend his date alone in his bathroom because he can't tear himself away from the mirror. A salesperson may miss work because she was up picking at tiny pimples until the early hours of the morning, and can't bear to have the resulting disfigurement seen the next day. Wearing a hat can make it hard to go outside on a windy day, eat in certain restaurants, or interview for certain jobs.

BDD-related behaviors can create problems for family members and other loved ones, and strain even the closest of relationships. Reassurance seeking is particularly likely to cause such problems—the questioning can be so incessant that friends and family can't tolerate it. Requesting others to join in rituals and avoiding daily activities or special occasions so rituals can be done can also be very hard on loved ones. Occasionally, the strain is so severe that friendship ends or divorce results.

Stuck to the Mirror: How Do I Look?

If there's any behavior that is prototypic of BDD—that reflects its essential nature—it's mirror checking. Most people with BDD have a special and torturous relationship with mirrors. The mirror reflects their greatest hope—that they look okay—and their deepest fear—that there's something hopelessly wrong with how they look, that they're defective and flawed in some noticeable and important way.

About 80% of people with BDD excessively check mirrors, spending a long time at one sitting, or checking repeatedly during the day. Many do both. Some who don't check excessively instead avoid mirrors, generally to escape the disappointment and frustration their reflection brings them. Some people alternate between excessive checking and mirror avoidance. This leaves few people with BDD who have a normal relationship with mirrors.

While checking is often done in a bathroom or bedroom mirror, virtu-ally any reflecting surface will do; mirror substitutes often become an im-portant part of the BDD sufferer's life. Store windows, car bumpers, windows, toasters, watch and clock faces, TV and computer screens, one's shadow, tweezers, and the backs of spoons all become vehicles of hope and great disappointment.

Before I started my research, the importance of mirrors in the lives of BDD sufferers escaped me. In much of what had been written about the disorder, mirrors weren't even mentioned. But when I started talking with patients and learning about their experience, the importance of mirrors became increasingly clear. One of the first patients I saw brought this home to me when she described her panic attacks, which were triggered by the mirror.

This is what she told me. "At least 10 times a day I have the urge to look in the mirror, but I don't. I try to avoid mirrors, because I worry that if I look and don't like what I see, I'll panic and be debilitated. But there are many times when I just can't resist, and I go running—I just hope that what I see won't be exaggerated. About 50% of the time, I don't feel so bad. I even feel somewhat relieved. I don't look that bad, and the problem doesn't seem to be getting worse. I can go about my business. But about half the time, I look worse. Or I think something like 'You look okay today, but you won't next year.' Thoughts like these overwhelm me with anxiety, and I have a panic attack. I have trouble breathing, I get sweaty, and sometimes I feel dizzy. Sometimes I feel so bad I go to bed for the day. Sometimes I don't go to work."

The power of mirrors in this person's life was very clear. Since then, I've heard similar stories from many others. While most people don't have full-fledged panic attacks, most feel anxious and fearful around mirrors. What they see affects their mood and even their functioning. As Jennifer said of her skin, "It's the first thing I think of when I wake up in the morning. I immediately rush to the mirror, wondering 'How does it look?' How my skin looks in the morning completely determines how my day goes."

Many people check mirrors in the hope that they don't look as bad as they fear. They look to reassure themselves. Is my hair okay? Are my legs too fat? Is my makeup smeared? As one woman told me, "I check because I'm hoping to find a miracle—that I look okay." Others check to make sure their view of the defect is correct. As one man said, "I check to see that I'm right, and that the scar is still there. It always is—I'm not stupid."

The response to checking varies. Many people sometimes feel worse and sometimes feel better. How they feel depends on whether they like what they see, which may hinge on such things as lighting, whether the mirror is a "good" one, how well they've applied their makeup, or how their clothes look. Many others usually feel worse after looking. The mirror confirms their worst fear—that they really are ugly, the perceived defect really is hideous. Very few usually feel better. Jennifer's experience was fairly typi-cal: "Unfortunately, 80% of the time I think I look terrible."

When the mirror reflects an acceptable image, the relief is usually only temporary. Doubts return, along with the urge to check again. Do I *really* look okay? Maybe I really don't. I need to check again to be sure. As one person told me, "When I look in the mirror I can be reassured for a few minutes. But then I usually feel worse. The more I look, the crazier I get. Overall I feel worse and my anxiety increases. And sometimes I get stuck there inspecting myself and worrying. I can't leave. It's like I'm superglued."

Another person also became more obsessed, anxious, and depressed after looking in the mirror. "I got very caught up in the mirror," he told me. "I'd think 'Which way do my lips look the best? Which position is most natural, most attractive?' The mirror definitely contributed to my problem—it took it to another level of obsession."

These descriptions reflect research findings suggesting that increased body awareness and body focus tend to lower self-esteem. The more people concentrate on their bodies, the more critical they become. Feedback on one's body, such as that provided by mirrors, increases body awareness, which can intensify dissatisfaction with one's appearance.

Like many other BDD behaviors, the need to check mirrors can feel very "compulsive"; it's something that *has* to be done. "I can't resist checking," Amanda said. "I have an overwhelming urge to do it. I *have* to look to see if I look normal." The urge, or compulsion, is often preceded or accompa-nied by a thought, such as "How do I look? Do I look okay? Has it gotten any worse?" But mirror checking can also be "automatic"—something that's "just done" while walking past a window or store mirror. Many people check mirrors both "compulsively" and "automatically."

Little resistance and poor control over checking can lead to frequent trips to the closest mirror. A board member may leave a board meeting, a student may leave class. Some people have had to leave their interview with me. They felt so anxious and tense over whether they looked okay that they couldn't focus on our conversation.

What do people do when they check? Typically they inspect the supposed defect, often in excruciating detail. A college student told me, "I examine the front of my hairline to see if the density is decreasing. My hair used to be a half an inch further down. Even on a daily basis I could see the changes." The inspection may be done from different angles or with differ-ent lights to get as good a look as possible. "I look at myself a lot at special angles," Eliza told me. "I have three mirrors in my bathroom so I can get a better look."

Some people try to fix the perceived defect while inspecting themselves. They comb their hair, reapply their makeup, rearrange their hat, pick their skin, or pull on their nose. One woman tilted her head, squinted her eyes, and covered the lower part of her face. "It made me look more like my old self," she said, "the way I want to look." A 22-year-old man said, "I make funny faces in the mirror to change my face."

Other people don't need mirrors to check. They simply look at the body part. A librarian repeatedly looked at her arms during the day to see how hairy they looked, hoping to reassure herself that they were okay. A young man repeatedly checked his calves to see whether they were too thin, especially while showering, resulting in very long showers. Some people frequently analyze their appearance in photographs or videos. One man told me, "I'm constantly analyzing my face in pictures. I'm thinking 'How do I look?' or 'Is my hairline going up?' "

Such checking is usually problematic, taking time needed for other things. A physicist who spent two to three hours a day checking mirrors performed her job well but had to stay late each night to complete her work. A man who checked mirrors 40 times a day for 15 minutes each time was unable to work at all because of this behavior. Mirror checking can also interfere with relationships and social activities. It isn't unusual to get stuck in the mirror and not go out because of feeling too ugly to be seen.

Eating out can be especially difficult. One person asked me if I'd ever noticed how many restaurants have mirrors in them. "A lot do," he told me. "Or they have pictures with reflecting glass on them. It's easy to get distracted by checking out how I look." Going to museums can also be difficult. "When I go to museums," he said, "I count my freckles in the reflections of the paintings instead of looking at the pictures."

Occasionally, mirror checking triggers a suicide attempt. Seeing the defect reflected back can be too much to bear. The mirror itself can become the vehicle for an attempt, with broken shards of glass used to inflict self-harm.

One man didn't look in any mirrors for 11 years because seeing his skin was so frightening. He combed his hair and shaved in his mirrorless basement for all those years. "Looking at myself in the mirror is like looking at a scary picture," he told me. "Now I look in them, but I still try to avoid them as much as I can. Especially in restaurants. It helps to some degree. Looking is very painful and makes me angry. I think 'I can't believe this—how I look.' The mirror is the enemy. I curse the person who invented the mirror."

Grooming: Cutting, Combing, Teasing, and Tweezing

Each day, during his girlfriend's lunch break, Daniel met her in the parking lot of the company where they worked. Then they drove to a nearby park. While sitting in her car, he had her comb and style his hair so it would look fuller. She also applied expensive tonics that were supposed to stimulate hair growth.

"I had her do it at least once a day because I couldn't see my hair well enough in the back. She followed the directions better than I did. And looking in the mirror is really traumatic for me. This way I'd be sure it got done at least once a day. I'd also ask her if she saw any changes."

Daniel felt badly about asking his girlfriend to do this for him, but thought it was necessary. He had severe BDD and suffered tremendously. "Having her do it kept me going," he explained. His insistence that she groom his hair strained their relationship. "She wanted to leave me because I was so obsessed with my hair and because I insisted that she work on it every day. I talked about my hair all the time, for hours at a time. We constantly fought over it. The relationship eventually deteriorated to where I wanted to end it, too. But I tried to hold on to her because I needed her to do my hair. The main reason I was still with her was so she could do my hair and monitor me for hair loss."

While this behavior was somewhat unusual, Daniel wasn't alone in having someone important to him participate in his grooming rituals. Daniel also combed and styled his hair himself, and applied hair thickener and hair spray "to create an optical illusion" of having more hair.

One-third of people with BDD groom excessively. Often they do it in front of the mirror. They may do it at home, in the car, at work, at school, or in other people's homes. As one woman said, "I do it wherever I can." Some people excessively groom only before going out, whereas others do it regardless of their plans.

One woman spent several hours on her hair every morning—washing, setting, combing, and teasing it—making the bathroom unavailable to family members. She then continued to comb and tease it repeatedly throughout the day. She told me, "My hair looks horrendous if I don't do my hair ritual. It's too flat and not full enough." A young man performed a similar ritual. "I fix my hair many times a day while I'm looking in the mirror. I comb it, brush it, and spray it, thinking 'Please just look normal.' I do it with my real hair and with my hairpiece. I'd look like a monster if I didn't do these things." A college student washed his hair three to four times a day, trying to get it to look better. Another man, who thought his hair was too curly, first straightened it, then permed it, then straightened it, and finally shaved it all off, trying to make it look acceptable.

William had a particularly complicated grooming ritual he had to perform each morning. "First I wash my face and remove the dead skin. Then I wash my hair with shampoo and hair thickener, and then I brush it a lot to remove the frizz. Then I style it so it's a certain way. Then I do my beard: I brush it, style it, and dry it. Then I do my hair again—the whole routine. Then I do my skin again, then I put on hair spray, and then I trim my beard. I have to do it in a certain order. If I get out of order, sometimes I have to start it over again. My day is determined by the outcome of this routine. . . . I don't want to do it—I try to shorten it. I've tried for 30 years, but I can't. I *have* to finish it."

Some people cut and recut their hair, in an effort to get it exactly even or just the right shape, a behavior they may describe as "compulsive." Some carry scissors with them and cut at work or school. Others have haircutting "binges," cutting in a frenzied burst of compulsive activity. Haircutting can become so excessive that an extremely short haircut results.

Suzanne thought her hair was too flat, so she spent hours a day trying to cut it exactly right, hoping to improve the shape. She couldn't trust hairdressers, but she also acknowledged that by cutting it herself, she "butchered" it. Then for a time she wore what she called "strange hairdos," which was yet another effort to get her hair "just right." She then went through a period of curling and recurling her hair to give it bounce and shape. "I had to do it over and over again to get it just right, and I wouldn't stop. I wouldn't let anyone see me do it, because it was embarrassing. It made sense to me at the time, but I still realized that other people would think it was strange for me to spend so much time on my hair. It seems silly now, but at the time it was agony."

Diane compulsively cut her hair for up to eight hours a day. "I couldn't stop cutting it," she told me, "even though I had to take care of my children. I had to get it looking exactly even and right. I cut minuscule amounts so it wouldn't get too short, but it did get really short because of the time I was spending. I bought wigs because I was so embarrassed about how short it was—I was practically bald—but I cut the wigs too, and I spent all of my money on them. To tell you how bad it got, once I cut myself by accident with the scissors, and I was bleeding. I was so caught up in the cutting that I couldn't even stop to take care of the bleeding." When I asked her how she'd feel if she couldn't cut her hair, she answered, "I'd get so extremely upset that I'd have to be hospitalized. When I'm in a bad period, I wouldn't be able to stop even if the house was burning down."

Like Suzanne and Diane, some people with hair concerns avoid hair salons and barbers because they can't tolerate looking in mirrors, they fear their hair will be wrecked, or they're too embarrassed about their hair to have anyone focus on it so closely. But some people frequently go to the beauty parlor, even several times a week, trying to find a solution to their hair problem. One woman who did this said, "Every time I go I drastically change my hair style—I don't just get a trim."

Hair removal may also be done to excess. People concerned about excessive body hair may spend lots of time tweezing it, removing it from their face, their arms, or other parts of their body. Others have frequent electrolysis. Eyebrows may be repeatedly plucked to create the right shape. Some men shave for long periods of time, or repeatedly shave, to get their beard to look the way they want. Josh, who worried about supposedly asymmetric beard growth, couldn't leave his house without shaving again. Another man shaved many times a day to get rid of his supposedly uneven shadow, to the point where he bled.

Other people apply and reapply makeup. "I use a lot of makeup, and I take a long time to put on my eyeliner and lipstick," Emma said. "I'm in agony if I can't do this. I need my fix! After I do it I feel a little less ugly. But then I worry that I've smeared it, and I keep checking mirrors to see if I have to fix it. I'd guess that I reapply my makeup as often as 30 times a day."

Like other BDD-related behaviors, grooming is characterized by varying degrees of resistance and control. A teenager who spent two hours a day fixing her hair, combing her eyelashes, and reapplying her eyeliner told me, "I can't resist this behavior, even though it drives my parents crazy. I've tried but I can't."

Although people who groom sometimes feel they improve their appearance, this often isn't the case. The teenager I just described said that she sometimes felt better—when she got her hair to curl the way she wanted it to—but usually she felt worse. If anxiety is diminished, the relief is usually only temporary.

Grooming rituals are especially problematic when staying at other people's homes. Some people with BDD in fact avoid staying with friends or family because it's so difficult to cart their beauty products with them or fully enact their grooming routine in private. "I won't stay overnight places because I need my special makeup light," Anne Marie said. "I don't go away on weekends because of it." Others describe the embarrassment they'd feel spending hours at a time in someone else's bathroom. "I never visited my in-laws or my family because of my combing," one man told me. "I couldn't take up the bathroom for that long, and I needed to keep my problem a secret from them. I think it's one of the reasons my wife left me—we could never visit her family."

The Batman Mask
and Other Forms of Camouflage

John was a 34-year-old electrician who thought he was good looking except for his skin. "I like to blend in with the crowd," he said. "But I can't with white skin." He'd had this concern since the age of 12, when he dreaded going to gym class and the beach because people would see his skin. Over the years, his preoccupation became increasingly painful. To decrease his self-consciousness, he wore long sleeves and pants at all times. "But that isn't enough," he told me. "Other parts of my skin are still exposed."

John's solution was to use a skin bronzer. "I put it on all the exposed areas of my body. I *never* go out without it," he said. In fact, he was wearing the bronzer during his interview with me. "I spend at least an hour a day trying to paint a perfect picture, so no one knows it's makeup. I look jaundiced, but that's better than pale. It helps me get to work, and it makes my life bearable."

At the same time, it created some problems. "First of all, it's much too much of an effort to paint this perfect picture every day," he said. "And it's very expensive. I'm too embarrassed to buy it in a drug store, so I order it through a catalog. But the hardest part of it is how it affects my girlfriend." This part was difficult for John to talk about. It was clearly a very painful subject.

"I couldn't be spontaneous with her, because I had to put the stuff on first, and it always took a long time. We couldn't just go out and do something. I didn't even tell her about it for a few years. The hardest thing I ever did was tell my girlfriend about it. . . . . It's why I never moved in with her. It would be too degrading to put it on in front of her.

"It's especially hard wearing the stuff in the summer, because it runs," he continued. "I'd love to go to a baseball game or the beach . . . but I can't. What put me into the deepest, darkest depression of my life was when I was outside in the summer watering the lawn with my girlfriend, and the hose split. I got covered with water, and the bronzing stuff ran. I've never been so humiliated in my entire life. I got very depressed, and I had to go into the hospital for my depression.

"It must be hard for you to understand how desperate I felt," he said. "Maybe this will help. After the hose accident happened, I realized I needed a better solution for my problem. So I decided to take some tanning pills. I knew it was a dangerous thing to do, because I was told they can damage your liver and gallbladder. But I was so desperate, I took them anyway. I had terrible stomach pain, but I kept taking them. A month later, I had to have my gallbladder taken out. I'm convinced it was because of the tanning pills. Before I had the operation, I made sure I put my bronzer on. Before the operation, all I could think about was how I'd look on the table, not that I could die!"

Eighty-four percent of the people I've seen have, like John, used camouflaging to cope with their appearance worries. I use "camouflaging" to refer to attempts to minimize or conceal a perceived defect in appearance so it's less visible and noticeable to other people. Some people use bronzers or other methods to change their skin color. More commonly, they camouflage with hats, other types of clothing, their hair, or makeup. Some wear wigs; others adopt a certain body posture, such as constantly jutting out a supposedly small jaw, or turning the "bad side" of their body away from others. Camouflaging methods are numerous and varied.

You may recall Bill, the man who wore a baseball cap pulled down over his forehead to cover "pockmarks" on his nose. He removed his hat only when he was alone in his own room. Bill had considered using makeup to cover the pores but didn't because he couldn't tolerate looking in the mirror to apply it—seeing the pores made him much too anxious. He also used his body position to hide the pores. "I hold my head in a certain way," he said, "turned to the right, so the bad side of my nose is turned away from people. And I always keep the lights turned down so the pores aren't so visible. But the only time I feel really good is on Halloween. When I give out candy to the neighborhood kids, I wear a Batman mask, which completely covers the pores. It's the only time I feel okay being around other people."

A 65-year-old man, who'd had severe BDD for nearly 50 years, told me the same thing: "If I wore a mask my problems would be over, but I can't do it in this world. I love Halloween, because I'm free for a fleeting moment."

Hats are used to cover various types of perceived defects: typically thinning hair or other hair problems, perceived abnormalities of the forehead, eyes, eyebrows, skin, nose, or some other feature. Joe had worn a hat in nearly all situations for the past 15 years. "Just about the only time I take it off is when I sleep," he said. "I've taken it off in front of my girlfriend only a couple of times. I felt so nervous about the thinning I couldn't keep it off for very long."

The hat had its advantages and disadvantages. On the one hand, it alleviated Joe's anxiety enough so he could work part time as a truck driver. Wearing it at work wasn't a problem. But wearing it in certain social situations was. "My girlfriend likes to go to a nice restaurant every once in a while," he said. "She's always asking me to take my hat off so we can go. She gets really dressed up, and I look stupid wearing this hat. But I can't do it. I feel so ashamed of my hair that I can't take it off, and I always back out at the last minute. Once I did go without it, and I ended up leaving in the middle of the meal, which was really embarrassing. I was so nervous, I was sweating in the restaurant over how my hair looked, and I couldn't stay. We've gotten into some big fights over this. I realize how strange it must look in certain places," he continued. "People probably even talk about it sometimes. But it's better for them to think I'm eccentric than ugly."

"I always wore this blue beanie in high school," a 27-year-old graduate student said. "A friend asked me why I was wearing it. I was wearing it to flatten my hair and put it in a certain shape. I was also trying to hide it. I recently tried wearing it again, and I looked like a bag lady."

Wigs are another attempted solution for a perceived hair problem. Like hats, they're used to cover hair that is considered thin or unattractive in some other way. Some men with BDD join hair clubs and buy expensive hairpieces, which they generally don't like. Some buy hairpiece after hairpiece, trying to find the right look.

Camouflaging with clothing is also common. Luisa intensely disliked her legs—especially her thighs. She thought they were "flabby, misshapen, and dimpling." To hide them, she wore "big, shapeless clothes." She almost never wore shorts or a bathing suit. "I'm so embarrassed by how my legs look, I can't bear to let other people see them," she said. "I always keep them covered." Another woman was very preoccupied with her "fat" stomach and only wore clothing that made her stomach look flatter. Pleated skirts were completely taboo, because she thought they accentuated her stomach size.

Jessica hated her "flat-chestedness." She was once teased about her breasts in junior high school and had been mortified over them ever since. She wouldn't wear certain bathing suits, and always used padded bras to appear larger. She kept searching for the perfect bra, one that enhanced her breast size but also looked natural.

Men do similar things, trying to appear larger, smaller, or taller. Some wear long shirts to cover their crotch; others wear shoes with lifts. Some men wear only long-sleeved shirts or pants, even in the heat of summer, to cover "thin" wrists or arms or "misshapen" knees. One man told me, "I've never gone out of the house in a short-sleeved shirt in my entire life, not even in the summer." And men with "reverse anorexia," who think their body build is too small, often wear bulky clothing or several layers of clothes to look larger. One man I interviewed was wearing six shirts.

But clothing solutions, too, are often unsatisfactory, because they can lead to frequent clothes changing and endless shopping for the perfect cover. One woman "compulsively" changed her clothes. "I change them 4 or 5 times a day because they don't look right. They don't hang right. They make my legs look too fat and my shoulders look too broad. I get very anxious and I think that people are analyzing my appearance, so I have to change them. Sometimes I change them even when I'm home alone. I keep checking my body in the mirror and changing until I look right. It can take up a lot of time."

Body parts are sometimes used to camouflage other body parts. Hair may be combed to cover an area where it seems particularly thin. Bangs may be pulled down to conceal a supposedly short or misshapen forehead. Men may grow a mustache or beard to hide a supposedly uneven lip or a scar. One person's camouflage can be another's BDD: what one person might perceive as excessively thick bangs another might consider the perfect cover for perceived forehead scarring.

Hands and body posture are also often used to conceal the disliked area. One man sat and stood only in certain positions so his shirt wouldn't rest against and reveal his "love handles." An unusually attractive woman stood in a certain way at her wedding so the congregation wouldn't see her face.

Camouflaging methods are virtually limitless. Makeup, dark glasses, and tinted car windows are other forms of cover. Lights may be kept low or turned off. Some people never sit near a window because they fear the light will illuminate their flaw. Some prefer winter, not only because they can cover themselves with clothes, but also because there are fewer hours of daylight during which the defect can be seen.

The intent of camouflaging is to decrease anxiety and emotional distress, especially when around others. Many people with BDD feel this approach is somewhat successful, that its benefits outweigh its disadvantages. Even though applying makeup, for example, may take too much time and can be expensive, some of my patients have told me they'll never give it up.

But camouflaging has its limits, not only because it can be so time consuming but often because it's considered only partially successful. Men who wear makeup worry that others will see it. Men and women alike may feel "fraudulent" because of their camouflaging techniques. "I don't like wearing all this heavy makeup," a young woman told me. "I feel like a fraud. And my breast implants make me feel unnatural and fake."

A young man who thought his nostrils were too wide camouflaged them with his hair, completely covering his face with long bangs. The problem was, he had trouble seeing. Bill's Batman mask wasn't an adequate long-term solution to his problem, either. And John's experience with his bronzer and tanning pills is a poignant example of the limitations of camouflaging.

Buying Beauty Products and Clothes:
"I Have to Find Something That Works!"

The cosmetics industry fuels our economy and promises us cleanliness, sex appeal, youth, and eternal beauty. What would we do without these products? We all need such things as soap and shampoo, and many of us feel we couldn't possibly survive without makeup, hair gel, and conditioners. Purchasing such products is a necessary part of our lives—a ritual as routine as buying our groceries or drinking our morning coffee.

But for some people with BDD, this gets carried to an extreme. Lots of time and money are spent buying products needed for grooming and camouflaging. One woman spent more than $100 a week on various shampoos and conditioners. "I go out many times a week to buy beauty products—mostly hair products," she said. "I can't walk out of a drug store without one. I keep looking for the perfect product."

Others buy expensive makeup from mail-order catalogs. Sandy got hers from California. "It costs me an arm and a leg, but I have to cover the white area on my face. I've tried every product that's sold in drug stores and cosmetic counters. None of them work. They wear off, and they come off in the rain. I have to have something that will stay on. And it got too embarrassing to keep buying all those things. The salespeople in the drug store must have thought I'm nuts!"

Ken often went to the drug store, searching for a cure for his acne. He spent hours examining the different products, and sometimes spent more than $100 a week on them, even though he couldn't afford it. He described his behavior as compulsive—he couldn't resist doing it, and felt extremely anxious if he didn't go. Several times, when his funds were low, he was so desperate to find something that worked that he shoplifted skin products.

Clothes shopping, too, can be expensive and time consuming. While some people avoid shopping because the mirrors or trying on clothes makes them so anxious, others shop excessively, trying to find something that will improve their appearance, distract others from their flaws, or provide the perfect cover. "I spent so much time shopping, and I was so concerned with clothes," Maureen said. "It was like an addiction. It was a way to cope with my ugliness. I needed clothes to make me look good."

The urge to buy—the hope that *this* product or outfit will solve the problem—overpowers the rational argument that nothing else ever has, and this won't either. Ken said of his acne soaps and medicines, "Some are better than others, but I haven't found any miracles." Nonetheless, he felt compelled to keep buying them, hoping for a solution to his painful problem.

Skin Picking: "I Can't Stop Destroying My Looks"

When Pamela came to see me, she began by saying, "I'm a picker." Pamela considered her skin picking the most troubling aspect of her BDD. "I can't stop destroying my looks," she said. "I have this compulsion of picking at my face at any tiny blemish. I try to remove any ugly things on my face. . . . I feel addicted to this compulsion."

Pamela was a 25-year-old music student with no obvious skin lesions. She'd picked at her skin for the past eight years, trying to remove small blemishes and imperfections that to her were "hideously ugly." To decrease her chance of getting pimples, she also picked to remove any dirt that she feared might be under the surface of her skin. Pamela usually picked for several hours a day but sometimes for up to 12 hours at a time. Occasionally, she stayed up all night picking.

I asked Pamela to describe her picking to me. "The way it usually goes is that first I check a mirror," she said. "I check in school with a pocket mirror, I check in store mirrors, or I check in my bathroom mirror at home. I hope to find a miracle when I check, but I never do—there's always something wrong with my skin. I see a tiny blemish, and I start obsessing that my skin looks ugly and that other people will notice it. I think, 'I see a bump there! People are going to notice it! I have to get rid of it!' I get very self-conscious and I start. The worst time for me is the morning, when I'm getting ready for the day, and at night before I go to bed. Sometimes I get totally caught up in it, and I don't even think of anything else.

"When I can't pick, I get shaky and anxious—I *have* to do it! I'm drawn by the mirror—I *have* to look and see how I look, and then I *have* to start picking when I see anything wrong, even though I know no one else will probably see it. I can't resist. Then, afterward, I check to see how I look. Usually, I look so terrible that I isolate myself. . . . I pick hoping to make my skin look better, but I usually make it worse."

Pamela's picking caused notable lesions that required dermatologic treatment. "The treatment helped my skin heal, but it didn't help me stop the picking," she said. "One dermatologist told me to just stop doing it. If only it was that simple! I've tried to stop a hundred times, but I can't. I've tried cutting my fingernails, and then I wore artificial fingernails and bandaids to avoid doing more damage to my face. It really didn't work."

Pamela attributed her recent breakup with her boyfriend to her picking. "I could no longer hide my need for privacy to pick—I was much too embarrassed to tell him about what I was doing. And the picking took a lot of time—I ran out of excuses about where I was and why I couldn't do things with him."

Twenty-seven percent of the people I've seen pick their skin. This relatively high frequency isn't surprising, given that skin concerns are so common in BDD. People with BDD who pick are usually concerned about minimal acne, scars, or scabs, or such things as "large" pores, "bumps," "small black dots," "white spots," "ugly things," or other supposed imperfections. They pick to make their skin look better—to make it smoother, clearer, more attractive. Some try to remove dirt, pus, or "impurities" from under the skin. While many use their hands to pick, pinch, or squeeze, others use tweezers, needles, pins, razor blades, staple removers, or knives.

For some people, picking is a relatively inconsequential aspect of their BDD. But for many, the picking is in and of itself a serious problem; some consider it their major problem. One woman attributed her suicide attempt and psychiatric hospitalization to her belief that she had "ruined (her) face because of picking." Another woman I know of needed psychiatric hospitalization largely because of her picking and eventually committed suicide.

Skin picking has been described in the professional literature, particularly the dermatology literature, for many years, but it's been little researched. Traditionally, this behavior has been considered a type of "neurotic excoriation," a broad and antiquated term used for more than 100 years that doesn't specify the cause of the picking or indicate treatment approaches. Not all people who pick their skin have BDD. Skin picking can occur as a symptom of obsessive compulsive disorder or a number of other psychiatric disorders. In some cases, it's simply a habit rather than a symptom of a disorder.

To determine whether picking is a symptom of BDD, people should be asked why they pick. Do they pick to remove or minimize supposed defects or imperfections in their appearance, such as pimples, bumps, acne, or scars? If so, and if the other criteria for BDD are met, the picking behavior can be considered a symptom of BDD and is often a clue to the diagnosis.

But often the picking is kept secret. Many people are very ashamed of this behavior and reluctant to reveal it to others. One adolescent who was referred to me because of his picking talked at length about other, more minor problems and didn't mention his picking at all. When I finally asked him about it, he acknowledged that it was his major problem but that he'd been too embarrassed to bring it up.

But some people talk about it quite openly. One young woman I saw not only talked about it with others—she even picked her friends' skin. "I can't stand to see anyone with things on their face," she explained. "I have to make their face smooth! When I see them, I pick off the little imperfections. They're my friends, so they let me do it." Another woman told me, "I look for anything to pick. I want to pick my friends' skin because I pick my own and there's nothing left. I especially like to peel other peoples' backs when they're sunburned." She also liked to peel paint off walls, paper off jars, and dried glue off her hands.

People with BDD who pick are similar in many ways to those with BDD who don't pick. But there are some interesting differences. Although skin concerns are common in both groups, those who pick are more likely than those who don't to be concerned with their skin (close to 100% versus about 50%). They are also more likely to excessively groom and camouflage, perhaps because they sometimes do create actual skin defects that they feel they need to cover. People with BDD who pick their skin are also more likely than those who don't pick to have actual skin defects, as opposed to none. Sometimes the minimal defects lead to the picking, and sometimes they result from the picking. Often the defects both lead to and result from the picking, a vicious cycle in which the presence of a minimal defect leads to picking behavior, which then creates more defects and more picking. Sometimes, skin defects are clearly present and noticeable as a result of picking.

Those who pick their skin are also more likely to be treated by a dermatologist: approximately two-thirds versus fewer than one-third. Although such treatment is sometimes needed to treat the skin damage that can be caused by picking, it usually doesn't decrease BDD symptoms (the skin-related preoccupations and associated picking). As I'll discuss further in Chapter 13, picking behavior often diminishes with serotonin-reuptake inhibitors.

Questioning: "Do I Look Okay?"

Many people with BDD never breathe a word to others about their appearance concerns—largely because they'd be much too embarrassed to mention them. As a college student said about her face, "People must notice it's long, but I haven't asked. I'd be *much* too embarrassed! And if people said they didn't notice it, I wouldn't believe them anyway. I'd think they were just trying to be nice."

But about 40% of people with BDD question others about how they look. Often, this consists of requests for reassurance: "Do I look okay?" "Is the problem noticeable?" The purpose is to allay anxiety and be reassured that the supposed defect isn't as bad or as noticeable as feared.

Some BDD sufferers instead try to convince others of the reality or ugliness of the defect. A question isn't asked; rather, a statement is made. "Can't you see this on my face?" "Can't you see I'm ugly?" A third variation on the theme is repeated requests for help in improving the defect—for example, questions about how to straighten "excessively curly" hair, or repeated requests for cosmetic surgery.

Kevin, who was preoccupied with his "large" lips, "small" legs, and "sparse" body hair, asked his mother 5 to 10 times a day whether he looked okay. "I need to know I look decent, so I ask my mother, 'How do you think I look?' I call my friends and ask them too, and I have huge phone bills because of it. They always say I look fine. Sometimes I feel better, and sometimes I don't. When I'm feeling really bad, I think they're just trying to be nice."

A 44-year-old homemaker who worried about a small scar on her face realized her worries were irrational, but questioned others because it was comforting. "I want the reassurance," she told me. "It's a reality check." She repeatedly asked her husband, "Do you see it? How bad is it?" She also sought reassurance at cosmetic counters to "get an objective view." As she explained, "My husband loves me, so he might have a biased view of how bad it is."

A young man who feared he was losing his hair and that his body build was too small repeatedly asked his father, "Dad, do you think I'm losing my hair? Do I look big enough?" He was also concerned that his penis was too small, and he frequently asked his father whether the chart of penis sizes he'd gotten from a book was accurate.

Many people confine their questioning to family members or close friends. But others ask strangers or doctors. One woman who had been in therapy for several years spent most of her therapy sessions asking her therapist if her nose looked all right. "It's just about all she talked about," her therapist told me. "I'd try to steer her away from the subject, but it was useless. She was so obsessed—and so upset—that she couldn't stop talking about it. No matter what I said, she couldn't be reassured that she looked fine. She thought I was just being nice."

Sometimes people with BDD don't directly question others because they're afraid they'll be considered vain. Or they worry that others will think the question strange, especially if that's what they've been told in the past. Instead of directly asking, they bring up the topic in a more indirect way. A man who was concerned with his body build explained, "I wanted to ask other people how I looked, but I didn't want them to know I cared so much about it. I thought it would seem like a sign of weakness that I was bothered by it. Instead, I hinted around the subject, talking about appearance or body size in a more general way, hoping to get them to say 'You look big.' "

A teacher directly asked her husband about her "sagging" eyes, saying "Do you see it? How bad is it?" "But when I'm around friends or at social events, I can't directly ask," she said. "It would be too embarrassing. So I switch into philosophizing. I talk about things like how society overvalues appearance, and all the cosmetic surgery that's done. I'm somehow hoping I'll be told I look okay."

Another woman had the urge to question others how her nose looked but didn't. "I don't want to directly ask because they'll probably think the question is strange. I think I'm distorting how bad it looks, and I don't want people to know I care so much about it. Instead I ask them if they think I look like other people, like certain actresses. I'm hoping they'll say I look like the ones with good noses."

Sometimes, the intent is to get others to confirm that the defect is bad. One woman tried to get her husband to comment positively on other women's breasts, which was a way of affirming that hers were unattractive. "The point was to get him to agree with me because I'm right." Another woman dragged her three children to the mirror each day, pointing to invisible marks on her face and insisting that they agree that they saw them and how awful they looked.

Some people use photos to convince others of how much they've changed and how bad they now look. One of the first people with BDD whom I met handed me a several-year-old photo within a few minutes of my meeting her. "Can't you see how much I've changed?" she asked. She implored me to agree with her, pointing out how much hair had fallen out, how much fuller her cheeks used to be, and how different her eyes were—how lifeless and dull they'd become. She described at length how the photograph clearly demonstrated these changes, although I couldn't see them. A young man showed me a year-old photo of himself, pleading with me. "Can't you see how I've changed? Physically, I've changed *drastically* in the past few years. My whole face is different! Can't you see that?!" He seemed desperate for me to agree with him. At the same time, I sensed he feared I might.

Some patients have tried to convince me that their view of the defect is accurate by holding their face at different angles or changing the lighting in the room. "Can't you see they're flat?" a young woman asked me about her cheekbones, turning her head and holding it at different angles.

Other variations of questioning behavior are asking others how to fix the problem—the best way to curl hair or how to pay for liposuction—or a discussion of the defect and the problems it's caused. Virtually all one man talked about was his hair—his belief that it was thinning, how his life would be different if it weren't, and how to fix it. These discussions dominated his conversations with his girlfriend.

Questioning often causes problems. It can take up a lot of time and be very difficult for family members and friends. Whereas mirror checking, grooming, and picking can be done in private, questioning can't be done without involving someone else. If the questioning is limited to once or twice a day, it's generally tolerable. But if it's more frequent, it can dominate relationships.

I've been told by many people with BDD that their spouse, girlfriend, or boyfriend left them because they spent so much time talking about, or asking about, their appearance. Other aspects of the disorder—such as avoidance of social situations—often contribute to relationship problems as well. But it's surprising how often the questioning is considered a major part of the problem.

Peter, a 40-year-old unemployed carpenter who disliked his ears, jaw, and eyes, discussed his appearance and questioned his wife so often that she left him. "All I did was complain about how I looked and talk about how I wanted plastic surgery," he said. "I didn't accept her reassurances. She considered it mental abuse. She ended up hating me because of my obsession and because I talked about my looks all the time. Once I drove her so crazy talking to her about it that she pulled a knife on me. She threatened me, 'If you think you need surgery, now you'll really need it!' "

A parent told me something that's been echoed by other family members: "The most frustrating part of it is that no matter what I say, it doesn't really help." Indeed, responding to requests for reassurance is a no-win situation. Saying the person looks fine doesn't help, but neither does telling them that something is wrong. If you say they look fine, they usually don't believe you. They think you're just trying to be nice or that you didn't get a good enough look at the problem. A handsome young man told me that he could "just tell" that his parents think he's ugly, even though they tell him he's handsome, because it's "their moral obligation." Another told me that "reassurance doesn't really help, because why did everyone laugh at me at camp and in the locker room?" And a very attractive woman said, "When people say I look fine and I get complimented, they overdo it, so I must be really ugly."

If the person with BDD does believe you, the relief is usually only temporary. The doubts soon return. Maybe the reassurance giver didn't get a good enough look. Maybe they're just trying to be nice because they're your friend. And the questioning starts again. As Julie said, "When my surgeon reassured me, I felt a little better, but only for a few minutes. It never lasted very long." And she'd go back to ask again. A young woman told me, "When people say I'm pretty, I like it. I need the feedback. But I feel good for only a few minutes. I see how I look, and I feel terrible. I know what I see." In this case, in which anxiety decreases temporarily, reassuring words may actually unwittingly increase the questioning behavior because the temporary decrease in anxiety reinforces and fuels more questioning. The BDD sufferer asks once again, looking for relief, even if only temporary.

Responding by agreeing with the questioner and saying that the defect is there and looks bad is usually even worse. This response is often given in desperation because reassurance hasn't worked. On the one hand, BDD sufferers may welcome the agreement because someone is finally telling them they're right; at the same time, their worst fear has been confirmed.

Another response that doesn't work is something like the following: "Well, now that you point it out I can see it, but it's really not that bad. Before you showed it to me I didn't even notice it." The person with BDD usually hears it differently. The "really not that bad" and "didn't even notice it" parts go unheard or are considered untrue. Responses such as these have the potential to plunge the BDD sufferer into a serious depression and can fuel even more desperate attempts to obtain surgical or other treatment. To summarize, the bind is this: no matter how you respond, it usually doesn't help.

As I'll discuss further in Chapter 15, the best approach is not to comment on the defect. I have my patients and their loved ones agree together that, overall, responding isn't helpful. When others don't respond by commenting on the defect, over time the questioning may diminish.

Comparing: "She Looks Better Than I Do!"

"I always look at other peoples' noses—mostly their pores—comparing myself to them to reassure myself," Bill said. "I see other people have pores and they're doing okay, so I should. But I can't reassure myself. I just get more down on myself." Another man compared himself with others and thought, "Why can't I have regular skin like that? Why can't I have normal skin?" "I compare to reassure myself by seeing someone else with the same problems," he said, "but I never see anyone else with the same problems."

Comparing is the most common BDD-related behavior of all. More than ninety percent of people with BDD do this. They frequently and silently compare their "ugly" body part with the same body part on others, thinking such things as "Do I look okay compared to her?" They seem to have built-in radar for the body part of concern, quickly focusing on it when they interact with others. As Mike described it, "I zero in on other peoples' ears and compare them to mine."

A woman I saw frequently compared herself to other women and also contrasted young people with old people to see if they had lines on their face. "I know every line and wrinkle on every person's face," she said. She usually felt that she looked worse than others, which triggered panic attacks. "I say to myself, 'I wish I could have that baby-smooth skin.' I think how lucky any older woman is who has no wrinkles." Another woman, who thought her breasts were too small, compared her breasts with those of every woman she saw. She said, "I panic when I see cleavage!"

As is true for reassurance seeking, BDD sufferers generally don't feel much better when they compare. In fact, they often feel worse. Aaron, who worried about his slightly receding hairline, told me, "I check out everyone's hair. And everyone looks better than me, even bald guys. At least other bald guys have a little hair left that looks good. Mine looks terrible—thin and stringy. I'm the one guy who can't lose his hair and keep any of his looks." He then added, "It's okay if other people are bald. They can look handsome, but I don't because I have a long face."

Aaron experienced the typical no-win situation. People with BDD generally think that other people look better than they do, which reinforces their feelings of defectiveness. A handsome young man told me, "I constantly stare at other people's noses and compare their's to mine—I'm an expert on noses. I think how bad I look and how good they look. I'm envious of good-looking people." "Do you ever see anyone who looks as bad as you think you do?" I asked him. "Occasionally I see people who look as bad as me, and I feel sorry for them," he replied. "I don't want people to feel sorry for me."

If people with BDD see someone who looks as bad as or worse than they think they do, they still don't feel much better about themselves. Somehow they interpret the situation in a negative way, thinking such things as "He doesn't have much hair, but he's laughing and seems to be enjoying himself. Why can't I?" Or "She looks as bad as I do, but she has a boyfriend. What's wrong with me?" A 40-year-old man said, "I stare at peoples' faces thinking 'He has freckles and he's talking to people. Why can't I do that?' " The situation is interpreted in terms of—and usually ends up reinforcing— the BDD sufferer's own perceived shortcomings.

"When I'm standing in line at the drug store or the grocery store, I talk to myself, trying to reassure myself that I don't look so bad and that I should stay in line instead of leaving," Jason said. "I look at other people and think they're uglier and worse off than me. But then my thinking takes a negative turn: I think things like 'It's true, he's really ugly, but he doesn't seem to care. He seems to be doing fine! What's wrong with me?' Or I check out all the successful people on TV—a lot of them aren't attractive, but they're smiling and seem happy, so I think maybe I can be happy too. But then I get down on myself because I'm not."

Comparing with people on TV or in magazines is relatively common. "The models have thicker hair than I do," Jordan told me. "As I look through magazines I think 'Why can't I look like that?' Then I feel even worse." "I have to buy *Cosmo* every month," a woman told me, "because I have to compare my body with the models'. I always feel worse when I do it, because they always look better than me, but I can't resist doing it. It's a monthly ritual; it's something compulsive that I have to do."

Comparing can take excessive time and make it difficult to focus and concentrate. It's hard to focus on a conversation, or instructions being given by your boss, if your attention is on the other person's physical attributes. One socially active woman couldn't really converse at social gatherings because she was so intent on analyzing other people's skin.

The comparing is done so surreptitiously that others don't realize how closely they're being scrutinized. I've never been aware that this behavior was occurring except in those rare instances when the person commented that I looked better than them. To my surprise, one person I saw early in my research told me that I had "a real cute nose." Never having received such a compliment before, I wondered what had motivated this remark. It was only after I'd seen more people with BDD that I realized how often comparing occurs, and that this woman believed that nearly *everyone's* nose looked better than hers.

Some people who compare assume that other important people in their life are also comparing them to others and finding them less attractive. This can wreak havoc in relationships. Linda compared her breasts with those of every woman she saw, and she assumed her husband was doing the same and was judging her as negatively as she judged herself. "It was a terrible problem in our relationship, because I'd think he was constantly looking at other women and thinking they were more attractive than me. I'd get insanely jealous and make all kinds of accusations. We even had to go into couples' therapy because it was such a problem. Now I realize that I was projecting my own behavior onto him. He wasn't comparing me with other women; I was!"

Doctor Shopping: The Sometimes Never-Ending Quest

I got a call one morning from a psychiatrist in Boston who needed some advice about a patient. "He's seeing all the ophthalmologists in Boston," he told me. "He thinks his eyes look cross-eyed, and he can't be reassured that they're not. He's seeing doctor after doctor. They all tell him he looks fine, but he won't stop doctor shopping. He wants to get his eyes fixed."

This story isn't that unusual. Many people with BDD seek nonpsychiatric treatment, often dermatologic or surgical. They see dermatologists for slight or nonexistent hair loss or skin problems, requesting various types of treatment. They see surgeons to have their lips thickened, jaws widened, ears pinned, or breasts enlarged. They see endocrinologists for supposedly excessive or insufficient body hair, dentists for braces, orthopedic surgeons for a supposedly crooked spine, podiatrists for "bent" toes, and urologists for penis enlargement. They may see doctor after doctor, trying to find one who will provide the desired treatment. Others visit nonprofessionals, seeking electrolysis, a hairpiece, or hair-growth tonics. There's no limit to the types of treatment requested.

"Seeing doctors is an obsession for me," Victoria told me. "I'm looking for something from them. I want to keep going until I find out the answer. I've seen all types—general practitioners, orthopedists, and podiatrists. I'm trying to find someone who can tell me why my feet are so misshapen. They all tell me that nothing's wrong with my feet. One doctor said my problem was that I had an obsession with body image. I agree that I have a body-image problem because I'm so obsessed, but I also need to find out what's wrong with my feet."

Doctors are sought for several reasons: to give a diagnosis for a BDD concern, to do testing to determine the cause of the perceived problem, to offer reassurance that it looks okay, or to give treatment. They may be asked to provide treatment after treatment, or to redo a procedure done by themselves or another physician that the patient wasn't satisfied with.

Jennifer had seen at least 15 different dermatologists. She visited each of them repeatedly, asking them over and over if her skin looked okay. "I saw some of them several times a week," she said. "I couldn't be reassured that my skin was fine. I wouldn't go away. I asked and asked them about my skin, and I begged and begged them for treatment. A lot of them refused to see me anymore."

Usually, reassurance is wanted from the doctor, but if he or she isn't available, the office staff may be asked instead. One person was certain all the staff in her surgeon's office thought she was "crazy." "I go there all the time to ask if I look okay. They look the other way when they see me coming. I know I'm driving them out of their minds."

Dwayne had seen 5 dentists, 4 dermatologists, and 16 plastic surgeons. He disliked "everything" about his appearance, which he described in the following way: "I must be an alien from another planet because I look so strange. I was totally obsessed with getting surgery. It's all I talked about. My girlfriend threatened to leave me if I got it. None of the doctors wanted to treat me. The dentists said braces wouldn't help me. One of the dermatologists said I should just wash my hair more. Fifteen surgeons refused to treat me because they said I looked fine. One of the surgeons said it was a good thing I didn't have much money, because I'd be mutilated if I did. I finally got a nose job from one surgeon, but it didn't make me look any better."

Dwayne was so desperate for more surgery that he was thinking of going to another country to get it, or threatening suicide if a surgeon didn't agree to do it. He was also considering getting into a car accident so he could destroy his face and have it completely reconstructed. "That way," he said, "insurance would pay for it."

Mac had been turned down for surgery many times because the surgeons said he looked fine. "But I kept going back to them, and going to new surgeons, trying to find one who would do it. I know when they saw me, they said, 'Oh no, it's him again!' " Finally, in desperation, Mac had tried to break his nose so a surgeon would agree to operate. As he explained, "That way, something would have to be done."

A Japanese psychiatrist has referred to people with BDD who obtain repeated surgery as "polysurgery addicts." This description fit a 52-year-old homemaker, who'd had 10 different surgical procedures. "I kept trying to make myself look okay," she told me. "I had surgery after surgery, but I was never really happy with the results. My solution was to get more! I was addicted to plastic surgery."

Dieting

While dieting is a common behavior, as well as a feature of eating disorders, it can also be a symptom of BDD. I first became aware of this when reading about BDD before I'd begun my own research. I found the case of a young man from Germany who thought his cheeks were too "rosy and round"; to make them thinner, he severely starved himself.

Since then, I've seen a number of people who've dieted for similar reasons. One young man severely starved himself in the hope that losing large amounts of weight would erase wrinkles on his face. Another dieted to make his face less wide.

Other people with BDD diet for more conventional reasons. They try to flatten their stomach or reduce the size of their thighs or calves. Some people avoid certain foods, such as salty foods, or take water pills to decrease preceived eye puffiness, stomach bloating, or facial swelling. Other people eat special diets, trying to make their skin clear. Men who think their body is too small eat special diets to become larger. One man who did this, however, didn't allow himself to become *too* large and muscular because he feared that in comparison to the rest of his body his penis would look too small.

Weight Lifting, Aerobics, and Other Forms of Exercise

Excessive exercise is another BDD-related behavior. Some people run or do aerobics to decrease cellulite or the perceived flabbiness of their thighs, or to make their arms or legs slimmer or larger. Others do sit-ups to flatten their stomach. Like other BDD behaviors, these behaviors are done excessively and carried to an extreme. As a 30-year-old woman said, "My whole day is planned around exercise."

Exercise often doesn't have the desired effect, and some people think it makes them look even worse. One woman did what she called "extreme exercises" to decrease supposed facial bloating. "But the exercise didn't have the desired effect," she said. "In fact, it made my legs look bigger and worse. I became obsessed with my legs while I was waiting for them to decrease in size."

Many men with the reverse anorexia form of BDD, who think that their body build is too small or that they're not muscular enough, excessively lift weights. Some use anabolic steroids, synthetic derivatives of the male sex hormone testosterone that have muscle- and tissue-building effects. Steroids have many problematic side effects, including sleep disturbance, mood disturbance, acne, a rise in cholesterol and blood pressure, and impotence, as well as more severe side effects including severe depression, hallucinations, and liver disease. Anabolic steroids may be addictive, and their use is very risky.

Nick, a 32-year-old former car mechanic, had considered using steroids but wisely didn't. But he carried weight lifting to an extreme and severely damaged his body. He believed his body was too small, which he related to feelings that women didn't find him attractive or "enough of a man." To increase his size, he ate large amounts of food, weight-gain powders, and special vitamins. He also wore extra shirts and padded his clothes. "But the main thing I did," he said, "was lift weights. I lifted for hours a day. In retrospect, I realize I looked fine before I started to lift, and I'm sure everyone else thought I looked fine, too. I looked normal. I was 195 pounds; I wasn't fat, but I wasn't overdeveloped. Now I realize I probably looked even *better* that way. But at the time, I thought I looked too small. I was obsessed with looking bigger. I wanted to be stronger and more masculine. I wanted to be the biggest person on the planet!

"I became *obsessed* with working out. I spent a lot of the day lifting. I *had* to exercise before I left the house. I had to get the feeling and the look of bigness before I went out. I was trying to keep up with my friends who were using steroids. And I did get big—I got a lot of reinforcement for it. People would compliment me. Sometimes I even felt high while I was lifting. But I still felt I wasn't big enough. I had to get even bigger."

Lifting became the focus of Nick's life. "It's embarrassing to talk about this," he said. "I'm ashamed of how it interfered with my life—I stopped working because of it, I dropped out of life. . . . I couldn't concentrate on my work because all I was thinking about was lifting. I actually stopped working because I couldn't get out of the house without exercising. I didn't see my friends—I just stayed in my basement lifting. I lost a lot of them because of it. Once, I got so upset thinking I wasn't big enough that I stayed in my basement for a month, lifting and lifting. I was desperate to be bigger—I couldn't get out of the basement! I was so depressed, thinking I'd never be big enough, that I thought I'd rather be dead. I couldn't let anyone see my body."

Nick injured himself so severely that he had to stop playing sports, and he wasn't able to work. He was often in pain, and even had difficulty walking. When I saw him, he was in physical therapy. "I totally ruined my body by lifting," he said. "I tore my muscles apart. The irony is that now I can't work out at all—not even a normal amount."

Distraction Techniques:
"A Good Tan Distracts People from My Ugly Jaw"

Another behavior characteristic of BDD is accentuating or improving certain aspects of one's appearance as a distraction. The thinking goes like this: by making an acceptable or attractive body part look even better, other people's attention will be directed to the attractive body part, rather than the defective one. This behavior may take the form of excessive grooming, having surgery, or wearing unusually nice or expensive clothes.

You may recall that Jennifer used lots of makeup to accentuate what she considered her more attractive features and thereby distract people from her skin. Another woman, who thought her breasts looked fine, was nonetheless considering breast augmentation to distract people from her "ugly" nose.

A man I saw excessively groomed his hair, which he considered one of his primary assets, to make it even more attractive and thereby distract others from his "sunken" eyes. "People will be looking at my hair instead of my eyes," he said. "I get a lot of compliments on my hair. It helps me feel less self-conscious about my eyes." And Arnie was obsessed with getting a tan—not to darken his skin, but to distract women from what he considered his "jutting" jaw. "I look a little better when I'm tan," he explained. "I get positive feedback from people, so I spend a lot of time in tanning salons. I figure a good tan distracts people from my ugly jaw."

Measuring

Measuring is another form of reassurance seeking. Am I the right size? Do I look okay? People who think they're too short may repeatedly check their height. Maybe I'm not such a midget! Women who think their waist is too large or too small may repeatedly measure its size. Muscle girth, breast size, and penis size may be measured over and over again.

One man measured his penis up to 10 times a day, even though a urologist had told him it was normal. When it seemed somewhat larger than usual, he felt better. But, when the measurement confirmed his fear that it was small, he felt devastated. When I asked him why he kept measuring it when he was so often disappointed with the results, he responded. "I measure it because I *hope* it will be bigger this time." This response echoes that of people who check mirrors, pick their skin, and seek reassurance: this time it *might* be different.

Reading and Information Seeking

Some people with BDD compulsively seek, buy, and read any relevant information about their perceived defect. Men with genital concerns may frequent bookstores and libraries, perusing every book and magazine they can find, searching for information about genital size. Is theirs really small? Or is it okay? This is yet another form of reassurance seeking and comparing. The important question that needs to be answered is "Am I okay?"

Some people with hair concerns read voraciously about hair growth. How quickly does it grow? Once it's lost, can it be regained? They search medical textbooks and seek information about agents purported to increase or speed hair growth. They hope to find information to fix the perceived problem.

Men and women with body size concerns may spend hours a day reading fashion magazines, weight-lifting magazines, and books on dieting or exercise. They compare themselves with the models, hoping to reassure themselves. Or they search for tips about how to look bigger or smaller, hoping to discover the diet or exercise regimen that will finally make them look the way they'd like.

Touching

Rosa frequently touched her hair to make sure it was puffed up. If it didn't feel right, she rushed to the mirror to fix it. Another woman constantly touched her face to "cool it off" so it didn't look so red. Zach frequently touched his lips, which he thought were too small, tense, and "never in the right position," trying to make them look more relaxed and natural. He also compulsively licked them hundreds—perhaps even thousands—of times a day. "I have to lick them to check them, and so they're not so dry and to make them look better. I try to resist, but I get more nervous and upset, and I can't talk to people unless I lick them. But when I do it I usually feel worse, because it looks so strange, and other people must think I'm really weird."

Frequent touching of the disliked body part is another form of body checking, which is done by a third of people with the disorder. Touching may also take the form of manipulating the body part to make it look better. A nose may be pushed up to look shorter or sideways to seem less crooked. Judy frequently touched her eye to make it more symmetrical with her other eye. She put so much pressure on it that she'd given herself a black eye.

Touching, like mirror checking and many other BDD behaviors, can actually fuel the obsession and is best avoided. One woman said, "Touching my face confirms that the defect is there and I feel worse, so I try not to do it." Sometimes it's a trigger for skin picking. Touching often increases emotional distress and may lead to further time-consuming and futile attempts to remove or improve the flaw.

Other Behaviors: Handwashing, Praying, and Doorknob Touching

There's no end to the behaviors that occur in BDD. Some of them don't clearly fit into any of the preceding categories. A woman I saw tensed and untensed her facial muscles to make them less "limp." Another person pushed on her eyeballs to improve their shape. One woman made paper cutouts of breasts, which she examined while obsessing about the size of her own. Another sunburned and peeled her nose to try to make it smaller.

Excessive handwashing, a classic symptom of obsessive compulsive disorder, can also occur in BDD. Hands are washed to avoid getting dirt on one's face, which might in turn cause acne. One woman tried to prevent acne by washing her face for hours a day, which sometimes damaged her skin. "The washing is a lot like the picking," she said. "I do them both to decrease my skin obsessions, but they actually create skin problems. A dermatologist told me to stop washing, but I couldn't. For about three years I was in a vicious cycle: I washed to get my face really clean to prevent acne and to get rid of the effects of picking, like the blood, and then I picked some more. Sometimes I stayed up all night doing this."

Several other behaviors typical of obsessive compulsive disorder also occur in BDD. These include excessive and ritualistic praying, and touching doorknobs. One woman, for example, repeatedly touched doorknobs to make her eyes brighter.

These cases illustrate the kind of magical thinking that can occur in BDD—that is, the belief that one's actions will cause or prevent a specific outcome in a way that defies commonly understood laws of cause and effect. They also illustrate the interesting overlap between BDD and obsessive compulsive disorder, which I'll discuss further in Chapter 12. And they're examples of some of the less common, varied, and creative behaviors that can occur in BDD.

These behaviors are unlimited. Claudia swallowed water a certain way so the skin around her mouth wouldn't drop and the lines wouldn't get worse. She also slept on her back so she didn't crinkle her skin and cause more wrinkles. Nicholas jutted his jaw out to compensate for his cheekbones, so they wouldn't look so prominent. To improve his acne, Tim got up in the middle of the night to put hot towels on his face.

To make his face look fuller, Frank slept without a pillow, ate lots of food, and drank more than 3 gallons of water a day. To change the shape of his face, Donald frequently crushed his jaw with his hands. Dennis, who worried about hair loss, searched his pillow each morning for hair, saved his hairs in a plastic bag, and developed complex math formulas to determine the rate of his hair loss. He paradoxically sometimes pulled out his hair, to see how easily it would come out. Somehow the evidence always confirmed that his fear was true.

·· *eight* ··

How BDD Affects Lives:
Social Avoidance, Problems at Work,
and Suicide

*"I've missed weddings, birthday parties, and funerals because of how
I look. I don't go outside, and I'm on medical leave from college
because of it. I'm an ugly duckling. I've been teased my whole life.
What's the point of living? I thought I was going to die after I
overdosed, and I was sorry that I didn't."*

Karen

Ian's Experience: "It's Ruined My Life"

"*I* look like a freak of nature," Ian told me. "I look like the Elephant Man. This is the cause of my problems. It's why I went to California. I was trying to look better."

Ian came to see me after his parents discovered that he'd had gone to California to get a tan. To obtain money for his trip, he had broken into houses across the country, stealing cash and credit cards. "I'm not a criminal," Ian said. "I've never done anything like this before. But I was hoping a good tan would distract people from my ugly face," he told me. "I look a little better with a tan, and I was desperate to get one.

"Maybe I was also sort of trying to get back at society, because people were making fun of how I looked," he added. Ian was also hoping to find a plastic surgeon who would agree to operate. "I was hoping to find a surgeon in California who would redo my whole face. The ones I saw here wouldn't do it because they said I looked fine and didn't need it. But I don't believe them. It's their moral obligation to say I look okay." When I asked how he would have gotten the money to pay for surgery, he replied, "I was thinking of robbing a bank."

Ian had been a good student, athlete, and musician in high school and had never gotten into trouble of any sort. He started having difficulties when he went to college. That was when his appearance concerns began. He went into the men's room one day after class during his freshman year and felt incredibly ugly. "I feel like my whole face has changed." he said. "I don't really want to say what it is . . . but the skin under my eyes has gotten darker. My face is too wide. My nose looks ridiculous. I have this tape that goes through my head that says 'I hate how I look.' I look in the mirror and it's not me. . . . I feel repulsed by what I see," he said angrily, covering his face with his hands. "It's made my life fall apart. I'm a devastated person because of it. It's ruined my life."

Because he thought he looked so ugly and felt so anxious in class, Ian stopped going to classes and spent most of his time alone in his room. "In high school I was considered good looking and was accepted," he said. "But in college, I started to look bad, and everyone there was Mr. GQ. I don't have to look great—I just want to look normal.

"All I thought about was my face. I didn't go to the dining hall to eat, and I didn't even know if I had classes. I thought about suicide every night," he said. As a result, Ian started failing in school. His professors and a dean met with him and encouraged him to go to class, but he couldn't. "They asked me what was wrong, but I couldn't tell them. I wanted to go to class, but I couldn't. My heart was willing, but my mind wouldn't cooperate.

"All of this happened because of the change in my looks. Why should I go to school or have a job and be productive when people will laugh and make fun of me? I might as well sit in my room." Ian also stopped socializing. He'd gone out on a date once in the past year and thought the woman had dated him because she'd felt sorry for him. "I don't go out with girls because I know they'll reject me. So I reject them before they have a chance. I've isolated myself from everyone."

Ian's despair got so severe that he attempted suicide after looking in the

mirror and thinking he couldn't go on living any longer. He was hospitalized and then moved back in with his parents.

Carl's Experience: "I Pull Myself Together"

While people with more severe BDD may, like Ian, be unable to function
because of their symptoms, others, like Carl, function well despite their
emotional pain. Carl was an intelligent man in his late thirties with a good
sense of humor. He worked as a partner in a law firm, where he'd been
very successful over the years. "I've been a fairly happy person, and I had a
good life," he told me. "But a year ago that all changed dramatically.

"I was looking in the mirror one morning, and out of the clear blue sky
I noticed unusual thinning of my hair, and I panicked. I feared I was starting to go bald. I looked hideous. I panicked because I thought that within
a year or two the whole front would be lost."

Carl started reading about hair loss in dermatology textbooks and seeing
dermatologists. "I even talked one of them into giving me minoxidil to
make my hair grow, which didn't do me any good. The other dermatologists I saw didn't understand why I was using it. I think about my hair 24
hours a day—it's on my mind all the time. It's like a feeling of hunger that's
always there. When I comb my hair or look in the mirror, my focus on it
becomes intense, and sometimes I have panic attacks."

In reality, Carl had a full head of thick, curly blond hair. He realized his
view was distorted. "I realize I look worse to myself than I do to other
people," he laughed. "I know I'm distorting how I'll look if I lose more
hair. I'll look worse to myself than to others. I'm distorting my perception,
but I also believe it. I can't help worrying about it. I'm very tuned in to
other people's hair and to changes in my own hair.

"I never really liked how I looked when I was younger. I always thought
I was the ugly one in my family," he told me. "Sometimes other kids called
me 'curly head.' But I gradually got to like my looks, especially my hair.
Now I feel I've lost the best part of my appearance." As a result of his
concern, Carl felt depressed, and it was hard for him to concentrate at
work. "It's affected every aspect of my life," he said. "I don't have enthusi-
asm for things, and I'm depressed. It's totally due to my hair."

Nonetheless, Carl managed to function well. "I do my best to pull myself
together for work," he said. "In the morning I purposely comb my hair
without my contacts in so I can't see myself. I try not to look at my hair

in my rearview mirror while I'm driving to work." The distraction of work actually helped him think a little less about his hair. He had to put in some extra hours at the law firm to make up for decreased efficiency, but he performed his job adequately. "But," he said, "I'm afraid that if I continue to lose my hair, I'll be too embarrassed to be around clients.

"Socially, it's caused me some problems," he added. "It affects my relationships because I'm so wrapped up in my hair. It's hard for me to empathize with other people's problems. I feel unappealing because I assume people are looking at me the way I do, which I realize they're not. I feel very self-conscious around women, but I force myself to go out. Even though I look terrible, I'm still asking women out on dates. I worry, though, that this will be an issue if I get into a serious relationship."

Although Ian and Carl had the same disorder, the consequences were quite different. Some people, like Ian, can barely function, whereas others, like Carl, function well. The consequences for most people are somewhere between these extremes. Most feel that their social life isn't as good as they'd like, and they may find it harder to do their job, schoolwork, or household duties. But they may compensate reasonably well, doing well enough that others can't tell that anything is wrong. When functioning is severely impaired, others may know that something is wrong but may not realize that BDD is the cause.

Many people with BDD withdraw from the world to at least some extent. Depression and anxiety are common. Accidents can occur. Occasionally, people do surgery on themselves, with disastrous results. Some people contemplate—and attempt—suicide. Some succeed.

Social Consequences: "I Stay Alone"

"There are traffic lights longer than my social life," Jake said wearily when he met with me. "This problem is ruining my life. It's like fighting demons."

Jake was preoccupied with his arms and legs, which he thought were too skinny, and his "pale" skin. "I have no sex life or love life. I'm almost completely socially avoidant. I hardly ever go out. If I do go to a night club, I feel suicidal. . . . I'm still in shock that I look so horrible after all these years. It amazes me that no one faints when I get on the subway!"

Jake had been married to someone he'd never liked, whom he later divorced. "I married someone I felt no desire for. She was an awful person, but she was the only one who would accept me. She was probably the worst woman in the whole world, but I didn't think anyone else would accept me because of how I look. I felt lucky to have anyone."

Samantha avoided swimming or any activities requiring shorts. She, too, was concerned with pale skin and with freckles on her arms, legs, chest, and back. "The color of my skin is dead looking," she said. "It causes problems in my social life. I miss parties sometimes, and if I go I can't focus on conversations because I'm thinking about my freckles and pale skin. I'm constantly scrutinizing other people's skin. I'm noticing what a nice color it is, or that they don't have any freckles. The only time I really tune into the conversation is when I hear anything about freckles or skin. Then my ears perk up.

"This problem also interferes with my sex life. My husband told me to make sure I told you. I feel very self-conscious, and I don't want him to see my body. I can't relax and enjoy anything. My husband can't understand me. He tries but he can't, and he gets angry about it."

Interference with relationships and social activities is the most common effect of BDD. Ninety-eight percent of the people I've interviewed have reported that at some point their symptoms negatively affected these things. Reluctance to go to parties, dances, clubs, weddings, class reunions, or other types of social activities is common. People with the disorder feel embarrassed to be seen, which leads to anxiety and self-consciousness in social situations, and they may appear quiet, preoccupied, and withdrawn. They're usually very focused on how they look and how others are appraising their appearance. Are they noticing it? Do they think I look bad? Are they going to reject me because of it? Or they're comparing with others. Such obsessive thoughts and doubts make it difficult to focus on a conversation, relax, or enjoy activities. As one man said, "Ninety percent of your mind is on your obsession—you have only 10% left over to focus on what someone is saying."

BDD behaviors can also contribute to difficulties in social situations. "When I first meet someone, I don't want to be seen," Jake said. "I'm morbidly self-conscious. Then I check out their arms and legs. I think they're lucky, or if someone looks worse than me I feel better for a short while. But not too many people look worse than me. *This* is what I'm thinking about when I'm with other people. I'm not listening to the conversation. I'm totally focused on whether they're noticing my arms and legs and how theirs look compared to mine."

People with BDD feel especially uncomfortable and anxious in situations in which the perceived defects are likely to be exposed. Swimming, the beach, or events requiring shorts or short sleeves may be avoided. People with facial concerns feel anxious in most situations and interactions with others. Many people report that their symptoms typically worsen when they're around other people, contributing to their discomfort and avoidance of others. As one young man told me, "My BDD bothers me less when I'm alone, so I stay alone."

Relationships may be strained or avoided altogether, and intimacy is often forgone. Feelings of isolation are very much a part of BDD. Spouses, boyfriends, or girlfriends usually have trouble understanding the self-consciousness and avoidance and may become irritated or even angry as a result. "My husband is very frustrated that I don't want to go places with him where I'll have to dress up," Maria told me. She avoided situations, such as parties or dances, in which she couldn't wear bulky sweatpants that covered her thighs. "He doesn't understand why I prefer to stay at home instead of going out or spending time with friends. He's afraid that we're starting to lose our friends because of it."

BDD often stifles intimacy. "I've not only avoided dating because of it," Martha told me, "I finally got a boyfriend, after 20 years of not having one, and my worries about my feet and thighs are interfering with our relationship. It interferes with sex—I'm afraid he'll reject me because of my appearance. It's a burden and a hindrance. I'm afraid I'll never get married because of how I look." Martha never told her boyfriend about her appearance concerns, even after they got engaged. "I'm much too embarrassed," she told me. "I discuss everything else with him, but not this." As a result of her self-consciousness, she tried to hide her body whenever she was around him. She undressed only in the dark, and she never allowed him to see her feet. "I wear socks at all times," she said.

Sally was able to be intimate with her husband. "But I can't exactly relax," she said. "I worry about my hair the whole time—is it getting messed up? Does it look okay? I jump out of bed right after sex to check my hair. My husband thinks I'm crazy!"

Arnie, who thought his skin was too white, had never felt comfortable with his girlfriends. "It's interfered with my love life and with any intimacy whatsoever. I wouldn't take any clothes off. I wouldn't even roll up the sleeves on a long-sleeved shirt!" Randy attributed his impotence to his BDD. "I'm constantly judging the size of my penis negatively. I'm probably misperceiving, but I think it anyway. The intensity of the feeling is severe. No wonder I'm impotent."

Some people attribute the breakup of a relationship, even divorce, to their BDD symptoms. You may recall Julie, whose first husband left her because of her BDD. "All I talked about was my nose," she explained. "All I talked about was wanting surgery. I was so preoccupied I could hardly take care of my kids or the household. We had no relationship."

Jonathan's wife left him because of his BDD. "She said that was the reason, and I think it was," he said. "And I don't blame her for leaving. I was totally obsessed. I'd spend weekends in bed, and I wouldn't go out with her because of my pimples. I got so wrapped up in the problem that she really didn't have a husband anymore. She called BDD 'the selfish disease.' "

Many people with BDD aren't in a relationship at all. Seventy-five percent of the people I've seen (who had an average age of 32) have never been married. Thirteen percent were currently married, and 13% were divorced. Many want to be in a relationship but aren't for various reasons—self-consciousness about the defect, fear of rejection, shyness, or low self-esteem.

Warren had never pursued a relationship with a woman he liked. "All of my relationships have been with women who pursued me," he said. "I've never been in a relationship with someone I liked because of my appearance. I've felt undesirable. I've stayed single so I don't inflict myself on anyone else." "I'd never ask a girl out," Paul told me. "I'm too shy, and I have the BDD problem. It affects all of my relationships, especially with girls. I totally avoid girls. I don't even think of being intimate with them. It paralyzes me socially."

Avoiding dating and social activities as a way to avoid rejection creates a vicious cycle, whereby social isolation grows. A young man who refused to ask anyone out because of his hair was certain that no woman would ever find him attractive or want to date him, let alone marry him. When I pointed out that in fact he might not ever date if he didn't ask women out and continued to avoid social gatherings where he might meet them, he was surprised. He had assumed the reason he wasn't dating was because women found him so unappealing. He didn't realize the extent to which he himself was creating his dateless situation by avoiding women.

BDD can also interfere with friendships. Friends may find it hard to understand why social events are missed or attended only after much urging and encouragement. They may be puzzled and frustrated by lateness and last-minute cancellations. Many a person with BDD has ended up spending an evening alone instead of with friends as planned.

"I can barely be with friends because I think they're thinking how ugly I am," a 28-year-old woman told me. "I haven't seen my friends in the past 20 years," another said. "The main reason is I'm afraid they'll see how I've aged and that my hair is thinner. I become really upset whenever I see people I haven't seen in a while. I think they'll notice how I've changed. It's gotten to the point where I totally avoid people. I've cut myself off."

Family get-togethers, weddings, and funerals may be anticipated with great trepidation and fear—or missed altogether. "I've missed a ton of social events because of my appearance," Guy told me. "To tell you how bad it is, I missed my two best friends' weddings! I felt too ugly to go. I've missed Christmas get-togethers. If I went, I wouldn't enjoy myself because of how I look. I've hurt other people because of it, by not showing up. My BDD is too overwhelming to go. I've humiliated my parents by not showing up at relatives'. It really bothers me. My family and friends never knew the extent to which I worried about this."

It's sometimes difficult to determine how much the BDD symptoms themselves are responsible for social problems such as these. Is it simply the BDD? BDD is so often accompanied by social anxiety and low self-esteem that it can be difficult to tease them apart. But people with BDD generally say that their BDD symptoms are the cause of their social problems or significantly contribute to them. When BDD responds to psychiatric treatment, social functioning usually improves, sometimes rapidly and dramatically and sometimes more slowly, especially if symptoms are long-standing and severe.

Social anxiety and fear of social rejection have been shown by researchers to be more commonly experienced by less attractive people and by those with a negative body image. While people with BDD aren't in reality less attractive on average than other people, they *think* they are. These research findings are consistent with what people with BDD say about how they feel in social situations.

Teresa summed up what so many people with BDD feel: "I feel so ugly and unpresentable that I avoid parties and dates. I feel too anxious when I'm around other people. I think they're evaluating how ugly I am and that they're thinking I'm ugly and disgusting. I feel like a leper. I've stayed in a lot in the past few years. This problem has utterly and completely limited my social life."

Effects on School and Work: "I Haven't Met My Potential"

"If I'm supposed to be in a meeting at work but I have blemishes, I don't want to go," Dan said. Alicia didn't work at all because of her appearance. "I'm too ugly," she said. "I don't want people to see me and comment negatively."

Three-quarters of the people I've interviewed reported that at some point their BDD symptoms significantly interfered with work, school, or other important activities. Like social difficulties, problems in this area range from relatively mild to severe. Most people find that their appearance pre-occupations and urges to perform BDD-related behaviors, such as mirror checking and grooming, make it harder to focus and concentrate. Efficiency is sacrificed. Grades or job performance may drop. Extra time may be needed to make up for time wasted on BDD-related thoughts and behaviors.

People with BDD may be late for school or work, or not go at all. They may be reluctant to interview for jobs because they assume they'll be rejected on the basis of how they look. Those with more severe BDD may never even try to get a job or may quit school or work. They may become financially dependent on others. Twelve percent of the people I've seen were on disability at the time of their visit, largely because of their BDD symptoms; an additional 3% were on disability for other reasons.

Elizabeth, a fashion designer in her thirties, had been concerned about her "rat's nest" hair for ten years, ever since she'd gotten a bad haircut. She thought that the shape wasn't right and that it looked a mess. "It's the first thing I think of in the morning: I think 'My hair looks so awful!' I have nightmares of having it cut. It *really* bothers me. It makes me feel desperate." Although Elizabeth had been widely acclaimed for her innovative work, she hadn't been able to work for the past four years. "I've always been told how much promise I have, but I'm so upset by my hair that I can't work," she said. "I've passed up lots of opportunities, all because of my hair. I can't work because I'm so depressed and demoralized. I don't want people to see how I look. I worry I'll *never* be pleased with my appearance."

Erica, a fourth-grade teacher, couldn't perform her job as well as she'd like. "Sometimes when I'm teaching I feel okay. But then I look in a mirror, and I get down and want to leave school. I start obsessing about my skin—it's what I think about for the rest of the day. It's like a carousel in my mind. The thoughts go round and round and never stop. 'Does my skin look okay? Is it red? Do I look rashy?' It's hard to focus on the students and their needs. By the end of the day, it's affected my teaching. I'm obsessing, and I feel agitated and depressed."

Reggie dropped out of his band because of his appearance worries. "I was too self-conscious to perform," he said, "and I couldn't groom my beard the way I wanted on the road. The other guys in the band thought I was crazy."

People with BDD sometimes avoid taking a job they'd really like. Jobs that involve a lot of interaction with others, especially if the defect will be exposed, are especially avoided. I've seen many people who had a solitary job, such as a night watchman. As one person told me, "I can't do any kind of job where I have to be up close to people. I don't want people to see my facial abnormalities. I think they're noticing how ugly I am, and I worry that they'll think less of me because of it."

Tony took jobs he didn't really like because he didn't want other people to see him. He had always longed to be a high school teacher and football coach, but he hadn't pursued these jobs because of his chin. Instead, he'd worked at office jobs where he sat in a back room doing solitary work. "I've been underemployed because of my appearance problem," he said. "I haven't met my potential or gone after the kind of job I've really wanted. When opportunities for advancement came along I turned them down because they always involved being around people more. I didn't want a job where people would see me. I would have felt too ashamed." Another man said something similar: "I could have a much better job if it wasn't for this problem. I haven't been able to get promotions to positions that involve more social interaction. I've stuck to more technical jobs. I would have liked to advance."

Use of camouflage can also interfere with work. One young man, who wore a hat to cover his hair, described the situation as follows: "I'm a pretty smart guy, and I should have a much better job than I do. But I can't look for a decent job with this stupid hat. I can't dress up in a jacket and tie and wear this ridiculous thing on my head!" Another man, who thought that his nose was crooked and covered his face with long hair, didn't look for jobs because he couldn't remove the curtain of hair from his face.

Poor concentration, not wanting to be seen by others, and depression can contribute to dropping out of high school or college. Sean, a 24-year-old student, was still enrolled in college but hadn't attended classes for the past three years. Instead, he'd been living with his parents. "First I started missing classes and school activities because my hair bothered me so much I couldn't go. I was too embarrassed over it. It always looks strange. It never looks neat or natural. It sticks up and looks bizarre. If I spray it, it looks greased down. Barbers ruin it, so I cut it myself and it looks ridiculous. I spend hours in front of the mirror combing it and trying to fix it. Once I had a perm, and it looked better for a while, but when it grew out I looked like a terrorist.

"First I started missing some classes, and my grades started dropping because I couldn't concentrate. But I was determined to blast through everything, and I pushed myself, but that didn't work. I started missing so many classes that I took a year off. I didn't tell the school officials why because I was too embarrassed. I tried to go back, but I couldn't concentrate so I dropped out again."

Rebecca had also missed many classes. "I wouldn't go to school. I couldn't concentrate because I'd be worrying about my skin or going to the mirror all the time to pick it. And when people saw me, I thought they were judging how it looked. I finally left college because of it. I was very active in high school, and I had lots of friends. But I couldn't leave my room in college. After I left school I stayed in bed for two weeks. . . . I let myself down by leaving. I want to go back in January, but I won't be able to succeed unless I'm feeling better. This problem is an obstacle to getting on with my life."

Students with BDD may find gym class particularly painful because their defects are more exposed or because they have to change their clothes or shower in front of their peers. Rita, who was concerned about her thighs, told me, "I always flunked gym because I wouldn't wear shorts." Doug skipped gym class because he thought his wrists and body build were too small and didn't want them to be seen. Another man had avoided all sports and skipped gym class because of his shame over his genitals. He eventually dropped out of high school and never returned because he feared having a required physical exam and being seen naked.

BDD can also interfere with caring for children and managing a household. Ann Marie spent so much time worrying about her facial creases and shriveled eyelids that she was unable to care for her young son. "I've neglected him," she said. "My appearance problems are so time consuming and energy consuming. My ex-husband has to take care of him." A 30-year-old woman told me, "I feel so extremely ugly, I can't get through my day. I'm not mentally or emotionally there for my kids. I'm removing myself from my family. My kids know something's wrong with me, but I haven't told them what it is. I want to lead a normal life so badly."

Other Types of Avoidance: Shopping, Bright Lights, and Leisure Activities

"I restrict going places," Jerry said. He was a 45-year-old man who'd had BDD for 20 years. "When I go out, I feel worse and uglier. It's hard to go to the store. I have to boost myself to go. I'm afraid I won't fit in. I constantly worry that people are scrutinizing me and criticizing me. I get incredibly anxious and panicked standing in line because I look so awful, and I think everyone is noticing how ugly I am. Emotionally, I feel like someone's holding a gun to my head. I try to convince myself it's not a big deal, but sometimes I leave the line in a panic, and I go and look at cookware because it calms me down."

Avoidance is a very common aspect of BDD. Many types of situations and activities may be avoided because of self-consciousness, depression, anxiety, or fear—public transportation, clothes and food shopping, restaurants, and other types of everyday activities. Robert avoided all these. "I'm afraid if people see me they might say to themselves 'Oh, gee, look at that guy. Isn't he gross looking?' I think people laugh at me. I avoid public transportation because of it. I can't get on the subway without hyperventilating. I stay in my apartment more. And I postpone grocery shopping. I usually go at night, because people won't see me on the way there, and there won't be as many people in the store."

Some people get their mail, shop, and perform other necessary activities under cover of darkness. Clothing stores and shopping malls may be avoided because of the plethora of mirrors. "There are so many mirrors there—you can't avoid them. Everywhere I look I see myself and how gross I am," one woman told me. "Sometimes I suddenly leave stores when I see my reflection." She eventually bought her clothes only through catalogs. Others keep their distance from mirrors when trying on and buying clothes. One man stood about 20 feet from the mirror when trying on clothes. "Or, if I get up close, I have to look at the clothes with my head down so I can't see my face," he said. "Otherwise I'll freak out."

Harry rarely went to movies, and when he did he tried to avoid being seen. "I always sit in the back row so people can't sit behind me and laugh at the shape of my head," he told me. Curt walked behind people and sat in the back of the class so the slight hair thinning on the back of his head wouldn't be seen. He also always waited for an empty elevator. Jesse avoided dancing, which he loved, because he thought everyone would look at his supposedly bowed legs.

Many people, especially those concerned about facial defects, avoid bright lights, which could illuminate the defect. "At parties, I'm very uncomfortable hanging out in the kitchen with bright lights," a 26-year-old computer programmer told me. "I prefer a darker room." Others avoid restaurants with bright lighting, or find a dark booth in the back, so their defect is less visible. Some people quit their jobs, or never accept one in the first place, if they have to work under fluorescent lights. In BDD-treatment groups I ran, the group members tried to avoid sitting next to the window, because they feared their defects would be more visible in brighter light.

Swimming and the beach may be avoided because the defect will be more exposed—large hips or thighs, small breasts, small body build, thinning hair, skin defects, or cellulite. In addition, camouflage and painstaking grooming can easily be ruined by wind and water: makeup runs, bronzers streak, and hair styles are destroyed.

Abby didn't travel because of her skin. "I used to travel a lot, and I loved it. But I might go to a climate that makes it worse, and I don't want to be seen. My skin makes me phobic. I recently passed up a great trip with my family that I would have gone on if my skin looked okay. The only place I travel is to dermatologists. I go running to doctors about my face whenever I break out even a little. I think I've gone to every dermatologist in Chicago."

Some people avoid the things they love most. Greg avoided sports, even though he'd been an excellent athlete and had played on several varsity teams in high school and college. Although he was muscular and in excellent physical shape, he feared that people would see his "small and puny" body build, and stopped playing altogether. Loni didn't play on her high school field hockey team because it would mess up her hair. "I missed a very important thing," she told me. "I loved playing team sports—it was what I liked best of all in high school."

Being Housebound

Being housebound is the most extreme kind of avoidance. One-third of the people I've interviewed have been completely housebound for at least a week because of their BDD symptoms. They didn't leave to go to work or school, or even to perform simple errands. Many more stay in for briefer periods, and others remain in far longer.

"I've stayed home for weeks at a time because of my beard," Josh said. "I was in my own world. I worried people were talking about it. It's the root of my paranoia." Kelly stayed in her house for three months. "I stayed in because I didn't want anyone to see me and how bad my skin looked," she told me. "My parents took care of me. This happened after I destroyed my looks by picking at my face at any tiny blemish. I felt unpresentable. My face is ugly. My skin is ugly. I didn't want anyone to see my face."

"I hide from people," Max told me, "especially after I get a bad haircut. I don't want to do anything. I just want to hide. There've been weeks when I didn't leave my house at all. I didn't go into town or shop or go out to eat because I was insecure. I ate my roommates' food and ordered out. I didn't even answer the door when someone came to the house. I was afraid.

I was petrified of running into people. I'm afraid they'll think 'Here's this guy who looks awful. I don't want to have anything to do with him.' "

Low Self-Esteem, Depression, Anger, Anxiety, and Panic Attacks

Many negative emotions typically accompany BDD—low self-esteem, depression, and anxiety. Although it may be difficult to determine whether these feelings *result from* BDD, many BDD sufferers believe they do. Others view them as part and parcel of their worries about their appearance and find it difficult to say which causes which. Sometimes they seem to feed each other: low self-esteem, depression, and anxiety worsen BDD, and BDD worsens these feelings.

Low self-esteem is a particularly common aspect of BDD. Ben's experience is typical: "I can't overcome my self-consciousness about my appearance. I don't know how to deal with it. I have an inferiority complex. My low self-esteem and sense of shame because of my appearance are a fundamental part of my makeup."

Research on self-esteem suggests that an association between BDD and low self-esteem is to be expected. Studies have shown a relationship between perceived appearance and self-esteem across the life span—the worse someone thinks they look, the lower their self-esteem tends to be. Physical appearance is important to the development of healthy self-esteem. In fact, studies indicate that of the domains of competence that appear to contribute most to general self-esteem—how much one likes oneself as a person overall—physical appearance heads the list. Thus, people with BDD—who *think* that their appearance is defective in some way—may have particular difficulty developing healthy self-esteem. Furthermore, it's my impression that because many people with BDD perceive the world to be giving them negative feedback, their self-esteem is further decreased.

BDD can also lead to anger. Anger has many sources: frustration over having the problem, not being able to improve it or stop a further deterioration in appearance, lack of control, a belief that others are being rejecting or mocking the defect. "I get angry because it isn't fair that I'm the one with the small penis," a college student told me. "And I get very angry at the people who laughed at me in the locker room in high school about my penis size." Some people with BDD smash mirrors when feeling extremely angry about their reflection. Others have violent outbursts.

Depression and anxiety are other common aspects of BDD. Many people believe that the BDD causes their depression, and indeed, the BDD usually starts first. The depression can be persistent and severe and become an important problem in its own right. Many people perceive their anxiety, too, to result from BDD. "I get so anxious over my physical flaws that it wakes me up at night. I wake up thinking about them and feeling panicked," an interior decorator told me. Another person felt anxious because he feared his ugly face made other people anxious and uncomfortable. "I want other people to be happy, and I worry they're not because of how I look."

Anxiety associated with BDD may be psychological, consisting of worry and fear, or it may be physical, with symptoms such as headaches and stomachaches. Panic attacks, which can result from BDD, have elements of both extreme fear as well as heart palpitations, difficulty breathing, lightheadedness, and other physical symptoms. "The stress of BDD has caused me to have a lot of anxiety and even panic attacks," Henry told me. "It's also caused me many stress-related physical symptoms—burning in my stomach, high blood pressure, headaches for which I've had brain scans. I've seen a lot of doctors for these problems, but I couldn't ever tell them what the cause was."

"My worries about my mouth exhaust me," Geoffrey said. "Sometimes I'm afraid to get up in the morning because my mouth will consume all my energy and take my time. That's why I'm so tired all the time. It's totally draining. I've had BDD for 16 years, and I honestly don't know how my body has withstood the enormous stress that this obsession causes me."

Unnecessary Medical Evaluation and Treatment

Another consequence of BDD is seeking and receiving unnecessary medical and surgical evaluation and treatment of the appearance concerns. Many are refused such treatment because the defect is so minimal that the physician considers treatment unnecessary. Several men I've seen have even been turned down by hair clubs. But some people nonetheless persist in their search for a doctor who will give them what they want. Some receive treatment after treatment—even surgery after surgery—hoping that the next one will finally provide the relief they so desperately seek.

This behavior can take the place of living. Abby, who told me she'd seen just about every dermatologist in Chicago, described this behavior as "just about all I do. The doctors I saw said my skin wasn't so terrible. Some of them thought I was crazy. So off I'd go to find another one. It's how I spend my days—going to skin doctors."

While usually successful in people without BDD, these treatments appear to only rarely succeed in people with BDD. Some people with BDD are very unhappy with the outcome and blame themselves or the doctor for having made a serious mistake. In other cases, preoccupation and suffering diminish temporarily, only to return. Or the bodily preoccupation may shift to another area.

Rarely, people with BDD who are dissatisfied with medical or surgical treatment are violent toward the doctor who provided it. In my experience, most people with BDD aren't violent, but I do know of several reported cases of violence, even murder or attempted murder, toward a physician who provided nonpsychiatric treatment that the patient thought had ruined their appearance. Occasionally, people with BDD sue, even though the treatment outcome appears acceptable to others. Large amounts of money may be spent seeking and receiving such treatments, to no avail. In some cases, life savings are depleted.

Self-Surgery

Some people with BDD are so desperate to fix their perceived defect that they attempt surgery on themselves. One colleague told me of a patient with likely BDD who thought the fingers on his left hand were too long, so he cut them off. Another colleague recalled a patient who was so upset about his skin, and who picked at minimal facial blemishes so excessively, that he picked through his skin and severely damaged his facial artery, a large blood vessel. As a result, he lost large amounts of blood and needed emergency surgery.

Another person was so desperate to improve the appearance of his nose that he did his own surgery, cutting his nose open and attempting to re-place his own cartilage with chicken cartilage.

While self-surgery appears to be infrequent, it's a dramatic manifestation of the severe emotional pain and extreme desperation that some people with BDD feel. More commonly, people with BDD say that they hate their defect so much they'd *like* to do surgery on themselves—for example, cut their nose off—but they refrain from actually doing so.

Bodily Damage

Bodily damage can occur in other ways. Harsh chemicals used on the face or scalp irritate and burn the skin. Excessive face washing leaves skin bleeding and raw. "Stuck-out" ears are superglued. To get rid of acne or white skin, severe sunburns are endured. Excessive weight lifting causes back strain or more serious harm to muscles and joints.

Ellie always had a very dark tan in the hope that her skin would look better, even though she often burned and knew excessive sun exposure could cause cancer. "My dermatologist told me to stop doing it, but I *have* to get a tan. I don't care if I get cancer. At least I'll look good in my casket. That's how screwed up this whole thing is."

Other people damage their body in frustration. While such behavior occurs in fewer than 10% of people with BDD, it does happen. Tara had gotten so frustrated and depressed over the appearance of her breasts that she'd cut them with glass from a mirror she'd smashed. "I hated them," she said, "and I wanted to die."

A young man hit his stomach when he got very upset over the "shriveled" skin around his navel. "This problem has made my life really unbearable," he said. "I say to myself 1,000 times a day, 'I hate my guts and want to die.' When it gets really bad, I take my anger and frustration out on myself."

Alcohol and Drug Use

A more common way of attempting to cope with BDD is by using alcohol or drugs. Usually the intent is to decrease the preoccupation, dull the emotional pain, and lessen anxiety and self-consciousness in social situations. The percentage of people with BDD who've had a problem with alcohol or drugs is quite high: I've found that 41% have had an alcohol or drug problem at some time in their life, and 12% had such a problem at the time I saw them.

An alcohol or drug problem can't always be attributed to BDD. Determining whether BDD is the cause of such a problem is a complicated clinical judgment that often can't be made with certainty. Nonetheless, some people believe that their drug or alcohol problem is largely attributable to their BDD symptoms.

Adam was one of them. He'd had a serious problem with alcohol and drugs for many years, and had been in and out of more than 30 detoxifica-tion and rehabilitation programs. "You might not believe this," he said to me, "but my alcohol and drug abuse problems were *totally* and *completely* due to my appearance problem. A lot of counselors have told me that's just an excuse, but I think they're wrong. It was a crazy way I tried to block the pain of my obsessions, and it never worked. I tried to numb myself to my perception of my body, but it didn't change. It actually made the pain over my appearance worries worse."

Rick's story was similar. "I slept too much and did alcohol and drugs as an escape, to try to forget my scars," he said. "Sometimes drinking de-creased my concern temporarily. But sometimes the alcohol could make my symptoms worse, and it became a problem in its own right. After his BDD responded to fluvoxamine (Luvox), he stopped using alcohol and heroin.

Emily described her experience as follows. "The only thing that brought relief was drinking. . . . My symptoms were totally debilitating, so in-tensely painful, and they were making me more and more depressed. Even though I was suffering so much, and drinking too much, no one knew I was suffering from BDD because I managed to look as though I was doing okay. I pulled it together, but the agony inside was totally overwhelming. I couldn't talk about it with other people.

"I finally went to my doctor and told him about the situation because I was worried about my drinking. He told me when I stopped drinking I wouldn't be depressed. But that wasn't true for me. I drank because of body dysmorphic disorder. . . . I drank and slept to deal with it. What causes me the most pain now is the effects of my drinking on my son. I wasn't there for him. That's the part that hurts me the most."

Accidents and Other Dangers

BDD can cause accidents. Janet had several of them because of her symp-toms. "I'm a mirror-driven person," she said. "I check all the time. The worst part of it is I check in the rearview mirror while I'm driving. A few years ago I had a car accident because I was looking in the mirror instead of the road." Many others describe near misses. "I check the rearview mir-ror, trying to reassure myself," a salesman told me. "I almost hit a tree once, and I almost ran over someone."

Some people, trying to stop this behavior, turn the rearview mirror away from them, or remove it altogether, but are then unable to see what's behind them—another setup for an accident. Others check a pocket mirror while driving instead of looking at the road.

One woman repeatedly hurt her back while bending into pretzel-like positions to obtain a better look in the mirror. She wasn't satisfied with a standard view—she needed to get an even closer look at a small scar on the side of her neck.

BDD can also lead to other kinds of dangerous behaviors, including breaking the law. Ian's breaking into houses was an example of this. Todd shoplifted from drug stores. "I don't like to do it," he said, "but I *have* to get stuff for my skin, and I don't have any money." He stole soaps, creams, acne medications, and other items he thought would improve his skin. Over several months, he'd stolen nearly $1000 worth of items. "I'm afraid I'll get caught," Todd said, "and I feel guilty doing it. But I can't resist. My acne is destroying my life. I have to make my skin look better!"

Hospitalization

Medical and psychiatric hospitalization as a result of BDD are relatively common. Hospitalization occurs for a variety of reasons, including accidents, following a suicide attempt, or because of suicidal thinking after medical or surgical treatment has failed to fix the defect. About half of the people in my study have been psychiatrically hospitalized. Thirty-five percent attributed at least one psychiatric hospitalization primarily to their BDD symptoms.

I met Lawrence in the hospital after he'd tried to kill himself. He was agitated, anxious, and depressed. This is how he described the reason he'd been hospitalized. "When I started graduate school in physics, I was troubled by not having many friends and also by a sense of my dramatically receding hairline. My hair had been very slowly receding for some time, but in the past month it became very quick. A few weeks ago I examined my hair and noticed excessive hair loss and decreased density in the front. Even on a daily basis I could see the change. Lots of hair came out in the shower in my hand.

"I worried about how I would have to present myself with my new appearance to my old friends. I also worried about how I could meet new people with my hair the way it was. My self-esteem plummeted, and I felt like a social failure. I couldn't concentrate on my studies. I started to wonder if people were talking about me or laughing at me.

"In the past week I started to panic. I felt very anxious. I was worrying more and more about how I looked and what other people thought of me. I worried that it would get worse and that I'd become bald. I couldn't stop thinking about it, and I felt I was falling apart. I was crying, looking at myself in the mirror. I thought I was collapsing, eroding, and I tried to kill myself."

When his family came to visit him in the hospital, Lawrence hadn't been able to tell them why he was there. "I'm much too embarrassed to tell them about it," he said. "I'm afraid they won't take it seriously. I'm afraid people will think it's trivial, silly, or pitiful. I'm afraid they'll see me as vain. And if I bring it up, I'm afraid they'll notice how bad my hair is."

Even when BDD symptoms are so severe as to lead to hospitalization, many people never discuss them. They keep them a secret not only from family but also from hospital staff. BDD symptoms are often never even mentioned in the medical record, even for patients whose main problem is BDD.

The Cost of BDD

The cost of BDD isn't known, but is certainly high. The economic cost includes medical costs for bodily harm and accidents, the cost of ineffective medical and surgical evaluation and treatment, and the cost of medical and psychiatric hospitalization. It also includes the costs of incomplete education, decreased productivity, lateness, and days lost from work, and the cost of disability payments.

Some people with BDD have significant financial problems because of these costs or because they spend so much money on wigs, clothes, and makeup. One woman was more than $10,000 in debt because she'd spent so much money on clothing and wigs.

Richard's experience illustrates how costly BDD can be. Richard had dropped out of school because he constantly went to the bathroom to check the mirror and couldn't concentrate on his studies. He tried several jobs, but quit each of them because of his symptoms. He then moved in with his family and went on disability.

Richard had made three suicide attempts, usually after looking in the mirror and feeling devastated by what he saw. Each attempt was followed by hospitalization. One overdose resulted in a long stay in an intensive care unit. In the six months before I saw him, he'd been hospitalized four times.

Richard had also had three operations on his lips, which were costly and ineffective. Two were followed by psychiatric hospitalization. "I had to be hospitalized because after the surgery my lips were black and blue and swollen," he said. "They looked deformed. I went wild, screaming and smashing things. I thought they were worse than ever, and I thought I'd done irreparable damage to myself."

Although Richard had suffered from BDD for only several years, the cost of his illness had been prohibitive—well over $100,000. But the greater cost of BDD is the human cost—the severe suffering and pain. Years lost to the illness can't ever be replaced. One man told me, "It's crazy because I've wasted so much of my life. I grieve for all the years this disorder took from me."

Suicide: The Most Devastating Consequence

The greatest cost of all is suicide—an irreversible act that reflects intolerable suffering and loss of hope. Luke attempted suicide after an acne medication failed to improve his skin. "It was my last hope," he said. "I got so upset that it didn't work that I had a nervous breakdown. I was constantly grieving over how I looked. I had to be hospitalized because I tried to kill myself."

Suicidal thinking is relatively common in BDD. Eighty-six percent of the people I've seen have had thoughts that life wasn't worth living or that they'd be better off dead. Nearly all of them attributed such thoughts primarily to their BDD symptoms. As one woman told me, "My appearance is the source of all the pain in my life. I feel hopeless about it. It's a feeling that I'll never belong anywhere or be happy. I feel unacceptable because of it, and sometimes I feel that life isn't worth living."

Juanita felt suicidal because of the hair she perceived on her face, arms, and legs. "It's *severely* upsetting. I fear I won't be able to lead a normal life—date, have sex, and do the other things that people do," she told me. "I feel like a freak, a bad person because I have a defect in my appearance. I fear that no one will ever love me—that I'll be an outcast. So what's the point of going on? I've seriously considered buying a gun to kill myself."

About a quarter of the BDD patients I've seen have actually made a suicide attempt, and the majority have attributed at least one attempt primarily or entirely to their BDD. Suicide attempts are sometimes triggered by looking in the mirror. "I once looked in the mirror," Gordon told me, "and I said 'That's it.' I looked so much worse than I ever had that I tried to kill myself."

In a study I did with Dr. Mark Zimmerman and Jill Mattia of Brown University School of Medicine, we found that of 60 outpatients with probable BDD, 57% had passive thoughts of death, 53% wished to be dead, 48% had thoughts of suicide, and 27% had a suicide plan. These percentages were all significantly higher than those for 430 patients without BDD from the same psychiatric outpatient setting.

While these numbers might seem high, they make sense. BDD symptoms usually involve a deep sense of shame, low self-esteem, and feelings of being unworthy, unacceptable, and unlovable. The symptoms often lead to isolation from others and the feeling that others don't understand. In addition, depression is common in BDD. Such feelings can culminate in the belief that life isn't worth living.

These high percentages speak to the unbearable pain and torment that many people with BDD experience. As Luke explained, "I hate myself and how I look. I think to myself that I can't live the rest of my life like this. I think it's possible that I may kill myself someday."

Although auditory hallucinations are rare in BDD, Karen had overdosed because she'd heard voices telling her to kill herself because she was so ugly. "These two voices inside me were talking to each other, saying, 'Look at all the pimples she has on her face. Look at her fat thighs. Don't you think she should kill herself? You're fat and ugly, and you should kill yourself.' It's all they talked about. They were laughing at me because of how I looked."

The rate of suicide in BDD isn't yet known, but some people with BDD do kill themselves. The psychiatric literature contains descriptions of people with BDD who comitted suicide because they were so distraught and despairing over their perceived ugliness. And I know of several people with the disorder who committed suicide. One was a beautiful young woman with skin concerns who picked her skin. Another was a young man who had been obsessed with his "misshapen" forehead.

Bill told me that there were some people with BDD I'd never be able to interview. When I asked why, he answered, "Because they're dead—they've killed themselves." He should know, because he had attempted suicide 15 times because of the pores on his nose. He could no longer cope with the torment of his perceived ugliness. Another man said something nearly identical: "I think many people have committed suicide because of BDD. I know, because it's so painful. I made two suicide attempts at the time my symptoms were severe. I felt very isolated, and I lost hope."

I have no doubt that in many cases successful psychiatric treatment prevents suicide. Juanita had a good response to fluoxetine (Prozac). She called me years later to say that she'd gotten married and had a good job. She was no longer suicidal over how she looked. Luke also had an excellent response to the same drug plus cognitive-behavioral therapy. After treatment, he was no longer tormented by his appearance. He went on to a successful career in television, and gave up thoughts of suicide. "It's the furthest thing from my mind now," he told me. "I have a great life. Thank God I got treatment. I owe my life to it."

·· *nine* ··

Gender and BDD Across
the Life Span

"I still think about how awful my back looks after all these years. I keep to myself because I don't want to draw attention to it. It's one of the things that's made me depressed."

Margaret, age 70

BDD and Gender

Is BDD more common in women or men? Is it different in the two sexes? We don't yet have definite answers to these questions, but what we do know is intriguing.

It's often assumed that BDD is more common in women. Aren't women more focused on their looks than men are? And doesn't society place a particularly high premium on attractiveness in women? Indeed, research findings from the general population indicate that more women than men are unhappy with their appearance.

One researcher found that his series of patients—who appeared to have relatively mild BDD—contained more women than men. Other researchers, however, have found that BDD is as common in men as in women. Of the several hundred people I've seen, 51% have been men. In a study done in France of more than 600 patients with obsessive compulsive disorder and related syndromes (e.g., trichotillomania), men and women were nearly equally represented among the 151 patients with BDD. A number of years ago, I reviewed all the published cases of BDD that I could find in the English-language literature as well as a large number published in other languages. In these published cases, the sex ratio was also approximately equal: 1.25 female to 1.0 male. Some researchers, however, have found that BDD may affect even more men than women.*

These data aren't adequate to give us as valid an estimate of BDD's sex ratio as we'd like. What's needed to determine it with greater certainty are large-scale epidemiologic surveys, in which the prevalence and sex ratio of BDD are determined in thousands of people. The studies I just noted were small and could suffer from various biases. In the meantime, until such surveys are done, we can be certain that BDD affects both women and men.

If future research confirms that BDD is as common in men as in women, this would suggest that BDD differs from normal appearance concerns in some fundamental way. While it's likely that BDD is on a continuum with normal concerns, it's also likely that there's something different about BDD, with biological factors probably playing a role. These factors may be similar to those of obsessive compulsive disorder, which also affects an approximately equal number of men and women. Sex ratio provides a clue that this is the case. If BDD were simply an extreme form of normal appearance concerns, it would probably be more common in women.

But it may be that the sex ratio differs according to the severity of BDD. Future studies may demonstrate that more women than men have mild BDD, because mild BDD may be closely related to normal appearance concerns, whereas as many men as women have more severe BDD.

What about gender differences? I and Dr. Susan Diaz of Brown University School of Medicine found more similarities than differences between men and women with BDD. In our study, men and women were similar in terms of most demographic features (e.g., age and marital status) and in terms of most clinical features, such as associated behaviors, severity of symptoms, and degree of impairment.

We also found that men and women are largely similar in terms of coex-

---

* Dr. Eric Hollander, of Mount Sinai School of Medicine, found that 62% of 50 patients with BDD were men, and a researcher in Japan who studied 274 patients with BDD seeking cosmetic surgery similarly found that 62% were men. Dr. Giulio Perugi and his colleagues in Italy found that 59% of 58 patients with BDD were men.

isting psychiatric disorders, including anorexia nervosa and depression. This finding is interesting because, in the general population, depression affects more women than men. Why women with BDD don't appear to have a higher rate of depression than men with BDD is puzzling. Although this finding requires confirmation, there are several possible explanations. One is that the same underlying biological and psychological mechanisms that cause BDD also contribute to the depression that accompanies BDD; because in our study BDD affected as many men as women, depression would be expected to as well. Another possible explanation is that, in at least some cases, the depression may be "secondary" to the BDD—that is, resulting from the distress and impairment associated with BDD. If this theory is correct, then it isn't surprising that men and women are equally likely to be depressed because they appear to experience similar degrees of distress and impairment as a result of their BDD symptoms.

The lack of difference between men and women in terms of the eating disorder anorexia nervosa is also interesting because anorexia generally affects far more women than men. An equal rate of anorexia in men and women has also been found in people with obsessive compulsive disorder, and it's one of the many things BDD and obsessive compulsive disorder appear to have in common (which I will discuss further in Chapter 12).

But there are some interesting differences between men and women with BDD. Women are more likely to have the eating disorder bulimia nervosa (see Appendix A for a description), whereas men are more likely to have a problem with alcohol or drugs. While the sexes are similar in terms of the number and areas of bodily concern, men are more likely to think that their body build is too small. I found a tendency for women to think they're too large and to be more concerned with weight, although this difference wasn't statistically significant. Another difference is that while men and women are equally likely to have hair concerns, men are more prone to fear that they're losing their hair. In addition, most of the people I've seen who worried about excessive body hair were women, whereas all of those with genital concerns were men.

These findings are interesting because they echo normal appearance concerns. Research findings indicate that women generally think their bodies are too large, whereas men tend to worry that theirs are too small. A study of college students, for example, found that 85% of the women wanted to lose weight, whereas only 40% of the men wanted to lose weight and 45% actually wanted to gain it. In the general population, concerns about balding are relatively common among men but not among women.

Another gender difference I found is that men are more likely to report that they were frequently teased about their appearance earlier in life, and they're more apt to use a hat for camouflage. Women, in contrast, are more likely to turn to cosmetics for cover.

Several treatment findings are interesting. Men are nearly as likely as women to seek nonpsychiatric treatment (dermatologic, surgical, other medical, and dental) for their BDD (70% of men versus 80% of women). However, women are more likely to receive such care (70% versus 51%, a statistically significant difference). In other words, men are more likely to be refused nonpsychiatric treatment for BDD. This difference is accounted for primarily by the fact that men are more often refused dental and other medical (but not dermatologic and surgical) treatment. The reasons for this finding aren't clear. It's noteworthy that men with BDD are as likely as women to receive cosmetic surgery; in the general population, women receive such treatment much more often than men.

The question of whether BDD in men and women differs is far from answered. Other researchers need to address this question to confirm these findings. In upcoming years, as more research is done, it will be important to continue to examine gender differences.

BDD Across the Life Span

BDD appears to usually begin during adolescence, but can start in childhood or adulthood. In the series of people I've studied, BDD began at an average age of 16.5 years. The standard deviation is 7.0 years, which means that the majority—two-thirds—were between 9 and 24 years old when their BDD began. The earliest age at onset I've found is age 4, and the oldest is 43. The distribution of age at onset is as follows:

Age 5 or less: 3%

Age 6 to 10:   10%

Age 11 to 15: 36%

Age 16 to 20: 32%

Age 21 to 25:   8%

Age 26 to 30:   6%

Age 31 to 35:   3%

Age 36 to 40:   1%

Over age 40:   1%

Case reports in the professional literature tend to agree with these findings. When I reviewed published cases of BDD, I found that the average age at which BDD began was 19 years. Other researchers have also found that BDD usually starts during adolescence.*

Some people have vivid memories of their early symptoms. A woman whose symptoms began at age 4, for example, clearly remembered specific situations at that age in which she intensely disliked her fingers and tried to hide them. Another woman had vivid memories of hiding behind her mother's skirt at the playground and not wanting to go to nursery school because she looked so ugly. And another told me, "At the age of five I looked in the mirror and said, 'I'm ugly.' To hide my ugly face, I wore sunglasses to kindergarten."

I've been interested in whether people with an early age at onset of BDD—before age 18—differ from those with a later onset. It could be hypothesized that those with an earlier onset would be more impaired as a result of their symptoms because they've suffered for a longer time. While my data reveal more similarities than differences, those with onset in childhood or adolescence are more likely to have been housebound (40% vs 11%) and psychiatrically hospitalized (70% vs 18%).

BDD usually begins gradually, but 25% report a sudden onset, going from no concern to a full-fledged concern in less than a week's time. A 21-year-old woman told me, "It started suddenly. I went into the bathroom one day, and I saw a mustache." In some but not all cases, the sudden onset of BDD appears to be precipitated by a negative comment about appearance or a stressful event.

BDD appears to be a chronic disorder. About 85% report that their BDD symptoms have been continuous and chronic rather than episodic; that is, they haven't been free, or nearly free, of their symptoms for at least a month at a time since they began. I ask the question, "What's the longest

---

* In the studies that have been done, age at onset was usually determined retrospectively rather than prospectively—that is, people who already had the disorder estimated the age at which the disorder began by looking back over time. Because memory can be faulty, this approach is subject to error. Nonetheless, many people with BDD have very vivid memories of their early symptoms, suggesting that retrospective recollections may be reasonably accurate.

Another complicating factor in determining age at onset is that onset of the disorder is usually gradual and sometimes preceded by a dislike of one's body that isn't severe enough to warrant the diagnosis. As one woman said, "I've had hints of concern since I was a child." Determining at what age BDD symptoms become clinically significant—that is, at what age the disorder begins—is sometimes difficult. Nonetheless, the ages at onset found in my own research and that of others are remarkably consistent.

time you've gone without worrying about your defect since the problem began?" By far the most common response is "less than a day." This answer reflects how unrelenting BDD symptoms often are; once they begin, usually during adolescence, they tend to persist. The average duration of BDD symptoms of the people I've seen is 16 years—an unusually long duration.

It does appear, however, that symptoms, while generally chronic, often wax and wane over time; that is, they're usually present, but they're more severe at some times than others. Severity may fluctuate for no apparent reason, or in response to stress or triggering events, such as skin picking or being in a social situation. Acne concerns are particularly likely to fluctuate, as the severity of the acne changes. I'll say more about the factors that worsen BDD symptoms in the next chapter.

A majority of the people I've seen—57%—have said that their symptoms have gotten worse over time. Only 20% reported that their symptoms improved. For the rest, symptom severity stayed fairly stable. If response to treatment is taken into account, the percentage who get better is much larger.

It isn't known why so many people get worse. This finding could reflect referral bias: people who come to see me are those who are still suffering, whereas those who've gotten better are less likely to seek help. It might also reflect the natural course of the disorder—that is, BDD may actually have a tendency to worsen over time. Long-term prospective studies that follow people over a long period, evaluating them repeatedly, are needed to more accurately determine BDD's course over time.

BDD in Children

"Johnnie, your hair looks so nice today!" the receptionist exclaimed as he walked by. "Oh, Johnnie, your hair looks wonderful!" one of the secretaries echoed. When Johnnie entered the psychiatrist's office, instead of sitting in the chair as directed, he crouched down and intently peered at himself in a thin strip of chrome on a chair. "What are you doing, Johnnie?" the psychiatrist asked him. Johnnie didn't answer. Instead, he tilted his head, examining his hair from different angles, patting it and smoothing it out. He also grinned at himself, examining and touching his teeth.

Johnnie was excessively worried about his hair, which he thought "wasn't right" or flat enough; his teeth, which he thought weren't white or straight enough; and his "pot" belly. He frequently checked mirrors and excessively brushed his teeth. He also frequently touched and groomed his hair, using special hair creams. If he couldn't get his hair to look right, Johnnie cried, dunked his head in water, and started his grooming routine all over again. "I wish the whole world was bald," he said, "including me, so I wouldn't have to worry about my hair."

Johnnie frequently asked his parents, "Is my hair okay?" "Am I fat?" His mother estimated that he spent at least three hours a day focused on his appearance and asking for reassurance. Johnnie was five years old.

We don't know how common BDD is during childhood. At the time of this writing, there isn't to my knowledge even a single published case of BDD in a child in the psychiatric literature, highlighting its underrecognition in this age group. But cases like Johnnie's make it very clear that BDD does occur in children. The children I know of with BDD had symptoms that were quite similar to those in adults.

BDD in children probably isn't rare, given that approximately half the people I've seen reported that their disorder began before age 16, and 13% reported that it began by age 10.

BDD in Adolescents

Adolescence appears to be a particularly vulnerable time for the development of BDD, but there's surprisingly little mention of it in the psychiatric literature and almost no published research on BDD in adolescents. The few published case reports and my clinical experience suggest that BDD characteristics in adolescents are similar to those in adults, with a focus on similar body parts and performance of similar behaviors. Degree of impairment, as in adults, can span a spectrum from mild to severe. And, as has been found for adults, preliminary findings suggest that BDD in adolescents may respond to serotonin-reuptake inhibitors. The following cases illustrate some of these features.

Holly was a shy and attractive 16-year-old high school student, who was reluctant to discuss her appearance concerns because of embarrassment. With encouragement, she finally did. "I think my problems first began with shyness," she said. "I felt very self-conscious and uncomfortable being around other people. But then, a few years ago, I started worrying about how I looked. First, it was my body shape. I thought my shoulders and hips were too broad and my waist was too small. Then I got a terrible haircut, and I started worrying about my hair—that it's ugly and never looks right. It's a real rat's nest."

Holly thought about these things for several hours a day, and frequently checked her appearance in mirrors and windows, trying to fix her hair. "I get down on myself about it, because I shouldn't be so concerned with my appearance," she said. "It's selfish and shallow." Holly also spent at least $40 a week on haircuts, permanents, and hair products—money she really couldn't afford to spend. She also wore loose-fitting clothes to cover her body. Although she greatly enjoyed swimming, she avoided it because she was so self-conscious about how she looked. "Because I look so bad, I feel I don't fit in anywhere," she said. "I'm avoiding my friends, and I hardly ever go to parties."

I met Kristin, a 17-year-old woman, in the hospital after she'd attempted suicide. She attributed her suicide attempt primarily to her appearance concerns. Since the age of 13 she'd been excessively preoccupied with her nose, which she thought was too large; her breasts, which she thought were too small; and her hair, which she thought "wasn't right." She described her concerns as "very, very distressing—an obsession. They're so horrible I get suicidal; it's why I overdosed. I couldn't stand the pain any more."

Kristin thought about her appearance "every second of every day," and she checked mirrors, store windows, and other reflecting surfaces for hours. "I also constantly compare myself to other girls, and I ask my mother a million times a day whether I look okay, but I really don't believe her when she says how pretty I am. . . . Sometimes people compliment me on my hair, but it makes me angry. I think they're saying they like my hair so they can avoid commenting on my ugly face and body." As a result of her appearance concerns, Kristin avoided social interactions and dating. She also failed some of her courses and eventually dropped out of school. To feel better about how she looked, she had a nose job, which diminished her concern with her nose but was then followed by increased concern about her breasts.

Eric is another adolescent with BDD. At the age of 14 he became preoccupied with the idea that he had severe acne, wrinkles around his eyes, and "stuck-out" ears—deformities that weren't discernible to others. Eric often checked himself in mirrors and kept lights dimmed so his "defects" wouldn't be visible. He also covered his forehead with his bangs and a baseball hat, and he wore makeup to hide his supposed acne. Eric had had many friends and had been a very good student and a star soccer player. But as a result of his symptoms, his grades dropped and he became increasingly self-conscious, depressed, anxious, and socially isolated. Eventually, after several years of symptoms, he was unable to attend school and became housebound.

Holly, Kristen, and Eric all responded to a serotonin-reuptake inhibitor. After several months of treatment, Eric returned to school and started playing soccer again and seeing his friends. Kristin worried less about how she looked, went back to school, and was no longer suicidal. And Holly stopped covering her body with oversized clothing and started swimming again.

It's interesting that BDD appears to usually begin during adolescence—a time when appearance concerns are often prominent and bodily changes dramatic. It has in fact been suggested that BDD may be a pathological response to the various physical and physiological changes of adolescence. From a psychoanalytic perspective, it's been hypothesized that minor skin changes of adolescence—for example, mild acne—could trigger BDD symptoms by further damaging a person's "vulnerable ego." From a biological perspective, it could be hypothesized that brain development during adolescence may contribute to the disorder's onset. Sociocultural factors that emphasize the importance of appearance and acceptance by others are also clearly important at this time. The causes of BDD and the mechanisms by which it's expressed may indeed be linked in some way to the biological, psychological, and social changes that occur during adolescence.

I'm sometimes asked whether BDD can even be diagnosed during adolescence, because this is a time when appearance concerns are so common. The answer is yes, it can. While it may sometimes be difficult to differentiate mild BDD from normal adolescent concerns, more severe BDD can easily be diagnosed in this age group. In fact, as previously noted, adolescence appears to be the time when BDD is most likely to develop.

As in adults, the diagnosis should be made when appearance concerns become preoccupying and cause significant emotional distress or interfere with functioning. The adolescent who gets depressed, has difficulty concentrating in school or whose grades drop, or who misses school, parties, or dates because of appearance-related concerns has concerns in excess of normal, which may constitute BDD.

Kristin's, Eric's, and Holly's concerns were clearly excessive and characteristic of BDD. Kristin avoided social interactions and dating, and she failed some of her courses and dropped out of school. Her suicide attempt and hospitalization were painfully clear signs that what she was experiencing wasn't just "normal adolescence" or something she'd "grow out of." Early on, Eric's grades dropped, and he became anxious and depressed. While these signs weren't dramatic, they signaled that something problematic and serious was occurring—that he wasn't just "going through a phase" or having normal adolescent difficulties. When he dropped out of school and stopped playing soccer, it became crystal clear that his concerns were a serious problem. While Holly's case was milder, the fact that she worried about her appearance for several hours a day and avoided friends signaled the presence of BDD.

All three adolescents also had some of the associated behaviors character-istic of BDD—mirror checking, camouflaging, reassurance seeking, and ex-cessive grooming. While not diagnostic, they provided additional clues to the disorder's presence.

It's sometimes difficult to diagnose BDD during adolescence because ad-olescents may be quite embarrassed by their concerns and reluctant to re-veal them. Holly felt that she was selfish and shallow because she was so focused on how she looked, and she was very reluctant to reveal her con-cerns to anyone. While adults also have these feelings, secrecy may be par-ticularly common during the teenage years because many adolescents hesi-tate to confide in and trust adults. Often, a trusting relationship with an adult must be established before adolescents are willing to divulge their concerns. The best approach to this problem is to simply ask. When adoles-cents show any signs of BDD, inquire whether they have any appearance concerns. If they do, the additional questions in Chapter 4 and Appendix B can be asked.

Although I discussed the consequences of BDD in the last chapter, it's worth considering whether the disorder might have any special effects on adolescents. There are reasons to think it might. Adolescents must negotiate a number of important developmental tasks: increasing their involvement with peers, becoming more autonomous and independent of their families, developing a stronger and more cohesive sense of identity, and coming to grips with their sexuality, to name just a few. How BDD might affect these processes isn't known with certainty because it hasn't been studied; again, prospective studies that specifically address such issues are needed. None-theless, it seems likely that BDD can interfere with these adolescent devel-opmental tasks.

Self-consciousness and social withdrawal can interfere with the develop-ment of healthy peer relationships—friendships as well as intimate relation-ships. Withdrawal from friends can be accompanied by an increased depen-dence on the family at a time when such dependence is usually decreasing. Indeed, some adolescents with BDD become dependent on their family members to do things for them that they would otherwise do for them-selves. They may spend more and more time with their family—particularly if they're housebound—and rely more on them for their social interaction. They may look to their family for financial and emotional support in cop-ing with the disorder. While some dependence on one's family is healthy, BDD can lead to an excessive dependency that interferes with normal devel-opment.

It's also my impression that ongoing untreated BDD that begins prior to or during adolescence can interfere significantly with identity formation, one of the central developmental tasks of adolescence. Identity is a broad concept that includes not only a sense of self, character, and personality, but also the establishment of goals, aims, anticipated career and life-style, as well as one's place in the community and the world. If this developmental task isn't successfully negotiated, doubt, insecurity, and aimlessness may result. People with BDD may develop a strong sense of shame and inferiority, about their bodies and themselves, rather than a healthy identity and good self-esteem. They often view themselves in terms of the defect: I am a person with an ugly nose; I am a person who is ridiculed and rejected by others.

BDD may be particularly likely to interfere with the development of healthy self-esteem and identity because of the importance of physical appearance to the development of self-esteem. Of the domains of competence that appear to contribute most to global self-esteem—how much one likes oneself as a person overall—physical appearance heads the list. Studies have shown that, among teenagers, physical appearance correlates most highly with global self-esteem. Thus, teenagers with BDD, who believe their appearance is defective in some way, may have particular difficulty developing healthy self-esteem.

In addition, adolescents with BDD may be so excessively and exclusively focused on the supposed defect that they ignore and don't develop their strengths. They may have difficulty in school and may avoid hobbies and other activities. Other aspects of identity formation, such as career goals, may be neglected.

Other psychiatric disorders that begin during adolescence have been shown to interfere with identity formation and similar adolescent tasks. Because the self-concept hasn't yet crystallized, adolescents may be particularly vulnerable to the influence of various disorders on identity and personality formation. Studies have shown, for example, that school phobia interferes with developmental tasks. One study found that young adults who suffered from school phobia in childhood were more likely than other adults to be dependent, and they had more difficulty completing school and earning a living. They were more socially isolated, were less likely to be in a healthy, intimate relationship, and had more problems in sexual adjustment. BDD may be particularly prone to have these kinds of effects because it's highly interpersonal in nature, perhaps increasing the risk to relationships. In addition, BDD appears to be a chronic disorder, making it more difficult to get back on track and resume developmental tasks. Indeed, a significant percentage of adults with BDD (41% of those I've interviewed) live with their parents; others are unemployed, haven't graduated from school, and aren't dating or socially interacting with others. Some do progress, but less than they'd like.

Early and successful treatment appears to minimize or even eliminate these longer-term effects. It allows the adolescent to get back on track, resume normal functioning, and progress with these developmental tasks. In addition to psychiatric medication and cognitive-behavioral therapy, many patients who haven't negotiated some of the developmental tasks of adolescence can benefit from psychotherapy that helps them reintegrate themselves into the world by establishing relationships and meaningful work. While family involvement can be helpful in the treatment of adults, it may be particularly important to involve parents or other caretakers when treating adolescents.

Research on BDD in children and adolescents is greatly needed. Despite the limitations of our knowledge, however, it's clear that BDD does occur in these age groups and that adolescents may in fact be particularly vulnerable to the development of BDD. Because of possible longer-term effects, it's particularly important to recognize, diagnose, and treat BDD in children and adolescents; the same treatments that appear effective in adults are also promising in younger people.

BDD in the Elderly

Mildred was 80 years old and had had BDD for nearly 70 years, since she was a teenager. "I've always felt homely and ugly," she began. "It's shameful to have these concerns, because they're so superficial. It shouldn't matter. . . . Now I realize how excessive and unrealistic they were. When I see pictures of myself, I think I didn't look so bad back then. It doesn't bother me so much now; it was at its worst in my teens and twenties. But I'm still too concerned with how I look."

Mildred had grown up in a small town in the Midwest. She described some of her early recollections. "There was one main street in town. It was a very small place. I remember sometimes crossing the street to avoid people because I was so ugly. I was always very self-conscious, and I thought people talked about me. I always had the feeling that my mother and her friends talked about how I looked. I remember that when I was very young one of my cousins commented on how homely I was. Now I think it was just sibling rivalry, but at the time I was devastated. I also remember being told that I looked like my mother. She wasn't a good person, and I thought she was unattractive. I hated it when people told me that I looked like her. I hated to be identified with her.

"I used to wish I were black so I wouldn't have freckles, and I used freckle cream. When people commented on my nice hair I felt bad because it meant I wasn't otherwise attractive. I disliked myself so much I can't imagine people liking me in any way. I didn't feel desirable in any way. My feelings about my appearance were all tied up with feelings of inferiority. I was convinced people thought I was ugly—that I wasn't likable or lovable.

"Seventy-five percent of my life has centered on how I look. I fought back. I tried not to let my appearance concerns interfere much with my life. But high school was an especially hard time. I missed parties, and I was very shy on dates. And I think I might have done different things with my life if I hadn't been so preoccupied. I did raise wonderful daughters, but I would have had more energy for them and for other things, like my music. I think my concerns also affected my personality. People thought I was aloof, but I cared so much about what people thought of me. I was very easily hurt, very sensitive.

"I feel very guilty about my focus on my looks, because it seems so self-centered. There are other things to think about. I've never even told my husband about it, even though we're close, because I think he'd think I'm foolish. I was in therapy for many years, but I never brought it up because it would have been too difficult. I was afraid my therapist would think I was superficial and concerned with unimportant things. I felt so ashamed, especially at my age. I feel I should have enough wisdom not to care about something so silly."

Margaret, who was 70, had also struggled with BDD for many decades. Her concerns, too, had begun when she was a teenager and persisted ever since. She'd been treated in her teens for scoliosis (curvature of the spine), which was severe and required surgery and the use of a brace. But after several surgeries, the scoliosis was much improved and hardly noticeable to others. Margaret, however, was still preoccupied with it. "It's been a concern ever since then," she said. "I think my back still looks very ugly. I think about it for hours a day. I can't wear certain clothes because of how it looks. I wear clothes that hide it, and I change them a lot, trying to find an outfit that makes it look better."

Margaret spent approximately 8 hours a day performing BDD-related behaviors: selecting her clothes each morning and changing them during the day, checking other people's backs, checking mirrors, and asking her husband whether she looked okay. "I still think about how awful my back looks after all these years. I keep to myself because I don't want to draw attention to it. It's one of the things that's made me depressed."

A woman in her sixties, who appeared far younger than her age, was obsessed with obtaining eye surgery to eradicate facial "lines" that resembled those of a 35 year old. She'd seen most of the plastic surgeons in town, and she spent hours a day examining the lines in mirrors and applying creams and makeup. She restricted her activities as a result, and rarely left the house without wearing sunglasses.

Given that BDD appears to be a relatively chronic disorder, it isn't surprising that it exists in the elderly. However, it isn't known how common BDD is in this age group. The average age of the people I've seen is the thirties; I've seen far fewer elderly with BDD. Does BDD "burn out" as people age, becoming less severe or remitting altogether? Conversely, can it become more severe over time, and can the elderly be particularly distressed and impaired because of the cumulative effect of suffering over so many years? Might they be particularly embarrassed about seeking help? Further research is needed to answer such important questions.

·· *ten* ··

What Causes BDD?
Clues to an Unsolved Puzzle

"I have no idea why I worry so much about how I look. I wish I knew."   **Anne**

"This problem is chemical," Bridget said. "I can't think of any reason for these gut-wrenching worries about how I look. It must be from a chemical imbalance in my brain." Cindy's explanation was quite different. "My mother has very, very thin hair. I worry I'll be like my mother. It also has to do with anger. When I get angry at my mother my blood vessels constrict, and my anger gets physically translated into a cold, tight scalp. This decreases the blood supply to my hair so more falls out. My scalp even gets sore afterward. My thin hair is related to turning anger toward myself."

"My mother is very pretty, and so is my sister," Alison said. "I constantly tried to look like my older sister. She's very feminine, and I idealized her. I wanted her nose, her long hair. I never accepted who I was. I was the ugly duckling, the odd-looking one. I was the runt of the litter."

"I started worrying too much about my skin at a time when I was really stressed," Caroline told me. "It began after I had to take a job working in a place I really didn't want to work. And I started worrying that my rear end was too big after a guy in my class commented on my big ass. My father had also started drinking at the time. But I think these things were mostly triggers. I think my worries have deeper roots, like how I was always put down when I was growing up."

"My father has bad skin," Jamie said. "I look more like my father than like my mother. I worried my skin might end up like his."

"Maybe I learned looks were important," Brad told me. "My family stressed the importance of looks. We always had to look our best and be well-manicured no matter what. . . . Everyone paid lots of attention to my brother—he was the champ of the family and my father's pet. I was always last on my parents' list. . . . I was always very sensitive. I was always sensitive to criticism and rejection. I'm a perfectionist. I've always been hard on myself—since day one. I have high standards. My parents expected a lot from me. I was always the black sheep of the family."

People with BDD have myriad and varied explanations for their symptoms. Some invoke biology—a chemical imbalance in the brain. Others give a psychological explanation, citing their upbringing, identification with a particular person, feelings such as anger, or personality traits such as perfectionism or sensitivity to criticism or rejection. Others blame society's emphasis on attractiveness. Some people attribute their symptoms to a comment or to stress in their lives at the time their concern began. Others have no explanation for their symptoms, but they search for one, trying to give their experience meaning. The explanations are varied and bear the stamp of each person's unique autobiography.

This chapter's topic—what causes BDD—is the most complex question I pose in this book. At this time, the cause of BDD remains largely unexplored, and there are no definite answers. This is the outermost edge of the BDD frontier. But even though we're at the beginning of our search in terms of hard data and facts, much fascinating terrain has been covered in terms of speculation and theory.

In past decades, most theories—a reflection of their times—had a psychological basis. BDD symptoms were assumed to have psychological meaning as well as a psychological origin. An example of this was the Wolf Man's psychoanalyst's suggestion that his nose represented his penis and that he unconsciously desired to be castrated and made into a woman. Furthermore, she thought that his nose preoccupation reflected an identification with his mother, in part because it began soon after he saw a wart on his mother's nose.

More recently, biological theories have been proposed. Very preliminary findings suggest that malfunctioning of the brain chemical serotonin might be involved. Might other brain chemicals play a role in causing BDD symptoms? Is BDD "hardwired" in the brain? Might recent findings about the biological origins of OCD (obsessive compulsive disorder) apply to BDD?

Sociocultural explanations have an obvious appeal. Magazines, television, and movies constantly convey the importance of appearance. We're supposed to look our best at all times. We're urged to fix any problems with our appearance, no matter how minor. Might these ubiquitous and powerful messages contribute to the development of BDD? Might cultural influences also play a role?

There are other mysteries as well. Why do certain people and not others get BDD? Why does one person focus on her nose and another on her legs?

Most likely, the cause of BDD has multiple sources; that is, factors from all these domains—neurobiological, psychological, and sociocultural—probably contribute to BDD's occurrence, as do both genetic and environmental factors. This theory is similar to that proposed for other psychiatric disorders and many nonpsychiatric medical disorders, such as high blood pressure. In the case of blood pressure, genetics plays an important role, creating a biological vulnerability. But psychological factors, such as stress, and sociocultural factors, such as diet, are additional risk factors.

While it's useful to think of risk factors in terms of categories—neurobiological, psychological or developmental, and sociocultural—these categories are to some extent artificial. Biological and psychological factors overlap and interact with each other in complex ways: biological givens, such as temperament (biologically based personality traits), affect how people interact with the world and influence life events; conversely, life events, such as repetitive severe trauma and other psychological factors can influence biology and actually change the brain. Trying to clearly distinguish biological, psychological, and sociocultural contributions to BDD from one another is complex and to some degree artificial.

At this time, theories about what causes BDD are largely speculative. Spinning theories and hypotheses is relatively easy; proving or disproving them is far more difficult. The "why" questions are always the hardest to answer. The cause of BDD is a puzzle that remains to be solved. Nonetheless, we have some intriguing clues to guide us.

Neurobiological Theories: Is BDD a Brain Disease?

How could excessive appearance concerns—which might seem clearly related to sociocultural factors, such as the influence of the media, or to psychological factors, such as low self-esteem—be rooted in neurobiology? How could BDD be a brain disease?

I start with this perspective because I think it's likely that neurobiology lays the groundwork for BDD—that biology makes BDD possible by creating a vulnerability to developing the disorder.

This hypothesis seems less strange when you consider that some patients posit a neurobiological basis for their BDD symptoms. "My obsession may or may not be related to my childhood experiences, but it mostly feels chemical—out of my control," Ron said. "It feels like something biological is driving it." Other people, after searching for a psychological explanation for their symptoms in therapy, are unable to find one. While it could be argued that this therapy outcome reflects unconscious resistance to uncovering a psychological reason for the symptoms, this seems unlikely to be the case for many patients.

A neurobiological basis for body image disturbance actually has a long tradition. The first writings on body image were by neurologists, who early in this century explored the neurobiology of several types of distorted body image. These included anosognosia (the inability to recognize or acknowledge impaired bodily functioning, such as paralysis) and neglect of one side of the body (e.g., shaving only one side of the face or using only one sleeve of a robe). In 1931, a neurologist reported that some of his patients had interesting reactions toward their left-sided paralyzed limbs, considering them "strange, ugly, disfigured . . . thickened, shortened, or snake like."

Such body-image disturbances are related to brain processes and are often caused by brain damage, such as a stroke, in the brain's parietal region. Injury to the occipital lobes of the brain—the primary visual processing area—can impair visual perception, including perception of facial images. And damage to another area of the brain, the temporal lobes, can result in a distorted view of body size and inability to identify previously known faces. Some patients with damage to this area can't identify their own face in the mirror. An example of the bodily misperception that can occur from brain injury is a 1947 case in which a man described a dog as a person with "curious hair."

An unusual case of BDD-like symptoms also points to the involvement of neurobiological factors in the disorder. A 21-year old man who became preoccupied with thoughts that his ears had become smaller, one foot was bigger than the other, and other appearance concerns was eventually found to have subacute sclerosing panencephalitis, a rare and diffuse brain disease that was presumably related to the BDD-like concerns. While very few people with BDD have an identifiable neurological disorder such as this related to their symptoms (I haven't seen any), this case illustrates that brain processes gone awry can lead to distorted bodily perception and excessive bodily preoccupations.

Another line of evidence implicating neurobiological factors in BDD is treatment response. Although a disorder's cause can't necessarily be inferred from its response to treatment, this provides valuable clues to the cause or pathophysiological mechanisms involved in a disorder. Preliminary evidence that BDD may respond to medications known as serotonin-reuptake inhibitors (SRIs) suggests that disturbed brain chemistry plays an important role.

Serotonin is one of the brain's natural chemicals, known as a *neurotransmitter,* that carries messages from one nerve cell to another, making the nerve cells communicate with one another and function. Serotonin is released from one nerve cell, crosses a space between nerve cells known as a synapse, and then fits into a receptor on a receiving nerve cell, like a lock in a key. This "unlocking" then triggers a variety of chemical reactions in the recipient nerve cell, making it fire an electrical impulse that gets transmitted to neighboring nerve cells by the same mechanism. This process occurs in countless interlocking nerve cell networks throughout the brain.

The chemical messenger serotonin is important in many critical bodily functions—including mood, cognition, sleep, appetite, eating behavior, sexual behavior, and pain. It plays an important role in a variety of psychiatric disorders, including depression and OCD. BDD, too, may involve dysregulation of serotonin. How does serotonin do so many things? Its multiple roles may be explained by the fact that there are many different types of serotonin receptors—we currently know of at least 15—located at diverse sites throughout the brain. Serotonin's effects on these receptors are heterogeneous and complex.

Because the interactions and overlap among brain neurotransmitters (chemical messengers) and their receptors are highly complex, it's likely that other neurotransmitters are also involved in BDD. One of these is dopamine, which appears to play an important role in delusional thinking. Dopamine may, in combination with serotonin, be particularly important in the delusional form of BDD.

The theory that BDD involves neurochemical abnormalities is given some support by BDD's many similarities with OCD. These disorders' similarities suggest that they may have a similar cause or share certain steps in the chain of steps required for their expression. Much more is known about the neurobiological basis of OCD than of BDD, and it's useful to look at what's known about OCD for clues. Data from a large number of studies suggest that OCD involves an abnormality in the serotonin neurotransmitter system. This "serotonin hypothesis" is supported by several lines of evidence, including treatment response. Many methodologically rigorous treatment studies have demonstrated that OCD responds better to the SRIs than to other medications, implicating the importance of serotonin. Exactly how the SRIs improve OCD, however, remains unclear.

Further support for the serotonin hypothesis in OCD comes from other types of studies, such as those examining the breakdown products of serotonin. Such studies generally show an association between improvement of OCD with a serotonin-reuptake inhibitor and acute alterations of serotonin and its metabolites in the brain. Studies known as pharmacological challenge studies, in which people are given agents that affect serotonin, also tend to support the serotonin hypothesis in OCD. Such agents may, for example, increase OCD symptoms and anxiety in patients with OCD but have no effect in normal control subjects. Although available data aren't entirely consistent, on balance there is substantial evidence implicating serotonin in OCD. However, the exact role of this neurotransmitter, and whether it has a central role in *causing* OCD, remains unclear.

Dopamine, a neurotransmitter involved in disorders of thinking and movement, may also play a role in the pathophysiology of OCD. When added to the serotonin-reuptake inhibitors, medications that antagonize— or counteract—dopamine have been shown to improve OCD symptoms in certain patients with OCD. It's been hypothesized that some forms of OCD involve an imbalance in the systems controlling serotonin and dopamine. This hypothesis may also apply to BDD, particularly its delusional form.

Data supporting the role of serotonin in BDD are far more preliminary than for OCD. I've already mentioned that BDD's apparent response to SRIs gives some indirect support to the serotonin hypothesis. A few other very preliminary reports also implicate serotonin in BDD. A case report published by Drs. Linda Barr, Wayne Goodman, and Lawrence Price of Yale University School of Medicine described a patient with BDD treated with clomipramine (Anafranil) and buspirone (Buspar) who underwent acute experimental dietary depletion of tryptophan. Tryptophan is an essential protein building block (amino acid) that is a precursor of serotonin. The tryptophan depletion was accomplished by having the patient eat a low tryptophan diet and drink an amino acid drink without tryptophan. This resulted in a dramatic exacerbation of her BDD symptoms, which was presumably mediated by a reduction in brain serotonin levels.

Consistent with this report, there have been several reports of BDD symptoms increasing with the use of agents that antagonize serotonin. One patient's BDD symptoms appeared to worsen after chronically abusing cyproheptadine, an allergy medication that antagonizes, or counteracts, serotonin. And LSD, which antagonizes some effects of serotonin, is well known to induce visual illusions, including bodily distortions, which may be present in BDD. Indeed, serotonin appears to modulate the visual system.

Might there also be neuroanatomical brain abnormalities in BDD? That is, can subtle abnormalities in certain structures of the brain be identified? Recent brain-imaging techniques have greatly advanced the search for abnormalities in brain structure and functioning in a variety of psychiatric disorders. Such studies haven't yet been done in BDD but are under way. Findings in OCD may again be relevant to BDD. Several studies using PET (positron emission tomography), a brain-imaging technique, have found abnormalities (increased metabolism) in areas of the brain known as the orbitofrontal cortex and caudate nucleus in patients with OCD compared with normal control subjects. Other PET studies of OCD patients found that after they responded to the serotonin-reuptake inhibitor fluoxetine (Prozac) or cognitive-behavioral therapy, previously abnormally increased activity in the caudate nucleus—a structure deep in the brain's core—tended to normalize. Neuropsychological studies of OCD also implicate abnormalities in these areas of the brain.

These findings have generated models for the basis of obsessions and compulsions, which suggest that there is dysfunction in a "circuit," or "loop," connecting certain areas of the brain to one another (the orbitofrontal cortex, the caudate nucleus, the thalamus, and other structures). Dr. Lewis Baxter and his colleagues at UCLA have hypothesized that in OCD certain structures in this loop (the caudate and other basal ganglia structures) don't "repress" or stop inputs from another area, the orbital cortex, as they should. It's as if a gate that should be closed is left open, allowing the brain impulses that generate obsessions and compulsions to repeatedly cycle through the gate and around the loop. This causes obsessions and compulsions to occur over and over. Effective treatments for OCD (the SRIs and cognitive-behavioral therapy) appear to somehow close the gate again, stopping this "reverberating circuit" and allowing it to work normally. Whether this fascinating hypothesis applies to BDD remains to be studied. The temporal and occipital lobes of the brain may also play an important role in BDD, as these areas contain cells that respond to faces, and they are implicated in other types of body image distortion.

Brain imaging and neuropsychological studies of BDD are currently being done, which should shed light on underlying brain mechanisms in BDD. Whether the findings will be similar to those in OCD remains to be seen. Of interest, the only study of which I'm aware that has directly related neuropsychological function to some component of body image found that size overestimation for the hip and thighs was correlated with errors in visual memory. Preliminary findings suggest that OCD may also involve visual memory errors.

Animal behavior gives us another fascinating window on possible neurobiological underpinnings of BDD. We don't at present have an animal model of BDD, yet the repetitive behaviors of some animals appear amazingly similar to those of BDD. Some animals, for example, excessively groom themselves. One form of excessive grooming is acral lick syndrome. Dogs and cats with this syndrome repeatedly lick their fur, causing skin lesions that may be severe. Some birds compulsively pluck their feathers, which seems similar to compulsive skin picking in BDD. Particularly fascinating are reports from several researchers that these abnormal grooming behaviors in animals may respond to SRIs—including clomipramine, fluoxetine, and sertraline—but not to non-SRI antidepressants or placebo.

These animal syndromes have been noted to have similarities with OCD, but they also appear strikingly similar to BDD because they involve excessive grooming and picking behaviors. Similarities between BDD and these animal syndromes provide further evidence for a biological basis for BDD. They suggest that, like OCD, BDD may involve normal neurobiological processes gone awry.

A preference for bodily symmetry, one of the concerns of one-third of people with BDD, may also have biological underpinnings. Some researchers have found that animals prefer symmetry, as opposed to asymmetry, in their mates. Male Japanese scorpion flies with the most symmetrical wings, for example, obtain the most mates. Female scorpion flies may prefer these suitors because they're more adept at killing their prey. People, like animals, seem to prefer symmetry as well. Studies have found, for example, that college students with more symmetrical features have more sex partners. This preference appears to have a neurobiological basis and may signal fitness, well-being, or, in animals, provide a way to recognize mates of the same species.

Yet another reason to think that BDD involves neurobiological underpinnings—which are likely genetically transmitted—is that most, if not all, psychiatric disorders appear to be at least partly neurobiologically and genetically based. Elegant twin studies of depressed individuals, for example, indicate that genetic factors play an important causal role in depression. Even the disorder that might be considered the most environmentally determined of all—post-traumatic stress disorder, which occurs after experiencing an extremely stressful event—is substantially determined by genetic factors.

Although largely speculative at this time, I would hypothesize that neurobiology provides a template for BDD; that is, neurobiological factors, which are probably genetically transmitted, make some people vulnerable to BDD and make its symptoms possible. It seems likely that psychological or sociocultural factors may combine with biological givens to increase the risk of, trigger, influence, or further shape BDD symptoms. The degree to which neurobiological factors account for BDD, whether they involve serotonin or other neurotransmitters, and which parts of the brain are involved in BDD remain to be discovered.

Psychological Theories: Is BDD a Mind Disease?

Kimberly's explanation for her BDD symptoms was psychological. "I never got positive messages from my family, even though I was the good daughter," she told me. "I was never praised, and I felt neglected. I wonder if that's how I developed such low self-esteem and my feelings that I look bad."

Might psychological factors also play a role in causing BDD? Might BDD result from identifying with another person, or from life experiences, such as teasing or rejection? What about the role of personality traits, such as perfectionism or sensitivity to criticism? Are BDD symptoms the expression or reflection of underlying psychological issues, such as problems in a relationship?

Psychological explanations for BDD have a long tradition. During the past century they've been considered by many authors to play an important role in causing BDD, a reflection of the dominant theoretical framework at the time. This framework—often referred to as a psychodynamic or psychoanalytic perspective—views symptoms as having psychological meaning and causation. Often, the cause is considered to be rooted in childhood experiences.

Some authors, for example, have suggested that BDD arises from the unconscious displacement of sexual or emotional conflict, or feelings of inferiority, guilt, or poor self-image, onto a body part. In other words, conflicts or feelings such as these are considered the underlying problem and the cause of BDD symptoms. This displacement process is presumed to occur because the underlying problem is too emotionally threatening or anxiety provoking to be dealt with more directly—thus, it is unconsciously displaced into the more psychologically manageable arena of appearance. It's been further posited that the body part of concern, such as the nose, may represent another, more emotionally threatening, body part, such as the penis.

It has similarly been suggested that BDD symptoms may unconsciously be used to "explain" dissatisfying relationships or failures in one's life. According to this theory, blaming your nose for your problems is less threatening to your self-esteem than admitting you're a failure.

Such theories are very difficult to prove or disprove. But in my view they don't alone provide a satisfactory explanation for BDD symptoms. The fact that many people respond well to medication or cognitive-behavioral therapy, without any attempt to treat presumed underlying psychological conflicts, suggests that such underlying factors aren't the primary or sole explanation for BDD symptoms. Some patients have been in psychotherapy or psychoanalysis for many years, searching for or working on resolving associated psychological problems, without successfully diminishing their BDD symptoms. Such therapy may be very helpful in resolving other psychological problems or life difficulties, but it generally doesn't appear to change BDD symptoms.

While this perspective may sometimes be helpful in understanding particular aspects of BDD, it appears inadequate to explain its cause.

It's likely, however, that certain psychological factors play a role in the occurrence of BDD—not as the sole cause, but perhaps as a risk factor for the disorder. Many, if not most, psychiatric disorders result from both biological and psychological factors, with biology laying the groundwork and psychological factors also contributing to the occurrence of the disorder. BDD is probably similar.

What psychological factors might contribute to BDD? The answer isn't known with certainty, but a few possibilities are worth considering. One is a history of frequent teasing. Degree of body image disturbance more generally has been shown to be related to teasing history. Dr. J. Kevin Thompson, for example, found that college women who reported more teasing during adolescence evaluated their body image as an adult more negatively. Individuals with an eating disorder report more past teasing than control subjects. Using sophisticated statistical methods, Richards found that teasing was *causally* related not only to general psychological dysfunction (depression and lowered self-esteem) but also to body dissatisfaction.

I've found that 60% of people with BDD report frequent or chronic teasing about their appearance during childhood or adolescence, focusing on the body areas of concern or on other aspects of appearance. I don't know whether this percentage is higher than in the general population; if it is, might frequent teasing increase the risk of BDD?

Might other life experiences that generate feelings of low self-esteem and rejection constitute psychological or environmental risk factors for the disorder? Several authors have proposed that "unharmonious" family backgrounds or "unfavorable" childhood experiences that lead to enduring feelings of being unloved, insecure, or rejected may contribute to BDD. Some people with BDD confirm this theory, stating that they believe that childhood experiences such as these contributed to their symptoms. They cite such things as parental expectations of perfectionism or feelings of having been unloved or neglected by their family. But not all patients report this.

The only systematic data pertaining to early family experiences of people with BDD come from the Parental Bonding Instrument. This scale is a validated and widely used self-report measure of patients' perceptions of parental care and overprotection before the age of 16. I found that average scores of 40 consecutive patients with BDD were notably lower than published norms on parental care and were in the average range on parental overprotection. These findings are consistent with how many patients describe their early life experiences, which often emphasize feelings of rejection and neglect.

Some people believe their family's or peers' emphasis on appearance contributed to their concern. One woman told me, "In my childhood people doted on my appearance. So I fear if I look bad, people won't like me." Another said, "Appearance was very important in our family, and it became very important to me. The only area of positive feedback from my parents was for my attractiveness. So destroying my appearance was the most destructive thing I could do." Experiences such as these could in theory lead to some of the cognitive distortions (distorted ways of thinking) that I'll discuss in Chapter 14—for example, that one's worth as a person is based only on one's appearance. Occasionally, BDD symptoms seem to begin with a parent's excessive preoccupation with their child's appearance—what might be called "BDD by proxy."

Some people with BDD, however, report none of these things. Whether particular family or other early life experiences contribute to BDD isn't clear at this time. While certain experiences, for example, experiences of rejection and neglect, may be risk factors for BDD, they are unlikely to be its major cause.

I'm sometimes asked about the possible role of trauma or sexual abuse in causing BDD. Very preliminary research findings suggest that trauma may be associated with BDD. Dr. Caron Zlotnick of Brown University School of Medicine and I have found that of 55 women with a diagnosis of post-traumatic stress disorder (PTSD; see Appendix A for a definition), a fairly high percentage—20%—reported clear-cut BDD, and many others reported other significant body-image concerns. In a study I did with Dr. Mark Zimmerman and Jill Mattia, we found that PTSD was more common among people with probable BDD (occurring in 13%) than among psychiatric outpatients without BDD. Because people with PTSD have experienced significant trauma of some sort, these findings suggest that BDD may be associated with a history of trauma. In the Zimmerman study, the type of trauma was unspecified; in the Zlotnick study it consisted of sexual abuse, although subjects may have experienced other types of trauma as well.

These preliminary findings suggest that a history of trauma may be associated with BDD. It makes sense that sexual trauma, in particular, might contribute to bodily shame or dislike of one's body. It hasn't been established, however, that trauma is *causally* related to BDD. In addition, it's clear from these studies and from clinical experience that not every person with past trauma develops BDD, nor has every person with BDD experienced trauma, such as sexual abuse. Experiences such as these are clearly not the cause of BDD, although they may prove to be risk factors.

And what about the role of other life events? Several patients linked their BDD symptoms with moving to a different culture. A man who moved from India gave the following explanation for his appearance concerns: "I'm obsessed about my penis and nose and eyes because I feel in general like an unattractive outsider. I'm not as accepted as I'd like to be." Another man from India gave a similar explanation: "I feel like a foreigner in every way— I feel different from others. I'm afraid I'll never have the all-American look."

It's also important to consider whether a previously noticeable physical deformity contributes to the development of BDD. Some people with BDD—although it's a minority—report that they had a more severe deformity, such as severe acne, scoliosis, or a facial gash from an accident earlier in their life. With time, their skin healed or their back was straightened, but their view of themselves didn't change. In their mind's eye, they would always be severely deformed. Body-image researchers refer to this as the adaptive failure theory. According to this theory, changes in actual appearance are not paralleled by a congruent change in self-perception of one's body. Research findings on the validity of this theory are mixed, but some studies have found that obese subjects' perception of their body size—as well as their thoughts, feelings, and concerns about weight—don't necessarily change with weight loss. After losing weight, they still don't see themselves as thin; a negative "vestigial" body image persists. One woman's comment about her BDD reflected this theory: "I'm like a person who lost 200 pounds and still thinks they're fat. I can't change my view of myself."

This theory hasn't been adequately studied and hasn't been studied at all in BDD. But it might apply to the development of BDD in some individuals with previous actual deformities, or explain why people with BDD are often dissatisfied with the results of cosmetic surgery.

Whether certain personality traits predispose people to BDD is a particularly interesting question. Personality traits are generally both "psychological or environmental" *and* "biological or genetic" in origin—for example, personality traits like submissiveness and extroversion are substantially determined by genetic as well as environmental influences.

Although some early authors viewed BDD as a symptom of an underlying personality disturbance, this is unlikely to be the case. People with BDD have a variety of personality traits—not everyone with BDD has the same type of personality. In addition, some people with BDD have no personality "disturbance" of any sort. It therefore is highly unlikely that BDD is *caused* by, or simply a symptom of, certain personality traits or problems.

But might certain personality traits *predispose* people to BDD and act as a risk factor for the disorder? People with BDD often consider themselves, and appear to be, shy, self-conscious, and hypersensitive to rejection and criticism. Their self-esteem is often low. Some people say things like, "BDD equals low self-esteem; this is just another expression of my low self-esteem." Or "The real problem here is shame. My appearance concerns all boil down to shame about myself."

As I'll discuss in Chapter 12, available data confirm some of these impressions. They suggest that people with BDD tend to be introverted and socially avoidant, and tend to score very high on "neuroticism," a measure of anxiety, depression, self-consciousness, anger, and feelings of vulnerability. In the BDD/depression study I did with Drs. Nierenberg and Fava, we found that people with depression (the atypical form) plus BDD scored higher on certain measures of rejection sensitivity than people with atypical depression without BDD. Those who also had BDD had significantly higher scores on questions measuring interpersonal sensitivity (emotional overreaction to rejection or criticism) and work or school impairment due to overreaction to criticism or rejection.

But the relationship of these personality traits to BDD is unclear. Do these traits *predispose to* BDD, contributing to its occurrence? Or, conversely, do they *result from* BDD? Or do certain personality traits and BDD simply *co-occur*, without one predisposing to or causing the other? One reason it's hard to answer this question is that both BDD and personality traits usually have their onset at a young age and are continuously present, making it difficult to answer this question on the basis of time course (e.g., which started first). But one piece of data suggesting that shyness might predispose people to BDD is my finding that in BDD patients with coexisting social phobia, the average age at which social phobia begins (13 years) is earlier than that of BDD (16.5 years), suggesting that introversion and social anxiety often predate BDD.

Another personality trait that might be associated with BDD is perfectionism or unusually high standards for oneself. Some people with BDD say that they want to look perfect and that they expect perfectionism in other areas of their life as well. "I have very high standards for myself," a college student said to me. "I expect much more from myself than from anyone else, in terms of my appearance and everything else. It's hard to live up to it."

I would hypothesize that personality traits such as these—shyness, social anxiety, low self-esteem, perfectionism, sensitivity to rejection and criticism—may predispose a person to BDD. In turn, it seems likely that BDD symptoms may strengthen some of these personality traits. For example, avoidance of social situations because of BDD symptoms might further increase social anxiety and shyness.

So far, I've been discussing whether certain biological or psychological factors might cause or contribute to the occurrence of BDD. It's also interesting to consider whether psychological factors might influence the *content* of BDD beliefs—the specific aspects of appearance that are worried about. According to this model, psychological factors or experiences might influence the specific body part of concern, or the theme associated with the concern, such as a fear of aging. For example, is a person more likely to worry about their nose, as opposed to their stomach, if that's what they were teased about in childhood? Are they more likely to worry about aging, as opposed to femininity, if a parent was very concerned about looking old? Might the content of BDD beliefs be influenced by identification with another person? Some authors have suggested that this is the case. A young man who was concerned about balding stated, "I'm afraid I'll end up bald like Uncle Joe." Others dislike a particular aspect of their appearance because they associate it with a particular ethnic group. One woman said that she focused on her hair because her grandparents had owned a beauty parlor, and hair was always very important in her family.

The role of psychological factors in BDD needs to be studied and better understood. In some cases such factors—such as identification with another person—seem to influence the *content* of BDD concerns. I would also hypothesize that psychological factors may also influence *whether* BDD occurs—that is, they may act as a risk factor for the occurrence of the disorder. Learning may also play an important role. I think it's likely, however, that psychological factors must act in concert with biological or genetic factors to bring on the disorder.

Sociocultural Theories: Mega-Makeovers and Perfect Thighs

"Mega-Makeovers: Go From So-So to Supersexy!"

"Perfect Thighs in This Lifetime?"

"Fast Fixes for a Bad Hair Day"

"3-D Abs: Work Your Front, Back, and Sides for a Great Middle"

These were messages I read while recently standing in line at the grocery store check-out counter. The most prominent message displayed on the magazine rack was that appearance matters and should be improved. The covers were adorned with beautiful women. You couldn't miss it.

Nor can you miss it on television, in films, or at the bookstore. We confront images like these everywhere. As one person with BDD put it, "You see models everywhere. How can you *not* think about how you look!" Advertisements and magazines reflect our society's incessant concern with appearance. The number of articles on beauty and diets in women's magazines has multiplied in recent decades. We spend huge amounts of money on diets, cosmetics, hair styles, clothing, and makeovers. A survey of working women published several years ago in a women's magazine found that some women spent more than $7,000 a year on their appearance. Increasing numbers of people, including men and teenagers, are having cosmetic surgery. The marketing of beauty has become a multibillion dollar industry.

Might society's incessant focus on appearance and beauty—and comparison of our own bodies with the sociocultural ideal—contribute to the occurrence of BDD? In support of this view is that sociocultural factors influence more normal and common body-image concerns. As J. Kevin Thompson has written, "The influence of our society and particularly the media is of paramount importance in attempting to explain the currently high levels of body image disturbance." According to this sociocultural model, we—women in particular—are indoctrinated with the message that we should be attractive. As the psychologist Judith Rodin has noted, current female sex-role stereotyping engenders a preoccupation with the pursuit of beauty and thinness—a message the media powerfully endorses.

But does the sociocultural model apply not only to normal appearance concerns but also to BDD? It's interesting to consider what people with BDD have to say about the influence of society and the media on their symptoms. Two-thirds of the people I've interviewed have reported that they believe this focus on appearance *increases* their BDD concerns. The constant messages about attractiveness, and the constant portrayal of attractive people on television, in movies, and in magazines, worsens their preoccupation.

But very few people have said that they believe this focus on appearance is the major *cause* of their BDD symptoms. They generally give other explanations or no explanation at all. Or they say that the media and society contribute to their symptoms but aren't the only or the major causal factor. As one woman put it, "Magazines play a role in BDD, but they're not the whole story because everyone sees them but everyone doesn't get BDD." Another agreed: "The media isn't the cause, but it feeds into it."

I would hypothesize, consistent with patient reports, that societal messages about attractiveness do trigger increased preoccupation in some people with BDD. These people obsess more about their appearance after seeing attractive people on television or in a magazine. This seems especially likely if they compulsively compare themselves with others.

I would also hypothesize that society's and the media's emphasis on attractiveness may contribute to the occurrence of BDD; that is, societal pressures and the media may increase the risk of the disorder. This theory is similar to that proposed for the eating disorders anorexia nervosa and bulimia nervosa. These disorders are partly biologically based, but their risk appears to be increased by a cultural ideal of thinness.

However, sociocultural pressures are unlikely to be the only, or the primary, cause. BDD has been described for more than 100 years, long before advertising attained its current power, suggesting that the media alone is not responsible for its occurrence. I would also hypothesize that if society's emphasis on appearance were the sole or primary cause of BDD, it would probably occur far more frequently in women than in men, which doesn't appear to be the case. In addition, BDD appears to respond to psychiatric medications, implicating the fundamental importance of biological factors.

If sociocultural factors contribute to, or increase the risk of, BDD, it would be reasonable to conclude that as we're increasingly exposed to images of physical beauty in the media, BDD is becoming more prevalent. Is BDD more common than it was a century ago, before advertising became such a powerful influence? We don't know. If it is, are societal factors responsible? Future research may shed some light on these questions.

Another interesting question is whether BDD occurs in different cultures and is similar across cultures. Is BDD culture specific—a "Western" disorder—or is it universal? And even if BDD is unlikely to be *caused* primarily by sociocultural factors, might cultural norms and preferences influence the *content* of BDD concerns? Like the question I posed for psychological factors, do sociocultural factors influence whether the concern focuses on the hair rather than the legs, or whether the nose is too large as opposed to too small? Does our society's obsession with a youthful appearance contribute to BDD concerns with aging?

To better answer these questions, cross-cultural comparison studies of BDD are needed. Although such studies haven't yet been done, Catherine Carter of Harvard University and I compared published case reports and case series of BDD from different countries (Japan, England, France, Germany, Italy, Russia, and the former Czechoslovakia). Comparing available case reports in this way has methodologic limitations—for example, is BDD defined similarly in different cultures? Nonetheless, our findings are interesting. They suggest that more similarities than differences exist across cultures—that there is a core, universal disorder (BDD) that may, nonetheless, have interesting cultural differences, especially in terms of the content of bodily preoccupation.

In our review we found that the sex ratio was similar in the different countries (approximately 60% men); the exception was France, where nearly 80% were women (although a recent study from France by Dr. Hantouche and his colleagues found similar numbers of men and women). Similar to what I've found in my research in this country, 85% of patients in our cross-cultural review had never been married (the average age of all cases was 25). Average age of onset was similar in different countries (age 22), with a chronic course of illness in 80% of cases. The most often cited body part was the nose, present in 45% of cases, with the eyelids the second most common concern. Eyelid concerns were mentioned only in cases from Japan and reflects the high percentage of Japanese cases in our series; I've seen few people with this particular concern in the United States. The face and cheeks were the next most common areas of concern.

Other similarities across countries were the presence of BDD behaviors, such as mirror checking and camouflaging, a high rate of being housebound, high rates of coexisting depression and anxiety, and social and occupational impairment that averaged between moderate and severe. The degree of insight most often noted (in two-thirds of cases) was in the range of fair to poor, with a fairly high frequency of delusional thinking.

Series of patients from Italy (seen by Dr. Giulio Perugi and his colleagues at the University of Pisa) and from England (seen by Dr. David Veale and his colleagues at Grovelands Priory Hospital in London) also suggest that BDD has more similarities than differences across cultures.

BDD's similarities across cultures are striking. While these findings require confirmation with more methodologically rigorous cross-cultural studies, they support a "universalist" point of view: culture appears to provide nuances and accents on a basically invariant, universal, expression of BDD.

Beauty, too, may to some extent be universal. While culture can influence what's considered beautiful, beauty is not simply in the eye of the beholder, or the eye of a specific culture. Scientists are finding surprisingly high agreement across cultures on what's considered attractive. When British researchers asked women from China, India, and England to rate pictures of Greek men, their ethnicity scarcely affected their preferences. Certain facial features—such as symmetry and smooth, unblemished skin—are considered beautiful around the world. It's noteworthy that these are common concerns of BDD sufferers.

In an intriguing twist, some researchers theorize that a universal preference for certain facial features may be innate—hard-wired into our collective brains over millions of years. Scientists have found that infants only several months old prefer to gaze at certain faces—those that adults consider attractive. Infants prefer attractive faces before they've had any significant exposure to cultural standards of beauty—before they've read Vogue or watched the soaps. Certain types of facial features, such as unblemished skin, may signal health and reproductive fitness, traits selected for by the evolutionary process. Thus, cultural views of beauty may be sculpted by evolution and biology. This theory echoes evidence that animal preferences for certain physical features, such as symmetry, are shaped by evolutionary processes.

But what constitutes beauty does vary to some degree from culture to culture. Culture affects what's considered the ideal—for example, plumpness or thinness—and this can change over time. Cultural preferences also influence whether a facial scar, for example, is considered ugly and defective or a sign of great beauty. Culture may also shape the content of BDD concerns. Just as a concern with the eyelids may be more common in Japan than in other countries, so is a fear that one's ugliness will offend other people.

Yet another important question is whether culture can influence the severity of BDD symptoms—and even whether the symptoms are expressed—in someone with the disorder. A woman in her late seventies described the following experience: "I've felt very ugly my entire life, ever since I was a child," she said. "The only time during the past 70 years that I haven't been preoccupied with how I look was for a couple of years when I lived in Fiji. Maybe it was because the culture was different. In that culture, whites were considered attractive and desirable. I wasn't concerned at all when I was there."

Triggers: Comments, Stress, and Other Possible Precipitants

"I started worrying about my skin when one of my friends in high school called me 'pizza face,'" Patrick told me. "I know he was only kidding, but it stuck in my mind. I started feeling very self-conscious about my skin." Scott started worrying about his appearance at the time his parents were getting divorced. "My parents split up unexpectedly," he said. "It was especially rough on me, because my father blamed me for the breakup. I remember in the middle of their divorce, when he was really angry about something, he said to me 'You're no longer my son.' I looked in the mirror and I thought I looked different. My whole face seemed to be sagging. I've never looked the same since."

Several authors have noted in the psychiatric literature that a chance remark about appearance may acutely trigger the onset of BDD symptoms. Examples given include "You certainly resemble your father," "You look very nice but you have got a small mouth," or "Why is your face half red and half white?" G. G. Hay, who wrote about BDD in the 1970s, reported that such a remark was at least partly responsible for the onset of BDD symptoms in 9 of his 17 patients. Several other case reports in psychiatric journals note the sudden onset of symptoms soon after a distressing event, such as a spouse's affair or abandonment by a boyfriend.

Can negative comments about appearance or stressful life events, such as parents' divorcing, cause BDD? Such factors do seem to sometimes play a role in the onset of the disorder. However, a negative comment about appearance or stress probably acts as a trigger or contributing factor, but not the only cause of BDD. In other words, such events seem to have the potential to precipitate the onset of BDD, presumably in someone who is biologically and/or psychologically vulnerable to developing the disorder. This is sometimes referred to as the vulnerability-stress hypothesis. According to this model, in a person vulnerable to developing the disorder, stress (which for BDD might include a negative comment about appearance) can precipitate the onset of symptoms. A high school teacher invoked this view when she said, "My concern about my nose was triggered by a comment about it, in a context of extreme sensitivity and low self-esteem."

One reason to think that comments or stress may act as a precipitant, as opposed to the major or only cause, is that negative comments about appearance and stress are very common. Who has never experienced significant stress? Who's never heard anything negative about how they look? Virtually everyone is teased or experiences severe stress at some point in their life, but not everyone develops BDD.

In addition, the majority of people with BDD are unable to identify a trigger of their symptoms, so a trigger doesn't appear necessary for the occurrence of BDD. Twenty-seven percent of those I've seen reported that a negative comment about their appearance triggered the onset of symptoms. In most of these cases, symptoms began abruptly and acutely, soon after the comment or stress occurred, as opposed to more gradually.

Precipitating comments are sometimes made directly to the person who subsequently develops BDD; in other cases they aren't directed at them, but are interpreted to refer to them. The comment is often clearly negative, such as "Get out of here! You're ugly!" In other cases the remark is more benign, such as "Your hair looks different today," but it's interpreted in a negative way. When one woman heard the comment, "You're red, white, and blue," which was referring to her outfit, she thought it meant that she had a red face, and she worried about it for the next 20 years.

Often the comment—like the "red, white, and blue" one—influences the content of the ensuing preoccupation. One man, for example, recalled his uncle telling him that he had an egg-shaped head and being called "egg head" by his peers. He subsequently worried about his supposedly egg-shaped head for 40 years.

Precipitating stressors are sometimes related to psychological themes that appear particularly relevant to BDD—for example, rejection by others.

Gail's BDD began right after her boyfriend broke up with her. "I was dating a man five years younger than me, and I was worried about being older than him. I was afraid he wouldn't want me because I was older. Shortly after he found out I was five years older, he broke up with me. I wondered if that was why, and I started being preoccupied with my appearance after that—that I looked too old."

In other cases, the stressor seems more general, such as marital or job stress. "My wife and I couldn't agree about whether to have children," Todd told me. "I was feeling guilty and stressed, and I started worrying about my face in that context." "The stress of work triggered my concern," Leslie said. "I had the sudden onset of obsessing and picking when things were really bad at work."

Some people report that surgery, dermatologic treatment, electrolysis, or other procedures precipitated their concern. As one woman said, "The electrolysis I had wrecked my face—now it's covered with scars." Another attributed her concern with her supposedly red face to a sunburn she'd gotten when she was 16. A 28-year-old man started obsessing about his face after he'd been hit by a softball, which he thought had permanently indented his cheek.

I've been struck by the observation that a precipitating comment is often recalled in great detail, with supreme clarity and a great deal of emotional anguish, even though it may have occurred decades earlier. The memory is sometimes accompanied by strong feelings of anger or resentment toward the commenting person. Reactions such as these seem to reflect an unusual sensitivity to negative comments, criticism, and rejection. Instead of brushing off and forgetting wounding comments, as many people do, people with BDD tend to feel them deeply, harbor them, and sometimes suffer enduring psychological pain as a result.

What Doesn't *Cause BDD*

There are a number of factors that do not or are unlikely to cause BDD. Some of them are the following:

- *Moral weakness* People do *not* get BDD because they are morally defective or weak. BDD is a psychiatric disorder with likely biological roots. It isn't caused by weakness of character. For this reason, trying harder isn't by itself an adequate solution to the problem.
- *Vanity* BDD isn't equivalent to or caused by vanity. Simply telling someone to stop being so vain won't end BDD symptoms.

- *Stress* While stress can worsen BDD symptoms, or appears to sometimes trigger its onset in someone vulnerable to developing the disorder, stress alone is not the cause of BDD. Diminishing stress may be helpful but by itself isn't adequate treatment.
- *Puberty* Some people are told that their BDD symptoms are caused by puberty. It's true that appearance concerns may develop or increase during puberty. But to say that BDD symptoms are simply due to puberty implies that they're normal and don't need to be treated. This isn't the case. By definition, BDD symptoms are more problematic than normal appearance concerns and need psychiatric treatment.

What Makes BDD Better or Worse

The question of what makes BDD symptoms better or worse is different from the question of what causes BDD, or what its risk factors are. Rather, once the disorder is present, and given that symptoms may increase and decrease in intensity, are there things that seem to affect its intensity?

BDD symptoms can wax and wane on their own, without being significantly affected by life events or stress. Often people can find no explanation for why their symptoms worsen or improve over the short run. They seem to have a life of their own. But many people say that certain factors seem to temporarily "turn up or turn down the volume" on their preoccupations and distress.

People with BDD report that the following factors can decrease the intensity of BDD concerns: exercise, seeing the body part look right, a "positive environment" (e.g., feeling accepted by others), camouflaging, being assertive, and distracting oneself with activities. As one woman said, "Work and other activities can decrease my concerns—when I'm impassioned about something, I focus less on my appearance." Patients with bipolar disorder (manic depressive illness) say that their BDD symptoms temporarily remit when they're manic. Some of these factors—for example, staying busy with activities—are helpful over the longer term. But others—such as camouflaging—actually perpetuate BDD symptoms over the longer term.

Many people with BDD report that certain factors can worsen their appearance concerns, the most common of which is seeing attractive people—in person, on television, in magazines, and in other situations. This is an example of how the media and comparing with others can worsen BDD preoccupations. Other factors reported to increase BDD symptoms are having the presence or ugliness of the defect confirmed by others, a "negative environment" (e.g., one in which the person is put down or undervalued), inactivity or unemployment, exposure of the defect to others, unflattering mirrors or lighting, haircuts, social situations, and stress. It's interesting that acral lick syndrome in dogs, which is similar to BDD grooming behaviors, can also be increased by stress.

People with acne typically report worsening of their preoccupation and distress when their acne flares. Compulsive hair cutters typically feel worse after a hair-cutting binge. Some women report that their symptoms worsen premenstrually. While social situations can make BDD symptoms more painful for many people, for a small number BDD symptoms are largely limited to social situations. As Zach explained, "When I'm by myself, my symptoms are hardly there. But as soon as I'm around people, I think they're aware of my mouth, and I'm no longer rational. I think that other people are noticing my lips. I become obsessed and anxious, and my rational thinking about them goes out the window." Social situations significantly worsened Zach's symptoms and also decreased his insight into their irrational nature.

It can be helpful to avoid some of these exacerbating factors—for example, making comparisons with others and looking through magazines at attractive people. But some of them should be faced. In the long run, exposing the defect and going to social events should actually decrease BDD symptoms.

It's fascinating to consider that some people report that they actually *look* worse in an exacerbating situation, such as a social situation. Their view of the defect seems to actually change. While such changes haven't been scientifically documented in BDD, they're similar to changes reported in some studies of normal college women and people with eating disorders. In these studies, research subjects overestimated their body size more after eating a meal high (or supposedly high) in calories or carbohydrates than after a low-calorie or low-carbohydrate meal. Data such as these suggest that exposure to feared situations can lead to a temporary worsening of perceived body image.

Concluding Thoughts

Most likely, a chain of steps is required for the development and expression of BDD. As appears to be the case for many, if not most, psychiatric disorders—as well as many medical diseases—BDD probably results from a combination of factors. Preliminary emerging clues suggest that biology may lay the groundwork for BDD and that psychological and sociocultural factors may also contribute to its occurrence. Symptoms most likely result from a complex interaction between genetic and environmental factors.

Neurobiological factors probably provide a template, making the BDD *process* of preoccupations, excessive worry, and ritualistic behaviors possible. This process appears similar to the obsessions and ritualistic behaviors of OCD and may involve similar brain abnormalities involving serotonin, other brain neurotransmitters, and certain brain structures. Perhaps neurobiological and genetic factors also increase risk for BDD by conferring an unusual sensitivity to the effect of stressful life events or negative comments about appearance.

Sociocultural and psychological factors—including psychodynamic processes, personality traits, and life experiences—probably also contribute to this process in some way, increasing the risk of BDD's occurrence. Such factors might also influence the *content* of BDD preoccupations—the focus on the body and the exact location of this focus. It's possible that neurobiological factors may also influence the content of BDD concerns, as reflected by the high rate of symmetry concerns. If BDD and OCD are eventually shown to have similar neurobiological underpinnings, it's interesting to consider whether psychological or environmental factors might influence whether BDD, as opposed to OCD, develops.

Theories about the cause of BDD should account for its usual age of onset. Does BDD commonly begin during adolescence because of the rapid and dramatic appearance changes occurring at this time? Or because adolescents normally become more self-conscious, more interested in their appearance, and judge their appearance more negatively? Might the brain development and maturation that occurs later in life contribute to the onset of BDD at this age? The multifactorial model I've proposed suggests that all these factors may play a role.

To answer the question of what causes BDD—to move beyond hypotheses and speculation—much more research is needed. We need family history studies to elucidate whether BDD is linked to—and therefore might share causal sources with—other psychiatric disorders. Twin studies are needed to elucidate the role of genetic versus environmental determinants of BDD, both likely contributors. Brain-imaging studies and neuropsychological studies are in progress and are expected to elucidate brain processes in BDD and their similarities to those in OCD, depression, eating disorders, and other disorders. Ongoing treatment studies will provide indirect yet important evidence about the cause of BDD.

Studies of psychological factors, including life events, and cross-cultural studies are also needed. The role of earlier risk factors needs to be disentangled from those that occur later and appear to trigger the onset of BDD in some cases. Because BDD may be a heterogeneous disorder, with different forms, it may ultimately be shown that the causal chain of steps varies to some degree for different variants of BDD.

Of all the unsolved mysteries about BDD, its cause is the most enigmatic. As one of my patients replied when I asked what he thought might cause his symptoms, "I have no idea. It's a mystery to me. But I hope you figure it out soon and let me know when you do."

·· *eleven* ··

Aren't We All Concerned with How We Look? BDD and Normal Appearance Concerns

We'd All Like to Look Better

Most of us care about how we look. Like it or not, appearance does matter. This is why BDD strikes a chord with so many people. BDD echoes normal appearance concerns.

Research studies confirm that most of us do want to look acceptable, if not attractive, to others. In a nationwide 1986 survey by Thomas Cash and his colleagues of 30,000 respondents published in *Psychology Today* magazine, only 18% of the men and 7% of the women who responded had little concern about their appearance and didn't do much to improve it. The vast majority thought about, paid attention to, valued, and actively worked on their appearance. Adolescents, especially females, reported the strongest appearance concerns.

There's good reason for this. Studies have fairly consistently documented that physically attractive people—both adults and children—are viewed more positively and generally are more popular with their peers than those who are unattractive. In adolescence, attractiveness influences dating. Attractive people tend to have certain other social advantages, like eliciting help and cooperation from others. In addition, the stereotype "what is beautiful is good" has been documented and confirmed by researchers. That is, attractive people are generally initially viewed by others as having more socially desirable personality traits and as being happier and more successful.

Beauty cuts both ways, however. Attractive people may also be considered more self-centered and can elicit envy. Research has shown that attractive women may be discriminated against when applying for or performing "masculine" jobs, and some people attribute the successes of attractive women to good looks. Further complicating the issue is that factors like facial expression influence views of attractiveness, and our judgments of attractiveness may change as we get to know others better. On balance, however, this body of research suggests that our society tends to view attractive people more positively and treat them better than unattractive people in a variety of ways. It also clearly documents that appearance matters.

Many other important research findings on appearance have come to light in recent years. These studies have found not only high rates of concern about appearance in the general population, but also high rates of dissatisfaction with appearance, and high rates of distorted body image. These findings raise important questions about BDD, which I'll address in this chapter. Does a high percentage of the population have BDD? How can BDD be distinguished from the normal concern with appearance that's so common? What is the relationship between BDD and normal appearance concerns?

Not only do most people care about how they look, but a significant percentage of the population *dislikes* some aspect of their appearance. And the percentage seems to be rising. A 1972 survey by Ellen Berscheid and her colleagues published in *Psychology Today* found that 23% of women and 15% of men were dissatisfied with their overall appearance. The 1986 *Psychology Today* survey previously mentioned found even higher levels of dissatisfaction: 38% of the women and 34% of the men were generally dissatisfied with their looks. Not only did the numbers rise, but the percentage of men greatly increased. Women, however, were still more unhappy than men with all body areas except their face and height.

Other studies support these findings. A study by Hesse-Biber and her colleagues in college students, for example, found that more than one-third of women and one-tenth of men were unhappy with their body. Another recent survey found that nearly one-third of teenagers worry that they weigh too much. Yet another showed that 81% of ten year olds had already dieted at least once. In general, studies indicate that women generally want to be thinner, whereas men are just as likely to want added bulk.

Further research findings document a high rate of *distorted* body image in the general population, involving both the body as a whole and specific parts, typically the waist and hips. Using a movable caliper technique, J. Kevin Thompson found that more than 95% of the women he studied overestimated their body size. Their estimates were typically one-fourth larger than their actual body size. Of interest, these same women accurately judged the body size of other people.

Similarly, the Cash *Psychology Today* survey found that 47% of females and 29% of males who were actually normal weight classified themselves as overweight. Men were equally divided between those who felt they were too heavy and those who believed they were too thin. Studies indicate that adolescents also tend to overestimate body size. Generally, women distort more than men, and distortions are greater when people are asked how they *feel* they look than when asked how they *think* they look.

So it appears that a large percentage of the population is concerned about, dislikes, and even has a distorted view of their appearance. Judith Rodin has referred to these widespread concerns as "normative discontent," a term that reflects the pervasiveness of unhappiness with one's body. BDD echoes these normal and common appearance concerns. In some ways, the concerns of people with BDD are similar to what most of us experience.

Indeed, the difference between BDD and normal appearance concerns may be largely a matter of degree. Most likely, dissatisfaction with appearance spans a continuum, from mild to moderate to severe and even disabling. BDD may be at the severe end of this continuum of concern and dissatisfaction with appearance. BDD-related behaviors may also be conceptualized as more extreme versions of normal behaviors. Grooming, checking one's appearance in the mirror, and dieting are things most people do. When done in moderation, they're common behaviors. But people with BDD carry them to an extreme.

In support of this continuum hypothesis, there's a "gray area" between mild BDD and normal appearance concerns. In some cases it can be difficult to say where normal concern leaves off and BDD begins. Does an adolescent girl who worries that her breasts are too small and who feels shy around boys as a result have BDD? Does a man with slightly thinning hair who feels anxious around women and is reluctant to ask them out on a date as a result have BDD? Cases of severe BDD are easily distinguished from normal concerns with appearance. The adolescent who won't go to school or go out with friends because of a few pimples on his face and the man who quits job after job because he thinks his buttocks are asymmetrical clearly have BDD. But what about milder concerns? How do we differentiate them from BDD? Appearance concerns are very common, and the boundary between mild BDD and normal appearance concerns is fuzzy.

The same dilemma applies to certain other psychiatric disorders that echo normal and common concerns. The boundary between normal grieving and depression, for example, is sometimes unclear. Grief after the death of a loved one is very common and expected. In some cases, it may be difficult to distinguish between a high degree of normal grief and excessive grief that is pathological and requires psychiatric treatment. It isn't difficult to differentiate moderately severe or severe cases from normal. But in milder cases, it's more difficult.

But while this "gray area" also applies to certain other psychiatric disorders, the distinction between mild BDD and normal concern may be especially unclear, given that concern with appearance is so common, if not nearly universal, especially during adolescence. In addition, cultural factors influence how the body is viewed and how much attention and concern its imperfections receive, making the boundary between normal and abnormal even less obvious.

At this time, our best guide to differentiating BDD from normal appearance concerns is the DSM-IV criteria for BDD: preoccupation, distress, and impairment. To meet criteria for BDD, the person must be preoccupied. Everyone with BDD whom I've seen has worried about their appearance for at least an hour a day. I'm reluctant to make the diagnosis in anyone who worries for less time than this, because their preoccupation may not be excessive enough to warrant a psychiatric diagnosis. But the hour-a-day guideline isn't fixed in stone and needs further empirical validation.

Appearance concerns must also cause clinically significant distress or impairment in functioning to be considered BDD. Many people with BDD experience both. One potential drawback of this definition is that "clinically significant" is a somewhat imprecise term that involves informed judgment. The opinion of a mental health professional can be helpful in determining whether appearance concerns are clinically significant. In most cases of BDD, however, the degree of preoccupation, distress, and impairment in functioning is clearly greater than what most people experience. Most people may have BDD-like concerns, but most people don't have BDD.

It's interesting to hear what people with BDD have to say about how their BDD concerns differ from the normal concerns of other people, or from normal concerns they have about other aspects of their own appearance. In making this differentiation, they often use preoccupation, distress, and impairment as their benchmarks.

Kathleen was concerned with her "wide" nose, her "fat" stomach, and the "grotesque" veins on her legs. She considered her nose concerns to constitute BDD, but she considered her stomach and vein concerns "normal." I asked her to explain the difference. "With my stomach and veins, it's different," she told me. " I can accept them and put them into perspective. My nose takes up much more of my time. I think about it a lot, and it's getting in the way of my life. My stomach and legs bother me, but they don't cause me such intense anxiety and pain. They don't keep me from socializing. My nose drives me out of my mind."

Melanie described the difference between her concerns and those of other people in a similar way: "My concern is totally obsessive—it's on my mind for hours a day—and it makes me miserable. Other peoples' appearance concerns don't make them so depressed, stop them from walking out the door, or make them unable to laugh at a joke. My concerns take all of my concentration, and they take over my life."

Kathleen's and Melanie's BDD concerns echoed normal concerns, but they were more intense and severe. They worried too much, and they suffered. I've interviewed many people with BDD who had some additional normal concerns about their appearance, which they could usually easily differentiate from their BDD concerns.

Thus, BDD appears to differ *quantitatively* from normal appearance concerns, lying at the severe end of a continuum of appearance preoccupation and dissatisfaction, differing by degree. But does BDD also differ from normal concerns in a more substantial and fundamental way? Is it also *qualitatively* different from normal appearance concerns?

The answer to this question is probably yes. BDD does seem to differ from normal appearance concerns in a number of ways other than severity. One difference is that most research findings suggest that BDD affects an approximately equal number of men and women, whereas studies of the general population indicate that more women than men dislike their appearance.

In addition, many surveys of the general population have found that weight—or aspects of appearance related to weight, such as the abdomen or hips and thighs—are the body parts most often disliked. For example, in the 1972 *Psychology Today* survey that I previously mentioned, 48% of women were dissatisfied with their weight, 50% with their abdomen, and 49% with their hips and upper thighs. Only 11% were dissatisfied with their face. Among people with BDD, however, I and other researchers have found that facial concerns are most common. While people with BDD can be preoccupied with *any* body part, they're more often concerned with their skin (usually facial skin), hair, or nose than with their hips or thighs.

Dr. James Rosen of the University of Vermont, however, has found that concern with nonfacial body parts, such as the stomach and hips, are more common than facial concerns, perhaps because his patients had less severe BDD.

Another difference (which might be considered a qualitative difference) between BDD and normal appearance concerns is that some people with BDD are preoccupied with normal-looking, or even attractive, body parts while having no concern about aspects of their appearance that others would be expected to dislike. Jennifer was so concerned with her skin—which looked fine to other people—that she was oblivious to her 25-pound weight gain. When it was brought to her attention, she didn't care about having gained the weight. I suspect, and surveys suggest, that most women would have been concerned about this change, and many would have gone on a diet. Evan, who was about 60 pounds overweight, didn't care about this—rather, he worried about his asymmetrical chest hair, which others couldn't perceive.

Another apparent qualitative difference between BDD and normal concerns is that available data suggest that BDD symptoms often diminish with medication. We wouldn't expect normal appearance concerns to decrease with medication, because the medication normalizes a "chemical imbalance"; if a chemical imbalance doesn't exist in the first place, medications wouldn't be expected to have any effect.

These differences between BDD and normal concern suggest that BDD may be qualitatively different from normal concern, with different psychological and biological processes coming into play. This seems especially likely in those with delusional BDD or delusional referential thinking. Biological studies (e.g., brain imaging) and other studies are likely to help us solve this puzzle.

The qualitative and quantitative hypotheses are not incompatible. It's possible—even likely—that BDD is *both* qualitatively and quantitatively different from normal appearance concerns. BDD may be on a continuum with normal appearance concerns—differing quantitatively, as a more severe version of normal concern. But it's likely that at some point on this continuum, qualitatively different psychological or biological mechanisms (e.g., involving the brain chemicals serotonin and/or dopamine) begin to come into play. This model is similar to that for high blood pressure: higher blood pressure is on a continuum with lower blood pressure, differing quantitatively, or by degree. But at the higher end of this continuum, qualitatively different physiologic mechanisms come into play that pose dangers to one's health.

So, if appearance concerns are very common in the general population, does a large percentage of the population, or even most people, have BDD? We don't yet know the prevalence of BDD in the general population, because large prevalence studies haven't been done. The prevalence of BDD that's found in future studies will depend in part on where the diagnostic line is drawn between normal concerns and mild BDD. Very preliminary findings by Dr. Rosen and his colleagues, based on a small study sample, suggest that BDD may affect as many as 2% of the population. Although this finding requires replication in a larger population, it's interesting. It confirms the commonsense conclusion that most people don't have BDD, but also suggests that BDD is not a rare disorder.

A Disorder of Distorted Body Image

Body image—something we all have—is a complex and elusive construct. Various definitions of body image have been offered by authors and researchers over the years. A definition offered by psychologists Thomas Cash and Thomas Pruzinsky in their book *Body Images* is the following: Body image consists of the internal, subjective representations of physical appearance and bodily experience. Another useful definition, offered decades ago by Paul Schilder, is "the picture of our own body which we form in our mind; that is to say, the way in which the body appears to ourselves." Body image is our internal self-portrait.

Body image is an umbrella term for a large number of concepts. It consists of many dimensions and has been said to include such diverse concepts as position of the body in space, perception of bodily sensations, and attractiveness. When even more broadly defined, it has been referred to as body ego, body schema, and self-concept. Body image has been said to embrace our view of ourselves, not only physically but also psychologically, sociologically, and psychologically. It has cognitive, emotional, behavioral, and perceptual dimensions. Body image is a core aspect of our identity.

The scientific literature on body image has a long and scholarly history, which has been explored by neurologists, psychologists, other social scientists, psychoanalysts, and philosophers. Luminaries such as Henry Head, Paul Schilder, Sigmund Freud, and Seymour Fisher have investigated such mysteries as how we distinguish self from non-self, and the cause of bizarre body-image experiences such as the phantom limb syndrome (the experience of still feeling the presence of one's limb following amputation) and neglect (the denial of the existence of parts of the body after brain damage).

Despite the long and rich history of body-image research, body-image disturbance in BDD has been virtually unstudied. However, some research that's been done on physical-appearance aspects of body image appears relevant to our understanding of BDD.

The "Insider"/"Outsider" View

One important and consistent finding by body-image researchers—and one clearly relevant to BDD—is that there is only a weak association between subjective body image and measures of objective attractiveness. The view from the "inside" (self-perception of physical appearance) doesn't match that from the "outside" (social perception of physical appearance) very well. In statistical terms, these two views of physical appearance typically share less than 10% variance. As Cash has stated, beauty is no guarantee of a favorable body image, nor is homeliness a decree for a negative body image.

This common mismatch is a central aspect of BDD; people with BDD view their appearance—in particular, their "defective" body area—very differently than others do. In addition, I've found that there's no association between the occurrence of BDD and actual overall attractiveness; BDD occurs in people of varying overall attractiveness, some of whom are very attractive. Furthermore, I've found no association between the actual appearance of the perceived defect per se and severity of BDD symptoms—in other words, severity of BDD symptoms is just as great in those with no defect whatsoever as in those with a present (although slight) defect. Just as in the rest of the population, "insider" and "outsider" views clearly differ in BDD.

Body Image, Depression, and Self-Esteem

Body image researchers have also discovered that in various populations—both patients and nonpatients—body-image distortion and dissatisfaction are associated with depression, low self-esteem, and general psychological distress. (What a person *actually* looks like, however, has little relationship to self-esteem.) Several researchers have found that the greater the extent of body-image distortion (e.g., size overestimation), the stronger the depression and the lower the self-esteem. Female adolescents and adults appear to suffer from these problems more than males. As Thompson cautions, most of this research has been conducted with college students, and it isn't clear how generalizable the findings are to other groups. Nonetheless, the results have been fairly consistent.

Researchers in the United States and Japan have similarly found that male and female adolescents who consider their bodies less attractive have lower self-esteem and higher depression ratings than those with a more favorable body image. Findings from the previously mentioned *Psychology*

Today survey appear to confirm these findings in adults. This study found that more than 90% of people with positive feelings about their appearance, fitness, or health reported favorable psychological adjustment (i.e., a positive self-concept, life satisfaction, and the absence of loneliness and depression). In contrast, negative evaluations of appearance, fitness, and health were associated with lower levels of psychosocial adjustment.

Another link between emotional distress and dissatisfaction with appearance comes from a dermatology study which found that patients with acne scored far lower than the general population on measures of general emotional well-being. Amazingly, patients with acne reported poorer emotional adjustment than patients with malignant melanoma, a type of skin cancer. The authors hypothesized that the low scores of acne patients were due to the lowered self-esteem that acne can cause.

In these studies, the direction of causality is generally unclear. Do body-image distortion and dissatisfaction cause depression, low self-esteem, and poorer psychological adjustment? Or do these latter factors cause poor body image? Or are the body image and other psychological factors simply associated, without a causal connection? Despite this lack of clarity, the association between poorer psychological adjustment and a dislike of, or a distorted view of, one's appearance is clear.

These results are consistent with what we know about BDD. A high percentage of people with BDD have depression. In addition, average scores on the Beck Depression Inventory in untreated people with BDD are high. Although self-esteem ratings in a large series of people with BDD aren't yet available, many report very low self-esteem and consider it a prominent aspect of their BDD. In a study I participated in of women hair pullers, conducted by Jennifer Soriano, Dr. Richard O'Sullivan, and their colleagues at Harvard Medical School, we found that women hair pullers with the lowest self-esteem were more likely to also have BDD.

The Burden, Pain, and Isolation of Actual Disfigurement

Erving Goffman and other researchers have vividly and movingly described the burden, emotional pain, and social isolation of those who are stigmatized by visible physical deformities. Such disfigurements may result from birth defects, illnesses, accidents, or other causes. In reading this literature, I've been struck by how similar the experiences of many of these people are to those of people with BDD. This makes sense. Because people with BDD think—and may be completely convinced—that their defect looks unattractive, even grotesque, it's not surprising that their experience might be similar to that of people with actual disfigurement. Indeed, some people with BDD describe themselves this way: "I'm the third ugliest person in the world," "I look like a burn victim," "I look like the Elephant Man."

Research suggests that people with facial disfigurements are very aware of their deformities and other people's reaction to them. They feel stigmatized. They may assume that all of the behavior of others who interact with them is a reaction to their appearance. This awareness of being obviously deviant in a negative way profoundly shapes their self-concept and self-esteem, which may be quite low. The visibly damaged often feel a profound sense of shame and vulnerability to exposure, devaluation, and rejection. They may feel deeply defective and not quite human. These experiences are very similar to those of many people with BDD.

Vigilance about appearance, and the fear of being ridiculed or rejected, is a constant concern. Disfigured people generally need more energy to prepare for going out in public and must cope with emotional hurdles in social situations in which the defect will be visible. When they do go out into the world, they may hide the defect by disguising it. They often try to fade into the background rather than stand out "deviantly" in the crowd. They struggle to maintain self-esteem and achieve acceptance by others. McGregor describes one reaction to facial disfigurement as "social death"— that is, badly disfigured individuals cut off their relationships with the world and go into a closet existence. Strikingly similar feelings, fears, behaviors, and isolation are experienced by many people with BDD, especially those with more severe BDD.

It could be said that an extra burden borne by people with actual deformities is that the world may actually respond to them less positively, or even with revulsion. But many people with BDD *believe* that this is how others react to them. They often think that the rest of the world shares their view of their perceived defect. A majority believe—and many are completely convinced—that people take special notice of their defects, are disgusted by them, and reject them because of how they look. They may be so absorbed in their perceived defect that they interpret virtually any kind of response by another person as a reaction to the defect. This misperception makes their experience similar to that of people with actual disfigurements.

The body-image literature also notes that people with actual physical deformities adapt quite differently to their physical defects. Environmental factors, personality, and other variables influence reactions to disabilities. This is also true in BDD, as some people are able to function relatively normally while others are disabled by their body-image concerns. It's been said that to psychologically overcome a disability, one must stop thinking about it all the time and get on with living. Paradoxically, to stop thinking about the defect is exactly what is so difficult in BDD.

The Domains of Body-Image Disturbance

Body-image disturbance—for example, in the eating disorders—is commonly considered to involve several domains: cognitive, emotional (affective), behavioral, and perceptual. While the precise nature of body image disturbance in BDD is poorly understood, it appears to involve all these domains.

Cognitive   Cognitive aspects of body-image disturbance in BDD include excessive preoccupation and self-consciousness, poor or absent insight, and referential thinking. In addition, a minimal or nonexistent physical defect is the focus of great concern, whereas an actual and very noticeable physical defect may be ignored.

Emotional (affective)   Emotional, or affective, aspects of body image disturbance in BDD include worry, distress, and fear. In addition, depression and anxiety commonly accompany BDD.

Behavioral   The distorted view of one's appearance that occurs in BDD often significantly affects functioning and frequently leads to avoidance of people and activities. In addition, the body image disturbance of BDD frequently fuels behaviors aimed at improving, hiding, examining, or reassuring oneself about the perceived defect.

Perceptual   A currently unanswered question is whether a perceptual disturbance is involved in BDD. It's my impression that in at least some, if not many or all, cases of BDD the answer is yes. Many people with BDD say that they actually *see* a physical anomaly—such as red marks on their face—that can't be observered by others. Or a minimal defect, such as a scar, is perceived to be huge and obvious. In addition, it appears that treatment with the serotonin-reuptake inhibitors sometimes corrects what seems to be a visual illusion. In a minority of cases, hallucinatory-like experiences may occur. One woman, for example, thought she heard other people call her "dog" as she walked by them; while such experiences generally aren't a prominent aspect of BDD, they are a type of perceptual distortion that can occur.

Perceptual Distortion of Body Image

Studies of perceptual distortion in the body-image literature are relevant to the question of whether a perceptual distortion occurs in BDD. Much of the research on the physical-appearance aspect of body image has focused on body image distortion—in particular, size overestimation—in eating disorders. A seminal study by Slade and Russell found that women with the eating disorder anorexia nervosa overestimated their body size, and by an amount more than normal control subjects. Subsequent studies using a variety of assessment techniques have generally confirmed these findings and have additionally found that people with bulimia also tend to overestimate their body size.

Many researchers, however, have failed to find a difference in body-image distortion in women with and without eating disorders. Overestimation of body size is not limited to individuals with eating disorders. Indeed, as previously mentioned, researchers have found that the majority of women studied misperceived and overestimated their body size to some degree. Thus, a large percentage of the population could be considered to have a distorted body image.

Although studies of the perceptual component of BDD haven't yet been done, my impression is that at least some people with BDD experience a perceptual distortion. One man said, "There's a clash between what I see and what I think. I think my worries are ridiculous. But I *see* it!" A woman told me, "I sometimes think I don't see my face correctly, that I'm like my mother after she had her stroke."

I've asked some people with BDD to draw a picture of themselves. Although I haven't done this in a systematic fashion, their drawings are revealing. The self-portraits tend to portray the disliked aspects of appearance in a prominent, distorted, and negative fashion, suggesting that perceptual distortion may be present. One woman, for example, who disliked her hair, drew herself as a stick figure with a huge mass of messy hair. This was how her hair actually looked to her. Another woman drew herself with what looked like a hair mask on her face. This is how she saw herself when she looked in the mirror. Another man, when asked to draw a picture of himself, drew only his nose—not one view of it but three! In addition, he covered all three noses with large open circles, which were the pores he perceived.

Another piece of evidence supporting the hypothesis that at least some people with BDD experience some type of perceptual distortion is that with response to a serotonin-reuptake inhibitor, some people report that the defect has disappeared. They no longer *see* it! The red spots are gone. The excessive facial hair has disappeared. They now see more hair on their head. One young man told me, after responding very well to fluvoxamine (Luvox), that his hair now looked fuller to him. He thought it was actually growing back. He wasn't sure how to explain this, but it was a definite change that he could see.

A young woman told me that within several days of responding to fluoxetine (Prozac), the excessive and dark hair disappeared from her face. "It's gone?" I asked her, amazed. "Yes, I don't see it anymore. It isn't there," she replied. "Where do you think it went?" I asked, very pleased with the change but also wondering how such a thing could have happened. "How could your face have changed so quickly? How do you think this might have happened?" "I don't know," she replied. "But it's gone." "Is it still there and looks the same, but you no longer think it's ugly, or does it actually *look* different to you—you actually don't *see* it anymore?" I asked her. "It's *gone*," she replied. "I know what I see. It's not there anymore." When she decreased her dose of Prozac, the hair reappeared.

Indeed, some people whose defects disappeared when they took a serotonin-reuptake inhibitor saw the defects again when they lowered their dose or discontinued the medication. One person told me that the holes in his teeth disappeared every time we increased his clomipramine (Anafranil). He didn't *see* them anymore. When we decreased the dose slightly to avoid side effects, the holes came back. This cycle repeated itself many times. He, too, insisted that his teeth changed visually. It wasn't that the holes were still there but he decided they weren't so ugly or that he could tolerate them better. They actually closed up.

One possible explanation for these experiences is that serotonin appears to influence vision. Animal research shows that serotonin-releasing neurons innervate the primary visual (occipital) area of the brain as well as relay stations along the brain's visual pathways between the eye and the occipital area. Serotonin seems to modulate and regulate the flow of information through the interrelated structures of the visual system. One hypothesis is that serotonin may protect animals from overreacting to unimportant sensory input. Might serotonin also protect humans from overreacting to unimportant visual input—that is, to defects in appearance that most people don't notice or consider minimal?

A patient whose BDD responded to phenelzine, a type of antidepressant known as an MAO inhibitor that also affects serotonin, had a similar experience: "I used to think I looked like Herman Munster or Lurch," he said. "I really believed it! Now I realize my vision was distorted. In the past, I was convinced. Now I know I was distorting. With the medication, my perception of myself is clearer. I see myself more accurately."

Additional Insights and Thoughts
About Body Image and BDD

What else do we know about body image in BDD? Results from the MBSRQ (Multidimensional Body-Self Relations Questionnaire) shed some light on this question. This self-report rating scale, developed by Cash and others, is a comprehensive and widely validated measure of various aspects of body image. On the appearance evaluation subscale, people with BDD generally rate their overall appearance negatively—as either mostly dissatisfied or very dissatisfied. This overall rating appears unduly influenced by the rating of the defect; they often rate other aspects of their appearance as acceptable or attractive.

Another piece of data similarily suggests that people with BDD judge their "defective" areas very negatively and inaccurately while evaluating other aspects of their appearance less negatively and more accurately, and that their negative ratings of the defect unduly impact their ratings of their overall appearance. I ask everyone with BDD who sees me the question, "*Excluding* your defect, how would you rate your attractiveness?" People with BDD tend to judge their attractiveness fairly accurately when excluding their defect. Most of the respondents to this question (62%) rated their appearance as average. Twenty-nine percent rated themselves as attractive (above average), and 21% as unattractive (below average). But when asked to rate their overall attractiveness *including* the defects, self-ratings usually worsen. A rating of average, for example, may drop to below average. One woman rated her overall appearance as 6 out of 10, where 10 equals very attractive, when excluding her defect, but when including the defect dropped it to 1 out of 10. My ratings on this question are quite different from, and more positive than, self-ratings. Many people explain the decrease in their rating by saying that the defect "takes over"; they weight it more heavily than other aspects of their appearance. As one man said, "Overall, my looks aren't too bad. I'm not ugly. But because of my nose I look ugly. All I can focus on is my nose."

These findings suggest that people with BDD generally judge their appearance accurately when they don't judge their perceived defects. But when they include their defects in their self-appraisal, their judgments become excessively negative and distorted. The perceived defect appears to dominate their views of their overall appearance.

The fact that people with BDD overfocus on their perceived defect is illustrated by self-portraits in which they emphasize the perceived defect while giving only cursory attention to other body parts. Examples are the woman who drew a massive and detailed head of hair while portraying the rest of her body as a stick figure, and the man whose self-portrait consisted only of three views of his nose.

Overfocusing, or selective attention, might lead to a type of visual distortion, in that focusing on one particular aspect of appearance gives that area visual prominence; other aspects of appearance fade into the background and may even be ignored. The view becomes unbalanced. By emphasizing the defect, it becomes unduly negative. One woman told me, "I can't even see my own face. All I see is my defect." Another said, "I focus on the negative things, and they become too prominent. I lose my balance; I get tunnel vision. I put too much weight on one particular aspect and get bogged down in it."

Overfocusing might also contribute to, or create, the perceived defect. Overfocusing might cause a minimal defect to become very noticeable to the BDD sufferer. As one person put it, focusing on a small pimple would cause it to "grow to hideous proportions." A mountain is made out of a molehill. Another woman said, "Other people say they don't see it. Maybe I look too closely. It's like I'm looking at my skin through a magnifying glass." A man I treated similarly said, "It's like when I put my thumb under a microscope—that's how I see my skin. I'm like a walking microscope— my perspective is off. I can't see my whole face the way other people do."

Another possible mechanism by which some people with BDD come to judge their defect so harshly is that they have very high standards for themselves. They want the body part of concern, or their appearance more generally, to look very good, or even perfect. This theory is similar to Thompson's "self-ideal discrepancy" hypothesis, in which dissatisfaction is proposed to result from discrepancy between the self and an ideal. "I have a different skin standard for myself," a teacher told me. "It's very high. I have to be perfect in every way." Another person said, "My perfectionism and high standards for my appearance are related to the distortion. It's why I look worse to myself than I do to others." Cecilia implied something similar when she said, "It's different when it's *you*. You care more about things like your skin when it's *your* skin. Other people might not think it looks so bad, but that's because it's not on them." I've already discussed the additional possibility that some, if not many, people with BDD experience a perceptual distortion, whereby the perceived defect appears physically different than it appears to other people. While the mechanism by which people with BDD judge their appearance so negatively remains unclear, the fact that they do so is abundantly clear.

As is true for so many aspects of BDD, the body image aspects need to be further studied. Do people with BDD experience a visual illusion, and, if so, what is the nature of this distortion? How does it come about? Is greater perceptual distortion in BDD related to more severe depression and lower self-esteem, as has been found in body image studies of eating-disordered women and other groups?

There are many assessment instruments that measure various aspects of appearance-related body-image disturbance, both perceptual and subjective. These techniques should be used in studies of BDD. One limitation of existing measures of perceptual distortion is that many focus on size estimation. Studies of other types of perceptual distortions, which may occur in BDD, are also needed.

And there are other unanswered questions. How do people with BDD judge the appearance of others? Some say they don't assess others harshly—they only judge themselves that way. But others say they have very high standards for everyone.

What are the similarities and differences between the body-image distortions of BDD and those of other psychiatric disorders, such as the eating disorders anorexia nervosa and bulimia nervosa, schizophrenia, and depression? The body-image distortions that sometimes occur in schizophrenia generally differ from those of BDD in that they are "bizarre" (e.g., "I have a radio in my teeth that's playing all the time"). It appears that the body dissatisfaction and distortions that sometimes occur in depression aren't as prominent as those in BDD, or as clearly focused on specific aspects of appearance or accompanied by prominent and time-consuming ritualistic behaviors. But body-image disturbances in these disorders—with the exception of the eating disorders—haven't been well studied or compared to those in BDD. Studies are also needed that compare the experiences of people with BDD with those who have actual and severe physical deformities.

The time has come to further explore body-image disturbance in BDD. Now that we can identify the disorder and can with reasonable accuracy distinguish those who have BDD from those who don't, we can begin to shed some light on that elusive, internal self-portrait.

·· twelve ··

Anorexia Nervosa, Obsessive Compulsive Disorder, Koro, and Other Disorders—Are They Relatives of BDD?

"For the past three months I've been giving off a body odor. It smells like a swamp, dug up mud, a rotten smell; it comes from my guts. I can't go anywhere. I don't want to go with my friends, and I think I've lost them on account of that."　　　　**A Patient**

*T*his description of a rotten-smelling body odor that leads to social isolation has much in common with BDD. Reminiscent of BDD are the embarrassing preoccupation with a bodily concern, the fear that others perceive the problem when in fact they don't, and the resulting loss of friends.

The quotation refers to olfactory reference syndrome (ORS), an under-recognized syndrome characterized by a concern with emitting a foul body odor—often flatulence, sweat, bad breath, or an anal or genital odor. Is ORS related to BDD? Might they even be the same disorder? And what is BDD's relationship to other psychiatric disorders, such as anorexia nervosa, a disorder in which people think they're too fat when in reality they're too thin?

And what about the relationship between BDD and obsessive compulsive disorder or koro? Like BDD, OCD is an often-secret disorder consisting of obsessional thoughts that are difficult to resist or control. Instead of focusing on appearance, they focus on contamination or on sexual, violent, or other themes. And most people with OCD, like those with BDD, compulsively do things over and over that are hard not to do—washing their hands again and again or checking the stove or a lock 30, 50, or 100 times a day.

Koro is a fascinating syndrome that usually afflicts men and occurs primarily in epidemics in China. Men with koro fear that their penis is retracting into their abdomen, which will kill them. Understandably panicked, they implore others—family members or emergency-room doctors—to pull on their penis with various types of clamps and retractors.

Whether BDD is related to these other disorders is an interesting and important question. If it is, it would follow that the same treatment approaches might be effective for BDD. Or, because they would probably run together in families—as related disorders tend to do—we could predict that relatives of people with BDD would be at increased risk for a related disorder, and vice versa.

Although scientific evidence isn't available to definitively answer all the questions I'll pose in this chapter, it does allow us to come to some reasonable conclusions—for example, that BDD is not a form of schizophrenia. While BDD may be related to depression, BDD isn't simply a symptom of depression. Available data also suggest that BDD and OCD are probably closely linked. And BDD's relationship with koro? This is yet another mystery to be solved.

BDD: Symptom or Illness?

Before I discuss the relationship between BDD and other psychiatric disorders, I'll first briefly address a larger issue that's been debated over the years. Is BDD a separate psychiatric disorder, as it's presumed to be in DSM-IV, or is it instead a nonspecific symptom that can occur in a variety of disorders, such as schizophrenia, depression, and personality disorders? As Dr. Nancy Andreasen wrote in 1977, is BDD a symptom of an underlying disease, or is it itself a separate disease entity?

Table 7 presents three hypotheses on this issue:

Hypotheses 1 and 2 propose that BDD is a symptom, of either a variety

---

Table 7   Hypotheses on Whether BDD Is a Symptom or an Illness

Hypothesis	Medical Analogy
1. BDD is a *nonspecific symptom* that can occur in a *wide variety* of psychiatric disorders (such as schizophrenia, depression, or personality disorders)	BDD is like a fever
2. BDD is a symptom or form of another specific psychiatric disorder (not of a wide variety of psychiatric disorders, as proposed by hypothesis 1)	BDD is like the butterfly rash in lupus
3. BDD is a distinct diagnostic entity— that is, a *separate* psychiatric *disorder*	BDD is like diabetes

---

of illnesses (hypothesis 1) or of a specific illness (hypothesis 2). Hypothesis 1 proposes that BDD is like a fever, which is a nonspecific symptom that can occur in a wide variety of illnesses, from chicken pox to strep throat to cancer. Hypothesis 2 proposes that BDD is similar to the butterfly rash in lupus, an autoimmune disease. The rash occurs on the face and is a fairly characteristic symptom of lupus. Somewhat similarly, some authors have considered BDD a form of schizophrenia; in Japan, BDD is viewed as a type of social phobia. And in ICD-10, DSM-IV's international counterpart, BDD is classified as a type of hypochondriasis. In contrast, hypothesis 3 proposes that BDD is a separate disorder—like diabetes—rather than a symptom of another underlying disorder or illness.

Which hypothesis is correct is important for several reasons. If hypothesis 1 is correct, then treatment would presumably be directed at whatever the underlying disorder was thought to be. If in one person it were determined to be schizophrenia, the schizophrenia would be treated. If in another person it were determined to be OCD, the OCD would be treated. The BDD symptoms would be expected to resolve as the underlying illness did.

If BDD is a symptom of a particular other psychiatric disorder (hypothesis 2), then treatment would in all cases be directed at that one underlying disorder. But if BDD is a separate illness (hypothesis 3), then treatment would be directed at the BDD itself. Treatment directed at another coexisting illness—if one were present—wouldn't necessarily be expected to successfully treat the BDD.

What I've written about BDD to this point has implied that it's a separate disorder, and indeed it's classified as such in DSM-IV. But some authors have proposed that hypotheses 1 or 2 more accurately describe BDD's relationship to other disorders. G. G. Hay, a British psychiatrist, proposed hypothesis 1 when he wrote in 1983 that "dysmorphophobia is a symptom, not a diagnosis or an illness"; he believed that it could occur as a symptom of a "variety of psychiatric syndromes." Hay thought that the underlying illness could vary from a personality problem (such as a "sensitive" personality type) to schizophrenia to mood disorder.

It seems unlikely that this hypothesis is valid. First, BDD is a well-defined syndrome, with characteristic symptoms and behaviors, that has been consistently described around the world for the past 100 years. Its features aren't identical to those of any other psychiatric disorder, let alone a variety of psychiatric disorders. Also compelling is what patients say. Sixty-two percent of those I've seen have reported that BDD is their most severe and primary problem or their only problem, suggesting that BDD isn't simply a nonspecific symptom of other psychiatric problems or disorders. In addition, BDD can occur in the absence of other psychiatric disorders. If BDD were simply a nonspecific symptom of other disorders, it would be expected that symptoms of some other disorder, such as schizophrenia or depression, would always be present, which isn't always the case.

Furthermore, when BDD does coexist with another disorder, it shouldn't be assumed that the BDD is "secondary," or due to the other disorder. It used to be thought that if OCD and major depression coexisted, then the OCD was a symptom of the depression, or, similarly, that if panic disorder and major depression coexisted, the panic disorder was a symptom of the depression. This view is no longer considered tenable. If two disorders are present, one isn't necessarily a symptom of the other; both disorders should be diagnosed. BDD is no different.

Finally, preliminary data suggesting that BDD responds to a specific medication treatment— SRIs—but not to other medications casts doubt on hypothesis 1. With the exception of OCD, no other psychiatric disorder has been demonstrated to respond *preferentially* to the SRIs.

While all this evidence suggests that hypothesis 1 is unlikely to be true, we need better data on the cause of BDD to more definitively answer the question "nonspecific symptom versus disorder?" When we know its cause, and whether it's the same as that of other disorders, we'll be able to answer this question. Brain-imaging studies and other research findings will shed light on this issue in the coming years.

What about hypothesis 2 versus 3? Is BDD a symptom of a *particular* other psychiatric disorder, such as OCD, or is it a *distinct disorder?* Until we know what causes BDD, we need to approach this question by assessing similarities and differences between BDD and other disorders in a variety of domains, such as symptoms, age of onset, course over time, and treatment response. The more similar two disorders are in these ways, the more likely they are to be related. In addition, if two disorders commonly coexist with each other or with the same disorders, this is further evidence for their similarity. And if two disorders both occur at a relatively high rate in family members, this is further evidence that they may be related. If they're the same in all of these ways, they may very well be the same disorder.

Table 8 on the next page summarizes characteristics of BDD and other disorders, which we can use to weigh the evidence to evaluate whether BDD might be related to another disorder. Unfortunately, there are no direct comparison studies of these disorders with BDD, except for BDD and OCD. In the future, when more is known, such a table will ideally include a "cause" category, which will provide the best evidence on the relationship of BDD to these disorders. In the meantime, it appears that BDD isn't identical to any other psychiatric disorder but that it has similarities to some of them, especially OCD, which suggests that they are related.

Obsessive Compulsive Disorder: Obsessional Worries and Compulsive Behaviors

Nina constantly worried that she'd throw her children out the window or cut them with a knife. She frequently checked to make sure she hadn't harmed them and that they were okay. "The thoughts don't make any sense to me," she said, "I would never hurt anyone, especially my children, but I can't stop thinking them."

Mark constantly worried that he'd get sick from dirt or germs. He feared that his house would become dirty, which could make him and his family ill. To prevent contamination and illness, Mark washed his hands for several hours a day. He refused to allow visitors in his home, and whenever he, his wife, or his children entered the house he had them change their clothes and take a shower.

Obsessive compulsive disorder (OCD) is an often-debilitating disorder characterized by obsessions (intrusive, recurrent, unwanted ideas, thoughts, or impulses that are difficult to dismiss despite their disturbing nature) and compulsions (repetitive behaviors, either observable or mental, that

Table 8 Strength of Evidence for the Hypothesis That BDD Is Related to Other Psychiatric Disorders

	Symptoms	Male/Female Ratio	Age at Onset and Course	Co-occurrence	Family History	Treatment Response
OCD	Supports	Strongly supports	Strongly supports	Supports	Supports	Strongly supports
Social phobia	Supports	Strongly supports	Supports	Supports	?	Mixed
Eating disorder	Supports	Strongly refutes	Supports	Mixed	Refutes	Mixed
Depression	Mixed	Refutes	Refutes	Supports	Strongly supports	Mixed
Hypochondriasis[a]	Supports	Strongly supports	Supports	Refutes	Strongly refutes	Mixed
Schizophrenia	Mixed	Supports	Mixed	Strongly refutes	Strongly refutes	Refutes
Olfactory reference syndrome	Strongly supports	Supports	Supports	?	?	Mixed
Koro (epidemic form)[b]	Supports	Strongly refutes	Strongly refutes	?	?	Refutes

[a] The evidence more strongly supports a relationship between BDD and the variant of hypochondriasis with many similarities to OCD.
[b] Some cases of koro (the "nonepidemic" form) appear much more similar to BDD; some probably should be diagnosed as BDD instead of koro.

are intended to reduce the anxiety caused by obsessions). Obsessions and compulsions are also hallmarks of BDD. The most common OCD obsession is fear of contamination, followed by pathological doubt (e.g., a fear that the house will burn down because the stove wasn't turned off), need for symmetry, and aggressive obsessions. The most common compulsion is checking, followed by washing, symmetry (a need to order or arrange things "perfectly" or perform certain behaviors symmetrically or in a balanced way), a need to ask or confess, and counting.

OCD appears to be the disorder most similar to BDD. Reflecting their apparent similarities, BDD is included in the Y-BOCS Symptom Checklist, the most commonly used instrument to assess the presence of OCD symptoms. Indeed, many patients with OCD are misdiagnosed with BDD, reflecting their similarities.

Similarities between BDD and OCD have been noted for the past century. In the late 1800s, Enrique Morselli stressed the obsessional and compulsive nature of BDD symptoms. He stated that patients with BDD are frequently "caught by the doubt of deformity" and noted that they compulsively check their appearance. In 1903, Pierre Janet classified BDD symptoms within a class of syndromes similar to OCD, referring to BDD as the *obsession de la honte du corps,* or obsession with shame of the body.

BDD and OCD are both characterized by obsessional thinking and by doubting, worry, and anxiety. More than 90% of people with BDD and OCD engage in compulsive, repetitive behaviors that are intended to decrease anxiety caused by the obsessions. In addition to this similar *process,* the *content* of the two disorders can overlap. Both BDD and OCD can be characterized by a desire for symmetry (of a body part in BDD and of other things in OCD), a concern that something "isn't right" (a body part in BDD and other things in OCD), and a need for perfection. Both disorders are also characterized by checking (e.g., mirrors in BDD and locks in OCD), skin picking (to improve appearance in BDD and as a pure compulsion or to cleanse in OCD), and repeated requests for reassurance (about appearance in BDD and about other things in OCD—e.g., that someone wasn't harmed).

BDD and OCD symptoms are occasionally so similar that it's difficult to differentiate them, as Brian's experience illustrates. Brian was a high school student who was preoccupied with his "stupid-looking" hair, "long" nose, and mild acne. He also had classic OCD, including contamination fears. Brian spent hours a day in the mirror, combing his hair and picking his skin. To "prevent bad skin," he also engaged in time-consuming OCD-like rituals. For example, he repeatedly walked through his dining room until he could do it without stepping on "spots" on the wooden floor that symbolized his acne. While drinking out of a glass, he repeatedly lifted the glass until he could do it without catching a glimpse of bumps on the ceiling or "spots" (i.e., anything small, red, and round) in his environment that reminded him of his acne. When sitting down, he had to sit repeatedly, until he could do so without feeling an acne-like bump on the chair. Brian believed that if he didn't perform these OCD-like rituals perfectly, his acne would worsen. In addition, to prevent an "acne breakout," he forbade anyone—himself or his family members—to move the radio. Over time, Brian performed these rituals not to improve his skin but to prevent general harm from occurring—a classic OCD concern.

Brian's experience illustrates the extent to which BDD and OCD symptoms can be interwoven. His unusual path through the dining room, his drinking and sitting behaviors, and his magical thinking about the radio are more characteristic of OCD than of BDD. Yet these behaviors were a response to his preoccupation with his skin—a classic BDD concern. In addition, he initially performed these behaviors to prevent an acne breakout but later to prevent general harm, a symptom of OCD. In this case, it was difficult to determine where BDD left off and OCD began. It furthermore suggests that BDD and OCD may be closely related.

Because I was intrigued by the apparent similarities between BDD and OCD, I did a study with Dr. Susan McElroy of the University of Cincinnati School of Medicine and with Craig Gunderson and Drs. Gopinath Mallya and William Carter of Harvard Medical School in which we compared 53 consecutive people with BDD to 53 consecutive people with OCD. We found that the two disorders were similar in terms of most of the variables we examined: sex ratio and other demographic variables, age at onset, course of illness (often chronic), impairment, and lifetime rate of most of the coexisting disorders that we assessed. BDD and OCD also commonly co-occurred: 15% of OCD patients had coexisting BDD, and about a third of those with BDD had coexisting OCD. Illness severity scores (as assessed by the Yale-Brown Obsessive Compulsive Scale) were nearly identical. The two groups were also largely similar in terms of family history of psychiatric disorders. In addition, BDD's possible preferential response to serotonin-reuptake inhibitors and to cognitive-behavioral therapy is strikingly similar to OCD's well-documented preferential response to these treatments.

However, we also found some notable differences. People with BDD were less likely to have ever been married (13% versus 39%) and more likely to have had suicidal ideation (70% versus 47%) or made a suicide attempt (22% versus 8%) because of their disorder. Those with BDD also had an earlier onset of major depression (19 versus 25 years) and a higher lifetime rate of major depression (85% versus 55%) and social phobia (49% versus 19%). They also had a higher rate of alcohol or drug abuse or dependence in their first-degree relatives. These results suggest that BDD and OCD have many similarities and are probably closely related, but that they also have some notable differences and are probably not identical.

Another obvious difference between BDD and OCD is the content of the preoccupations. Although I just noted that the content is sometimes very similar, it's usually quite different. While BDD focuses on defective appearance, OCD often fixates on such fears as becoming ill, causing harm, and the possible occurrence of dire events. In OCD, the fear underlying such thoughts often is *"What if something terrible happens and I'm responsible?"* In contrast, in BDD, the underlying fear often involves feelings of shame and low self-esteem, and is often interpersonal in nature: *"What if I'm rejected or go unloved?"*

BDD and OCD also differ in that insight in OCD appears to usually be better than in BDD, a finding reported by Drs. Daphne Simeon, Eric Hollander, and their colleagues of Mount Sinai University School of Medicine. Dr. Jane Eisen of Brown University and I have also found this and have in addition found that referential thinking is common in BDD but rare in OCD. In addition, it's my impression that BDD rituals are less likely than OCD rituals to temporarily relieve anxiety and that they often increase anxiety. In addition, BDD appears to cause more social difficulties, including problems in intimate relationships.

A case report published by Dr. Linda Barr and her colleagues at Yale, which I described in Chapter 10, suggests that there may be physiological differences between BDD and OCD. The patient with BDD who underwent acute experimental dietary depletion of the amino acid tryptophan, which likely led to decreased serotonin levels, experienced dramatic worsening of her BDD symptoms as well as her depression. But her OCD symptoms didn't get worse. This finding suggests that BDD and OCD may have a somewhat different underlying pathophysiology and are not identical disorders.

I would conclude, on the basis of available evidence, that BDD is closely related to OCD but that the two disorders aren't identical. A reflection of this hypothesis, BDD is often referred to as an "OCD-spectrum disorder"— one of a number of disorders (including Tourette's disorder, hypochondriasis, eating disorders, and trichotillomania [hair pulling]) that share clinical features with OCD and are postulated to be related to it. I would hypothesize that BDD is one of the OCD-spectrum disorders that will be demonstrated to be most closely related to OCD, but that it will also be shown to have some important differences.

It's interesting to hear what patients with both BDD and OCD have to say about similarities and differences between their BDD and OCD symptoms. One patient often tells me that the symptoms seem so similar that he's certain that BDD and OCD are the same disorder. But, like many people with both disorders, Alex saw some differences as well as similarities. "They're similar because they both go over and over in your mind," he said. "They're both obsessions and they're hard to resist. But they have a different kind of pain. The OCD is more senseless—it's more crazy. There's a kernel of truth to the BDD. When I'm alone, the OCD is more frequent and more painful, and it drains me more because I worry about it so much. When I'm in public, the BDD and my fear of rejection are much greater than the OCD. I'm more limited socially by the BDD." Another man said something similar about BDD: "There's a social humiliation and isolation that doesn't happen with OCD."

Renee described her experience as follows: "My BDD concerns seemed more reasonable to me, whereas my OCD concerns had *no* basis in reality. They seemed crazy and senseless. . . . My BDD seems pettier than my OCD, and yet it affected my self-esteem more because appearance is so important, especially during adolescence. Even though my OCD was more severe than my BDD, the BDD hurt me more socially because people could see the problem; I couldn't keep it a secret. It's harder to discuss the BDD because it's harder to describe the sadness and loneliness that goes with it. . . . I felt worse and more self-conscious around people with the BDD than with the OCD."

Bill's comparison was similar: "They're alike in a lot of ways, but the OCD is irrational and senseless. The BDD is true; it makes sense. The BDD has a much worse effect on your social life. Everyone can see it. You can't hide it like you can hide OCD. . . . My OCD rituals gave me some relief— each check temporarily relieved my anxiety. The BDD rituals didn't relieve my anxiety even temporarily. The BDD made me suicidal."

Social Phobia: *Social Anxiety, Embarrassment, and Avoidance*

BDD also has many similarities to social phobia, an anxiety disorder characterized by an excessive fear of social or performance situations in which the person is exposed to unfamiliar people or to scrutiny by others and fears they'll do something embarrassing or humiliating. The excessive fear may occur in most social situations (generalized type) or in specific situations, such as speaking in public or eating or writing in front of others.

Natasha had felt extremely anxious and fearful in social situations since childhood. "I've always been really nervous around other people," she said. "Even in grade school. I'd miss school on days I had to give a book report in front of the class. I've never gone to parties because I'm afraid I'll do something embarrassing, like blushing or saying or doing the wrong thing." As a result of her social phobia, Natasha didn't date and had no friends. She spent most of her time alone at home.

Fear and anxiety in social situations, as well as avoidance of those situations, are also very common in BDD. In fact, in Japan, BDD is considered a member of a larger group of disorders (Taijin Kyofushu) that is similar to social phobia. Taijin Kyofushu is a common Japanese disorder characterized by the fear of offending or hurting others through one's awkward social behavior or physical defect. In support of the view that BDD is a type of social phobia, patients report that BDD symptoms often intensify in social situations, and occasionally are present primarily in social situations.

BDD and social phobia are both characterized by social anxiety and avoidance, fear of scrutiny, feelings of shame, preoccupation with others' views of the person, fear of negative evaluation, and fear of embarrassment, humiliation, and rejection. A difference, however, is that social phobia doesn't focus on appearance concerns and doesn't usually involve compulsive behaviors.

Some symptoms have features of both BDD and social phobia, underscoring their similarities. For example, a fear of blushing (erythrophobia) in social situations has features of both social phobia (fear of looking embarrassed) and BDD (fear of facial redness). As shown in Table 8, the sex ratio, age at onset, and course of illness are also similar. In addition, BDD and social phobia often co-occur. Treatment response has both similarities and differences. The medications with greatest demonstrated efficacy in generalized social phobia are the MAO inhibitors; in specific social phobia, medications known as beta blockers have been demonstrated to be effective. Although adequate studies of these medications are lacking in BDD, the beta blockers don't appear to be effective, and the MAO inhibitors seem of intermediate effectiveness (less effective than the SRIs but more effective than many other medications). As for BDD, SRIs have been shown in preliminary studies to be effective for generalized social phobia, and cognitive-behavioral strategies are also effective for social phobia.

To better evaluate similarities and differences between social phobia and BDD, studies are needed that directly compare people with BDD to people with social phobia. I and Dr. Joseph Penn of Brown University School of Medicine have done a variation on such a study in which we compared a series of people with BDD alone to a series of people with BDD *plus* social phobia. We found that the two groups didn't differ in terms of most of the variables we examined (demographics, clinical features, coexisting disorders, and level of functioning). Of interest, the two groups had similarly high degrees of introversion; the fact that the addition of social phobia to BDD didn't increase introversion scores highlights the high degree of introversion in many people with BDD. Treatment response of BDD symptoms (assessed in an uncontrolled fashion) was also similar in the two groups; those with coexisting social phobia were *not* more likely to respond to MAO inhibitors, as might be expected.

But we did find a few interesting differences between the groups: those with both BDD and social phobia, as opposed to BDD alone, were less assertive and had higher rates of lifetime alcohol abuse or dependence (51% versus 20%) and drug abuse or dependence (36% versus 20%).

Our finding of many similarities between the two groups is interesting, since the group with both BDD and social phobia might be expected to be more introverted, less likely to be married, and more impaired in their functioning. The relative lack of differences might be explained by the fact that most people with BDD have social phobia *secondary* to BDD (i.e., apparently due to BDD), which might obscure expected differences between the groups.

On balance, BDD and social phobia have many similarities, although they appear to have more differences than BDD and OCD. It's quite possible that BDD is closely related to both OCD *and* social phobia, and that all three disorders are related to one another.

Eating Disorders: Disturbed Body Image and Eating Behavior

Might BDD and anorexia nervosa be related disorders, or even variants of the same disorder? Their similarities make this a reasonable and intriguing question. I've in fact received letters from young women who assume they have BDD—yet, as best I can tell, they appear to have anorexia or another eating disorder. In some cases, the symptoms of BDD and the eating disorders closely overlap, making it difficult to differentiate them.

Anorexia nervosa, bulimia nervosa, and BDD all have at their core a preoccupation with the appearance of the body and a distorted body image. In anorexia, the distortion consists of thinking one is too fat, which leads to excessive weight loss, usually to the point of appearing emaciated and very malnourished. Yet the person with anorexia thinks she looks fine, or even—at a weight of 60, 70, or 80 pounds—too fat. People with bulimia binge on food in an out-of-control way and attempt to counteract the effect of the binges by vomiting, using laxatives or diuretics (water pills), excessively exercising, or other means.

BDD and the eating disorders are also similar in that both often involve compulsive behaviors such as mirror checking and body measuring. BDD sometimes involves unusual eating or excessive dieting—for example, when trying to make one's face less wide. BDD can also fixate on body areas that are typically focused on in anorexia and bulimia, such as the size of the stomach, hips, or thighs.

However, there are some differences. One difference is that people with BDD, unlike those with anorexia, actually look normal. People with anorexia really look emaciated—in some cases like concentration camp victims—but the more abnormal their appearance becomes, the better they think they look. As they lose weight, they often report feeling more satisfied and more in control of their body and their life. They typically defend their strikingly abnormal, skeleton-like appearance as looking right, or even too fat. If they camouflage their body with bulky clothing, the purpose is generally to prevent others from seeing how thin they are and telling them to gain weight. In contrast, people with BDD nearly always feel exceedingly distressed and out of control as a result of how they look. They camouflage out of a deep sense of shame and a desire to prevent further embarrassment by exposing the defect.

Another difference is that people with eating disorders typically focus primarily on overall body weight, whereas in BDD the focus is more often on specific body parts, often facial features. However, this distinction can break down to some degree, in that individuals with anorexia often also have more focused complaints—for example, the size of their stomach or thighs. And some people with BDD are concerned with their overall appearance, such as general ugliness or overall body build. "Reverse anorexia," which I previously described and which is considered a type of BDD, consists of a preoccupation that one's overall body size is too small.

As shown in Table 8, BDD and the eating disorders differ in terms of male-to-female ratio, with women constituting the vast majority (more than 90%) of people with eating disorders. However, the disorders have a similar age of onset and course of illness. With regard to co-occurrence, I've found that 10% of people with BDD also have an eating disorder, which is much higher than in the general population but lower than might be expected if BDD and the eating disorders were closely related. Dr. Hollander, however, found that 20% of 50 patients with BDD had a coexisting eating disorder. Available family history data refute the hypothesis that the disorders are related—both I and Dr. Hollander have found that only 4% of first-degree relatives of patients with BDD had an eating disorder.

Data on treatment response give mixed support for the hypothesis that BDD and the eating disorders are related. Although recent preliminary data suggest that anorexia may respond to SRIs, the response in anorexia appears to occur less frequently and to be less robust than it often is in BDD. And while bulimia responds well to the SRIs, unlike BDD it also responds to a wide range of antidepressant medications.

There's a gray area between BDD and the eating disorders, where the symptoms overlap and the correct diagnosis is sometimes unclear. Jean, for example, was preoccupied with her supposedly large hips. She occasionally dieted but didn't otherwise meet criteria for an eating disorder. Did she have BDD or an "eating disorder not otherwise specified"? If the concerns focus on the hips, stomach, or thighs but not on overall body weight, and the person doesn't have notably abnormal eating behavior or otherwise meet criteria for an eating disorder, I diagnose BDD. Most of the people I've seen with such concerns also had other classic BDD concerns, such as an excessive preoccupation with facial features. However, I don't diagnose BDD if the only preoccupation is body weight, because of my concern that an eating disorder may be the more appropriate diagnosis.* But some researchers do consider a concern with weight alone to constitute BDD. This issue remains controversial, and more research is needed to determine the correct approach in cases such as these.

A related question is whether the diagnostic hierarchy in DSM-IV is correct. This hierarchy states that BDD shouldn't be diagnosed if body-image concerns are better accounted for by another psychiatric disorder, such as anorexia nervosa. But might the eating disorders actually be a form of BDD? Many eating disorder researchers consider disturbed body image, not disturbed eating behavior, to be the core abnormality in the eating disorders. After all, people with these disorders eat abnormally because they don't like how they look. Perhaps the hierarchy should be reversed, and the eating disorders considered a form of BDD!

On balance, BDD and the eating disorders have many similarities but also some notable differences. They do not appear to be identical disorders. Until we know more about their relationship, it's best to consider them

---

* If a person's only concern is with body weight and being or becoming fat, and they also meet other required criteria for an eating disorder, the eating disorder, rather than BDD, should be diagnosed. Diagnosis becomes more complicated if abnormal eating behavior is present but criteria for full-fledged anorexia or bulimia aren't met. I often give the diagnosis of "eating disorder not otherwise specified" in such cases.

separate disorders and to try to carefully differentiate them in research studies. We have much to learn about the overlap of these possibly related disorders of disturbed body image.

Depression

Because BDD so often coexists with depression, it's reasonable to consider whether it's a symptom of depression, rather than a separate disorder (hypothesis 2). Several lines of evidence indicate that this isn't the case. First, preliminary data suggest that BDD responds poorly to electroconvulsive therapy (ECT, or shock therapy) and to antidepressants other than the serotonin-reuptake inhibitors, to which depression responds very well. In addition, patients not uncommonly report that ECT or an antidepressant other than a serotonin-reuptake inhibitor alleviates their depression but not their BDD, which wouldn't be expected if BDD were a symptom of the depression. Some say that the severity of their depression and BDD symptoms can worsen or improve independently of each other—another reason to think BDD isn't simply a symptom of depression. In addition, I've found that in the majority of cases in which BDD and depression coexist, BDD began more than a year before the depression, which is another clue that BDD isn't a symptom of depression.

Other apparent differences between BDD and depression include depression's more frequent occurrence in women than in men, later age of onset, and less chronic course. While feelings of unattractiveness might occur in depression as a reflection of low self-esteem, depression doesn't involve prominent preoccupations with specific aspects of appearance or prominent and time-consuming compulsive behaviors such as mirror checking and reassurance seeking.

But might BDD be *related to* major depression? As shown in Table 8, on balance the evidence is mixed. Strongest evidence comes from comorbidity and family history data. A very high percentage of people with BDD have lifetime major depression; conversely, there appears to be a surprisingly high rate of BDD among people with major depression (see Appendix C). In addition, I and my colleagues have found high rates of major depression in first-degree relatives of people with BDD. Through interviews with BDD patients (which is likely to underestimate the rates of illness in relatives), we found that 17% of first-degree relatives had major depression, which was higher than for any other disorder we assessed. And the intriguing case report by Dr. Barr and her colleagues, in which the patient who underwent acute tryptophan depletion experienced a worsening of both BDD *and* de-pression, suggests a relationship between these disorders.

In summary, available evidence indicates that BDD isn't simply a symp-tom of depression (hypothesis 2), but it does suggest that BDD may be *related to* depression. Psychiatrists James Hudson and Harrison Pope have hypothesized that there is a family of disorders—known as "affective spec-trum disorders"—related to one another, which share a pathophysiologic "step" in the causal chain of steps required for their expression. This hy-pothesis is based on the fact that a number of psychiatric disorders respond to antidepressants, and it is further supported by similarities in co-occur-rence and family history. Although more data are needed on BDD's treat-ment response, available evidence suggests that it, too, may be an "affective spectrum disorder"—related to major depression as well as to other disor-ders in the affective spectrum family, including OCD, eating disorders, and social phobia.

Hypochondriasis: Bodily Preoccupation and Illness Fears

In the ICD-10 Classification of Mental and Behavioural Disorders (an inter-national classification manual), BDD is classified as a type of hypochondria-sis. Hypochondriasis consists of a preoccupation with fears of having, or the idea that one has, a serious disease. The preoccupation is based on a misinterpretation of bodily symptoms and persists despite appropriate med-ical evaluation and reassurance.

Comparing BDD and hypochondriasis is complicated by the likelihood that hypochondriasis has different subtypes—one that's more similar to OCD and one more similar to somatization disorder (see Appendix A for a description). The subtype that's more similar to OCD is also more similar to BDD.

BDD and hypochondriasis are similar in that they both involve bodily fears and preoccupations, and sufferers frequently seek medical treatment. Repetitive body checking and reassurance seeking are also common to both. Moreover, the two disorders are similar in terms of male-to-female ratio, and they have a similar early age of onset and chronic course with waxing and waning symptoms.

However, the focus in BDD is on appearance rather than on illness. In addition, available data on co-occurrence and family history appear to re-fute the hypothesis that BDD is a symptom of, or even closely related to, hypochondriasis. In my series, only 3% of people with BDD had coexisting hypochondriasis, and Dr. Hollander found that 10% of 50 patients with BDD had hypochondriasis—rates far lower than those for many other disorders. In addition, Dr. Hollander found that no BDD patients in his series had family members with hypochondriasis.

A comparison of the treatment response of BDD and hypochondriasis is limited by the lack of controlled studies. Dr. Brian Fallon of Columbia University found in a preliminary uncontrolled trial of 16 patients with hypochondriasis that 10 had a good response to fluoxetine (Prozac). In addition, preliminary data suggest that hypochondriasis may respond to cognitive-behavioral therapy, similar to BDD. However, in another uncontrolled study, other researchers reported a good response to the non-SRI antidepressant imipramine, which doesn't appear effective for BDD.

Overall, it appears that BDD is not identical to, or a variant of, hypochondriasis. However, it's possible that BDD is related to the OCD-like variant of hypochondriasis, which is, like BDD, currently considered one of the OCD-spectrum disorders.

Schizophrenia

Some earlier authors considered BDD related to, or a variant of, schizophrenia. Schizophrenia is characterized by a constellation of symptoms, including delusional thinking, hallucinations, disorganized speech (e.g., incoherence), grossly disorganized behavior, and "negative" symptoms, which include such things as lack of emotion and motivation.

A number of authors, including M.V. Korkina and E.W. Anderson, considered patients with BDD to be schizophrenic. Others viewed BDD as an early sign of schizophrenia. Hay, for example, wrote in 1970 that BDD was "an ominous symptom" that was a precursor of schizophrenia. This theory was supported by a 1978 retrospective study by Drs. Francis Connolly and Michael Gipson, which found that patients with likely BDD who received cosmetic nose surgery were more likely to develop subsequent schizophrenia than patients who had nose surgery to correct a deformity caused by injury or disease.

But definitions of schizophrenia used in past decades were somewhat broader than that currently used; thus, it's possible that schizophrenia was overdiagnosed among people with BDD. In terms of symptoms, there are some similarities, such as the presence of delusional thinking and referential thinking in both disorders. But not all people with BDD are delusional or have referential thinking. More important, the delusional thinking that occurs in BDD usually isn't bizarre, as it is in schizophrenia, and other symptoms of schizophrenia (prominent hallucinations, disorganized speech, grossly disorganized behavior, and negative symptoms) are generally absent in BDD.

As shown in Table 8, the male-to-female ratio and a chronic course of illness are similar, but schizophrenia usually begins at a later age than BDD. Data on the co-occurrence of these disorders strongly refute a close relationship between them: in my series of patients with BDD, none were diagnosed with schizophrenia, although several had a disorder with similarities to schizophrenia (schizoaffective disorder; see Appendix A for a definition). Similarly, I found no relatives with schizophrenia.

Treatment response also appears to differ. Antipsychotic medications (neuroleptics) are the mainstay of treatment for schizophrenia and are often effective. Although some investigators have reported that delusional BDD may respond to a neuroleptic known as pimozide, I haven't found this to be the case (although it appears that BDD may respond to pimozide and other neuroleptics in combination with SRIs). Overall, available data suggest that BDD is not a variant of, or closely related to, schizophrenia.

Olfactory Reference Syndrome: The Distress of Perceived Body Odor

Nikki's life centered on her body odor, which no one else could smell. Since the age of 18, she'd believed that she smelled bad. At first, she thought she smelled like sweat; later she also worried about her supposedly bad breath. "I think I smell *really* bad," she said. "It's hard to describe it—it's a horrible smell sort of like an enchilada that everyone notices."

As a result, Nikki showered and changed her clothes five times a day. She used large amounts of soap, perfume, deodorant, and mouthwash, and she constantly chewed gum and ate mints. She repeatedly checked her breath by blowing into her cupped hand, and to get rid of the smell she ate a special diet and scraped her tongue and mouth until they bled.

She also thought that other people took special notice of the odor. "I know everyone can smell it from at least 20 to 30 feet away. Why else would they frown at me the way they do and make comments like 'It's stuffy in here?' Or why would they open the window or make a comment about soap when I'm with them?"

Nikki's preoccupation and referential thinking prevented her from working. She'd tried many jobs but quickly quit them when she thought people were talking about how bad she smelled. She became very socially isolated. She also saw numerous doctors and dentists without attaining relief. Eventually, as a result of her preoccupation, Nikki went on disability and became depressed and suicidal.

In olfactory reference syndrome (ORS), the body odor is thought to smell like flatulence, bad breath, sweat, an anal or genital odor, or even nonbodily odors such as ammonia or enchiladas. It's generally thought to come from the anus, mouth, skin, feet, armpits, or genitals. Just as other people can't perceive, or can barely perceive, the physical defects of BDD, they can't smell the body odor of ORS.

As in BDD, depression, avoidance of work and social activities, suicidal thinking, and suicide attempts are relatively common. Both disorders are characterized by referential thinking. When other people do such things as turn away, look disgusted, open a window, say the word "smell," sit at a distance, or hold a newspaper in front of their face, the behaviors are assumed to be a response to the repulsive odor.

Like BDD, ORS appears to often be chronic, and it appears that most people with the disorder are unmarried. In addition, people with ORS engage in many BDD-like behaviors—frequently checking for the presence of the odor, repeatedly questioning others about whether they can smell it, and camouflaging with excessive amounts of deodorant, perfume, or mouthwash. Showering and washing or changing clothes may also be done to excess. Believing that they suffer from a medical problem, help is usually sought from nonpsychiatric medical specialists—dentists for supposed bad breath, gynecologists for supposed vaginal odor, proctologists for supposed anal odor or flatulence, or surgeons for the removal of "smelly tonsils." As in BDD, such treatment tends to be ineffective.

On the basis of these similarities, some authors consider ORS to be a form of BDD, or they consider BDD and ORS variants of the same disorder. In Japan, both are considered a type of social phobia, reflecting the social avoidance and impairment that characterize them.

But BDD and ORS also appear to have some differences. Although the treatment of ORS has received very little investigation, a small number of reported cases suggest that ORS may respond equally well to a combination of an antidepressant and an antipsychotic medication (neuroleptic, with 5 of 8 cases responding), to a variety of antidepressants (7 of 16 cases responding), or to the antipsychotic pimozide alone (15 of 29 cases responding). While the paucity of treatment data on ORS makes it difficult to use treatment response as a clue to whether BDD and ORS are related, these preliminary data suggest that ORS's treatment response may differ from that of BDD. I'm aware of only two published cases of an SRI (clomi-pramine) in ORS, with one of two cases responding. In a small number of cases, a cognitive-behavioral approach similar to that used for BDD (expo-sure and response prevention) was effective.

Although no direct comparison studies of BDD and ORS have been done, it appears on balance that BDD and ORS have many more similarities than differences. Further research may demonstrate that they're the same disorder. Until we have such evidence, however, it makes sense to consider them separate, although probably closely related, disorders.

Koro: Panic over Penile Shrinkage

When koro strikes, men panic and rush to emergency rooms in droves. They fear that they will imminently die from penile shrinkage, and they implore family members and doctors to save them by pulling on their penis.

Koro, a Malay word for "the head of the turtle," consists of the erroneous belief that one's penis is shrinking and acutely retracting into the abdomen, which will result in death when the disappearance is complete. Intense dis-tress and panic spur the use of various mechanical means to prevent penile retraction: tying, grasping, or clamping the penis with plier-like devices. Koro occasionally occurs in women, who fear their breasts or labia will shrink. Real or fantasized violations of cultural rules for sexual behavior have been theorized to cause this syndrome.

Koro usually occurs in certain parts of Southeast Asia, primarily south-ern coastal China and among Chinese living overseas in Southeast Asia. However, similar symptoms have also been reported in other parts of the world, such as Indonesia, India, Thailand, and England.

BDD and koro share an intense, anxiety-provoking preoccupation with a perceived defect in appearance, and concern with the genitals is fairly common in BDD. However, Southeast Asian cases of koro differ from BDD in a number of ways. Men with koro believe that their body is acutely and dramatically changing, which I've seen only occasionally in BDD. In addi-tion, anxiety in koro is due to the fear that penile disappearance will result in death, which isn't a feature of BDD. Furthermore, unlike BDD, koro usually begins acutely, has a brief course, occurs as an epidemic, and often resolves with reassurance alone.

However, many cases of koro from the Western world lack these charac-teristic features and are more similar to BDD. In these cases, men worry that their penis is too small or shrinking, but generally don't believe that it will actually disappear into their abdomen, and few believe that penile shrinkage will kill them. The belief is sometimes more chronic (lasting as long as several decades) and doesn't occur in epidemics. Some of these cases are so similar to BDD that the diagnosis of BDD may in fact be more accurate than koro. While the epidemic form of koro that occurs in Southeast Asia differs in many ways from BDD, it's unclear whether it's truly a different disorder than BDD or a cultural variant of BDD. This is one of the many BDD mysteries that remains to be solved.

The Delusional Variant of BDD

The relationship between BDD and its delusional variant is controversial. As I've previously mentioned, the nondelusional form of BDD is classified in DSM-IV as a somatoform disorder (i.e., a disorder involving physical complaints), whereas the delusional form is classified as a separate disorder, a type of delusional disorder. Yet when I and my colleagues compared these two disorders, we found that they were similar in terms of nearly all the characteristics we examined, leading us to conclude that they may actually be the same disorder, with the delusional variant a more severe form.

Although our findings are preliminary, they suggest that BDD and its delusional disorder variant should probably be classified as the same disorder. In fact, a step in that direction was taken in DSM-IV: although they remain separately classified, they may also be double-coded. In other words, a person with delusional BDD may receive a diagnosis of both BDD and delusional disorder. While this is a somewhat awkward compromise, it underscores the possibility that BDD and its delusional variant may indeed be the same disorder but that more investigation of their relationship is needed.

BDD appears to span a spectrum of insight—from good insight, to poor insight, to absent insight (delusional thinking)—with the entire continuum constituting a single disorder. Thinking in BDD may fluctuate along this continuum, with nondelusional thinking sometimes becoming delusional, and vice versa. In addition, insight may improve with treatment. Observations such as these further support the hypothesis that the delusional and nondelusional forms of BDD constitute the same disorder, as it's unlikely that people whose thinking changes in this way have two different disorders. In addition, it's sometimes difficult to distinguish delusional from nondelusional preoccupations, which gives some support to the continuum model.

The delusional-nondelusional issue is relevant to other disorders, such as OCD, anorexia nervosa, hypochondriasis, and social phobia. Like BDD, these disorders appear to span a spectrum of insight, with insight sometimes fluctuating along a continuum. This is a particularly interesting subject that needs to be further studied and has important implications for the classification and treatment of a number of psychiatric disorders.

BDD and Personality

Another intriguing question is whether BDD is associated with certain personality traits. Are people with BDD shy, self-conscious, sensitive to rejection, or flamboyant? And what about a causal relationship between BDD and personality traits? Are people with certain personality traits more likely to get BDD? Or does BDD change personality?

People with BDD can have virtually any type of personality. Some are quiet and withdrawn, whereas others are outgoing, colorful, and adventurous. Some tend to be suspicious, whereas others are trusting. Some are constrained and careful, whereas others are impulsive, craving excitement and novelty. This list could go on.

Despite this variety, however, people with BDD often do seem to have a particular constellation of traits. They often describe themselves as shy, quiet, self-conscious, unassertive, having low self-esteem, and sensitive to rejection. In published cases reports, shyness and an obsessional personality style have been noted. And G. G. Hay, in a 1970 study, found that compared to control subjects, 17 subjects with BDD were more introverted, "obsessoid," hostile, and neurotic.

I've assessed personality traits in 66 people with BDD using the NEO-Five Factor Inventory, a questionnaire developed to assess five aspects of normal personality: neuroticism, extroversion, conscientiousness, openness to experience, and agreeableness. Neuroticism measures a variety of negative emotions and cognitions—in particular, anxiety, self-consciousness, anger, depression, and feelings of vulnerability. People with BDD as a group scored in the very high range on this scale, which isn't surprising, given that so many people with BDD say that they often experience unpleasant emotions such as these.

In terms of extroversion—a measure of gregariousness, warmth, assertiveness, activity/energy, and excitement seeking—the average score was in the very low range; as a group they were introverted, quiet, and reserved. This finding is consistent with the high rate of social phobia among people with BDD. I found that people with BDD scored in the low range on conscientiousness, a measure of disciplined striving after goals and will to achieve. They scored in the average range on openness to experience (aesthetic sensitivity, intellectual curiosity, creativity, and willingness to try new things) and agreeableness (altruistic, trusting, good natured, and agreeable as opposed to antagonistic, irritable, stingy, and critical).

In general, these findings agree with Hay's results, which found that people with BDD are "neurotic" and introverted, but they differ in suggesting that people with BDD aren't unusually hostile, since scores on agreeableness were in the average range.

It's worth emphasizing that the NEO scores are average scores, and that scores of some individuals with BDD are quite different from these averages. It's also worth noting that it's difficult to interpret these scores. They tell us, for example, that low extroversion *is associated with* BDD, but this doesn't say anything about the causal relationship between BDD and introversion.

I've also assessed the rate of personality disorders (see page 320 for a definition) in nearly 40 individuals with BDD. Two thirds had at least one personality disorder, with avoidant personality (characterized by social inhibition, feelings of inadequacy, and hypersensitivity to negative evaluation) the most common. Despite this high rate of co-occurrence, it seems clear that BDD isn't simply a symptom or reflection of a personality problem.

Like many aspects of BDD, the relationship between BDD and personality traits—both normal and problematic—has been little studied and needs further research. Questions about whether personality traits predispose a person to BDD, or whether BDD changes personality, are particularly important. In the coming years, as more research is done, our knowledge of this aspect of BDD will rapidly expand.

Concluding Thoughts

On balance, it appears that BDD isn't identical to, or completely subsumed by, any other psychiatric disorder. However, it has many similarities to, and is probably closely related to, a number of disorders, most notably OCD. It's also probably related to social phobia, the eating disorders, hypochondriasis, and olfactory reference syndrome. Because BDD is likely to be a heterogeneous disorder, with several different forms, it's possible that some forms of BDD are more closely related to certain disorders, such as OCD, and other forms to other disorders, such as the eating disorders.

One way to conceptualize BDD's relationship to other psychiatric disorders is to consider it a member of a "family" of related disorders. I mentioned that BDD is considered one of the "OCD-spectrum disorders," a family of disorders that appear closely related to OCD. BDD is also a candidate for the "affective spectrum disorders," a broader grouping of disorders that includes OCD and many of the OCD-spectrum disorders. The affective spectrum disorders are postulated to have a common pathophysiological abnormality based on their response to antidepressant medications, similarities in their co-occurrence with other disorders, and the family history of sufferers.

In the coming years, as we better understand the cause of BDD and other disorders, we'll have a clearer understanding of their relationship to one another. This understanding will lead to their more accurate classification, better diagnosis, and more effective treatment.

·· *thirteen* ··

Help for BDD Sufferers:
Overview and Medications

Patients' Responses to Treatment

Christina: A Quick Response to Medication

When I first met Christina, she was worried that her skin wasn't clear enough. "It has red blotches on it and too many pimples," she said. "I've gotten depressed because of it. Every time I talk to someone they look at my skin, and they're thinking how bad it looks. It's really hard for me to be around other people at work and school."

Christina was indeed depressed. She felt sad and anxious, was tired all the time, and couldn't concentrate. She thought about her skin for more than eight hours a day and believed that other people took special notice of how bad it looked. Although she was very conscientious, she had missed several days of school during the preceding weeks. "I couldn't get myself out of the mirror, and I didn't want other people to see me," she explained. She was also having difficulty doing her part-time job. She was avoiding other people at work and was very quiet when she was around them because she felt so self-conscious about how she looked.

Christina was reluctant to take medication but decided to give it a try. "If there's a chance it'll help, I'll try it," she said. "I generally don't like to take pills, but this is getting to be too much." She started fluvoxamine (Luvox), one of the serotonin-reuptake inhibitors. For the first few weeks nothing much happened. But during the third week, Christina thought she noticed that she was starting to obsess a little less and that she wasn't quite as depressed or anxious. During the fourth week, I received a phone call from her. "I just want you to know how much better I'm feeling," she told me. "I really noticed a change yesterday. I went out with friends instead of staying home, and I had a great time!"

Over the next few weeks Christina continued to further improve. By the eighth week on fluvoxamine, her symptoms were essentially gone. "I can't believe this has happened," she said. "I had this problem for so long, and now it's gone!" Christina had had BDD for ten years; this was the first time since her symptoms began that she'd felt well. She was now thinking about her skin for only five minutes a day. She was no longer in emotional pain and was no longer depressed. She was going out with friends and dating for the first time in years. She was also doing very well in school and in her job.

Christina also realized that she had been distorting how bad she looked. Her skin now looked fine to her. "I just wasn't seeing myself clearly before," she said. "I feel calmer, happier, and more confident. It's hard to believe the medication has made this much of a change, but it has. I feel the way I used to feel, before the BDD ever started. I feel great!"

Sophie: A Circuitous Path to Effective Medication

Sophie's path to recovery was more circuitous. She first insisted on having nose surgery. Although she was happy with the results for several months, she gradually became more and more dissatisfied and decided to have another operation. This time, she thought the surgeon had ruined her looks. "I was devastated," she told me. "The nose is the most important part of your face. I told him I wanted it smaller; I didn't say to make it *too* small!"

Sophie was then psychiatrically hospitalized because she was so obsessed with her "atrocious appearance" that she felt suicidal. She was treated with psychotherapy and desipramine, an antidepressant medication, without improvement. Lithium was then added to the desipramine, with no response. She then received an antipsychotic medication, haloperidol, which wasn't helpful either.

After she left the hospital, Sophie took other psychiatric medications and continued in psychotherapy. All she talked to her therapist about was needing to get her nose fixed. She eventually dropped out of therapy, because her nose problem was no better. Sophie then had yet another nose operation to "repair the damage" caused by the previous surgeries. This procedure was also unsuccessful. At her family's insistence, she decided to try a psychiatric approach again, although her previous treatment had been disappointing.

It took six months before Sophie would see me. She made several appointments but canceled them. "I feel too ugly to leave my house," she said on the phone. "I don't want anyone to see me." At the insistence of her family, she finally came in. When she did, she waited in a nearby bathroom, where no one could see her, instead of the waiting room. When her brother signaled that the coast was clear, she ran from the bathroom into my office.

Sophie agreed to try clomipramine (Anafranil), one of the serotonin-reuptake inhibitors. After six weeks she started feeling somewhat better. "I think the medication might be starting to help," she said. "I'm not thinking about my nose all the time. My family keeps telling me that I'm getting better—I'm not talking about my nose as much, and I'm not spending so much time in the mirror." After eight weeks on the medication, Sophie started leaving the house more, even taking walks into town and going shopping for the first time in years. "I can think about other things, and I can do more," she said. "I'm not totally wrapped up in my nose."

Sophie still had some remaining symptoms—she still thought about her nose for several hours a day and avoided some social situations. But as she said, "With this problem, even 50% better is a great relief." Sophie's family was also immensely relieved. "Her nose used to be her whole life. Now she has other things," they told me. "We're in her life again. We have our daughter back."

Alan: Response to Cognitive-Behavioral Therapy

Alan had tried several serotonin-reuptake inhibitors for his BDD but hadn't given them an adequate try because he was reluctant to take them religiously. He had also tried cognitive-behavioral therapy but hadn't responded to this approach. He'd had BDD for 20 years and had been disabled by his symptoms.

Alan's concern focused on his lips. He thought that they were large and ugly and that they offended other people. He frequently licked them to improve their appearance, covered them, checked them in mirrors, and tried to keep them in a more attractive position. He also avoided other people as much as possible. He came for treatment because he wanted to improve his social life, return to work, and get off disability, which he was receiving because of this problem. He wanted to give cognitive-behavioral therapy another try. He was a good candidate for this treatment, with his relatively good insight about his distorted view of his appearance and his high level of motivation.

Alan's treatment consisted of such approaches as telling himself that other people didn't see him the way he did and trying to resist his compulsive behaviors such as checking mirrors and licking and covering his lips. He also exposed himself to the social situations he feared; he and his therapist pushed him to talk more with other people, speak up in groups, and socialize.

After several months of 5-day-a-week treatment, Alan's lip licking, mirror checking, and mouth covering had virtually stopped, and it was easier for him to be around other people. He did, however, continue to feel very self-conscious in social situations, and his obsessions, although decreased, were still present for many hours a day. Although he'd made notable gains with cognitive-behavioral treatment alone, Alan decided to add medication to better treat his remaining symptoms.

David: Response to Medication plus Cognitive-Behavioral Therapy

David was feeling desperate. A 32-year-old disc jockey, he was at the point of quitting his job. He couldn't focus on his work because of his hair obsessions, and was often late because he couldn't tear himself away from the mirror in the morning. Even the expensive new hairpiece he'd bought to hide his slightly receding hairline didn't help him feel any better. "I don't like going out in public, and I've given up on dating," he said. "I don't want to date because someone will run their fingers through my hair and know it's a hairpiece. I can't focus on conversations because I think people are looking at my hair. At times I stay in completely; I don't even food shop."

In the week before he saw me, David missed work three times and had considered going to an emergency room because he was so panicked about his hair. "I hate myself and how I look. I'm really down on myself. I've even had thoughts of ending my life. I can't live the rest of my life like this. How can you live in your own body if you can't stand it?"

David started taking fluoxetine (Prozac) right away. He continued psychotherapy, which had been a helpful support but didn't diminish his BDD symptoms. As expected, the medication didn't work immediately, and the first month of treatment was rocky. David and I considered hospitalization several times. But with the support of friends and his family, he maintained his will to live. About a month after beginning treatment, David started to feel somewhat better. His hair preoccupation began to wane, and the thoughts were less painful. He was more willing to see his friends. David also found it easier to avoid mirrors, and he questioned others about his appearance less. He was no longer suicidal.

Cognitive-behavioral treatment was then added to the medication. His therapist worked with him to improve his self-esteem and helped him resist looking in mirrors and questioning others. He forced himself to socialize, putting himself in increasingly anxiety-provoking social situations. Finally, he even gave up his hairpiece and combed his hair in a style that accentuated his slightly receding hairline. He received many compliments on his new hair style, and his self-confidence greatly improved. He then discontinued behavioral treatment, continuing on medication alone, essentially symptom free.

Overcoming Barriers to Treatment: The First Steps to a Successful Outcome

Before they overcame BDD, David, Christina, Sophie, and Alan all took some initial steps, which made it possible for them to be successfully treated. First, they acknowledged that they had a problem—that they worried too much about their appearance and that their worrying was a problem for them: it caused them too much emotional pain, made them depressed and anxious, and interfered in some way with their functioning or caused difficulties for their family or friends.

They also recognized that they needed professional psychiatric help. Some of them had attempted other approaches—trying harder, trying to reassure themselves that they looked okay, surgery, and hair clubs. They finally acknowledged to themselves that such approaches hadn't worked and weren't likely to work. Although Christina and Alan didn't like the idea of seeing a psychiatrist or taking medication, they did. They realized they had nothing to lose and potentially much to gain.

There are, unfortunately, many barriers to getting effective treatment for BDD, which need to be overcome. Some of them include the following.

- *Overcoming lack of knowledge about BDD* Many people are unfortunately uninformed or misinformed about BDD, or even unaware of its existence as a psychiatric disorder and that it often responds to psychiatric treatment. Education about BDD is an essential first step to a successful outcome.

- *Overcoming embarrassment and shame*   Embarrassment and shame can be significant barriers to obtaining effective treatment. Many people never mention their BDD symptoms, even to a mental health professional, even though they consider them a major problem. They may instead talk only about depression, anxiety, or relationship problems.

- *Making the diagnosis*   Accurate diagnosis is a necessary step toward effective treatment. Unfortunately, BDD is still unfamiliar to some mental health professionals, and many people with BDD seek non-psychiatric treatment. Perhaps most important, the secrecy of BDD prevents the diagnosis from being made.

- *Overcoming trivialization of BDD*   BDD is easily trivialized. Why should someone care so much about how they look? The fact that the person looks okay only compounds the problem. It may lead to reassurance—don't worry, you look fine—rather than effective treatment. For BDD to be diagnosed and adequately treated, the symptoms must be taken seriously by family members and clinicians; BDD must be recognized as a serious psychiatric disorder that can cause severe suffering.

- *"Your appearance concerns aren't your real problem"*   This kind of statement is a common example of trivialization. When patients hear a statement like this, and are told that they need to figure out what their "real problem" is, they generally feel misunderstood. They may also feel angry, as did one patient who told me "I've been told that BDD isn't my real problem. It's very frustrating, and I get angry over it—they don't get it! There's no mystery about what my problem is—*my nose* is what bugs me. It's painful!" Or, to be compliant, they may no longer discuss their BDD and even leave treatment. As one patient said, "If you treat BDD as something other than the real problem, the patient will never bring it up again." Although people with BDD may have other problems as well, it's important that BDD be recognized as a real problem in and of itself that requires diagnosis and adequate treatment.

- *Overcoming stigma*   To some extent, psychiatric disorders are still unfortunately associated with a sense of stigma, which may lead to reluctance to seek psychiatric treatment. However, this view is changing. Psychiatric problems are increasingly being recognized as

medical problems that deserve treatment, thanks in good part to
the advocacy of consumer groups such as the National Alliance for
the Mentally Ill, the Obsessive Compulsive Foundation, and the
Manic Depressive and Depressive Association.

• *Overcoming reluctance to try psychiatric treatment*   Some people are
reluctant to try psychiatric treatment for a variety of reasons. Sometimes, it's the stigma they feel is associated with such treatment.
Sometimes it's fear, which is often based on a misunderstanding of
the treatment and possible side effects, or an insistence that surgery is the solution. Sometimes it's based on a desire to "do it on
my own," and a sense of failure if such treatment is needed. Education about the treatments for BDD often allays misfounded fears.
Understanding that BDD isn't a moral failing or due to weakness
of character may diminish reluctance to get adequate help. Receiving psychiatric treatment for BDD should be no different than receiving treatment for heart disease or any other medical problem.

For BDD to be effectively treated, these barriers must be overcome.
When they are, the stage is set for a successful—in some cases a lifesaving—
outcome. Sandy, who had an excellent response to Luvox (fluvoxamine)
told me, "I'm feeling fantastic, for the first time in 20 years. My appearance
is fine now—there's no cause for concern." Like many people I've treated
who responded to medication, Sandy "tested" the medication by trying to
bring her obsession back. But she couldn't. "The medication definitely
curbs the obsession. It released a logjam. My life felt like a stream that had
thousands of huge boulders and logs in it—the water couldn't flow through
smoothly. Now it flows with ease. I feel full of energy and creativity."

Overview of Treatment Strategies

Several psychiatric approaches (medications known as serotonin-reuptake
inhibitors [SRIs] and certain cognitive-behavioral strategies) appear to often
be effective for BDD. Available evidence suggests that the SRIs significantly
diminish symptoms in a majority of people with BDD, and many are also
helped by cognitive-behavioral approaches. A number of researchers, on the
basis of clinical experience as well as what are known as "open" treatment
studies, concur that BDD appears to respond to these treatment approaches
but not to others. Many clinicians have patients like Christina, Sophie,
Brian, and David, whose experience supports these conclusions.

Yet available evidence about treatment is limited from a scientific stand-point. Methodologically rigorous studies that might *prove* that these treatments are effective are still in progress. This is an awkward time to be writing about the treatment of BDD—awkward because we know some things about BDD's treatment response, yet there's much that we don't know. The scientist in me wants to be cautious—to emphasize that without scientifically adequate studies it's difficult to state what treatments are effective for BDD. At the same time, my treatment of many patients, many of whom have suffered for decades and who've responded well—sometimes miraculously—to these approaches leads me to advocate them. My excitement about them is nonetheless tempered by the recognition that they clearly require further research.

What follows is a brief summary of the key points that I'll be making:

- *Serotonin-reuptake inhibitors (SRIs)—antidepressant medications with antiobsessional properties—appear to be effective for a majority of people with BDD.*   With these medications, appearance-related preoccupations, as well as associated behaviors, usually diminish. Functioning often improves. Symptoms often diminish partially but may resolve completely.

- *If an SRI alone isn't adequately effective, certain combinations of medications may further improve symptoms, as may switching to another SRI.*

- *Cognitive-behavioral treatment consisting of exposure and response prevention (facing feared situations and resistance of compulsive behaviors) may also be effective for some individuals with BDD.*   With this approach, symptoms often diminish only partially but sometimes resolve nearly completely.

- *SRIs and cognitive-behavioral treatment—what I consider the "core treatments" for BDD—may be successfully combined.*

- *Other psychotherapeutic approaches may be useful when combined with an SRI or cognitive-behavioral treatment.*   Such psychotherapeutic approaches do *not,* however, at this time appear to be effective for BDD when used alone. These treatments include insight-oriented psychotherapy, supportive psychotherapy, and family therapy.

- *Available evidence suggests that surgical and other medical treatments are generally not helpful for BDD and may even worsen the symptoms.*

- *A number of other approaches appear to be ineffective for BDD.*   These include natural remedies, efforts to uncover a presumed trauma, and reassurance that the person looks fine.

- *The treatment of BDD needs to be further studied.* All these treatment recommendations, while based on the best scientific data currently available, require confirmation in more scientifically rigorous studies. Such studies are currently in progress, and much will be learned about BDD's treatment in the coming years.

Serotonin-Reuptake Inhibitors

Christina, Sophie, David, and many other people described in this book improved with medications known as serotonin-reuptake inhibitors (SRIs). The SRIs are a type of antidepressant that also counteract obsessional thinking and compulsive behaviors. They effectively treat depression; in addition, they effectively treat obsessive compulsive disorder (OCD). While *all* antidepressants effectively treat depression, only the SRI antidepressants also treat OCD, a disorder with many similarities to BDD.

In addition to effectively treating depression and OCD, the SRIs are effective for a number of other psychiatric disorders. These include panic disorder, bulimia, and binge eating disorder. Ongoing studies suggest they may also be useful in other disorders, such as social phobia, anorexia nervosa, and alcoholism. The SRIs are also used for nonpsychiatric problems, such as headache, obesity, and pain syndromes. Like other psychiatric medications, the SRIs are prescribed by psychiatrists and other physicians.

As shown in Table 9 on the next page, the SRIs currently available in the United States are fluvoxamine (Luvox), fluoxetine (Prozac), paroxetine (Paxil), sertraline (Zoloft), and clomipramine (Anafranil). The first four medications are sometimes referred to as SSRIs (*selective* serotonin reuptake inhibitors) because they affect the brain chemical serotonin far more than other brain chemicals.

Serotonin is one of the brain's natural chemicals that transmit signals between nerve cells. These chemicals *(neurotransmitters)* are the chemical messengers that make the brain's nerve cells fire and function. Healthy functioning of serotonin is important in many bodily functions, including mood, sleep, and appetite.

The SRIs increase the amount of serotonin at the junction between nerve cells by preventing its reuptake, or reabsorption, into the releasing nerve cell (neuron) and its subsequent breakdown. More serotonin is then available to act on neurons that are "downstream." This increased amount of serotonin between nerve cells in turn influences the activity of brain neurons. It appears that the SRIs may increase the overall activity of serotonin-releasing

Table 9   Serotonin-Reuptake Inhibitors

Medication	Usual Effective Dose Range (milligrams per day)
Fluvoxamine (Luvox)	100–300
Fluoxetine (Prozac)	20–80
Paroxetine (Paxil)	20–50
Sertraline (Zoloft)	50–200
Clomipramine (Anafranil)	100–250

neurons in the brain. They probably work by increasing serotonin availability at key areas in the brain. However, the serotonin system in the brain is extremely complex, and the SRI's overall effect on this system needs to be better understood. In addition, because different neurotransmitter systems are highly interconnected, the SRIs also influence other neurotransmitters in addition to serotonin. Furthermore, it's possible that the SRIs' effect on serotonin isn't what actually leads to decreased symptoms. This effect may simply be one step in a complicated chain of events.

The work of Dr. Lewis Baxter and his colleagues at UCLA on the effect of the SRIs in obsessive compulsive disorder is extremely interesting and sheds some light on how these medications might work in OCD. Because of BDD's many similarities to OCD, it's possible that the SRIs have similar effects in BDD. These researchers studied patients with OCD before and after treatment with fluoxetine (Prozac) alone or cognitive-behavioral treatment alone (specifically, exposure and response prevention). They found that each treatment *normalized* abnormal brain functioning. Before treatment, a type of brain scan known as a PET scan showed abnormalities in blood flow in certain areas of the brain that are characteristic of OCD; after either of these treatments, PET scans showed that brain functioning became normal. The normalization occurred only in patients who responded to treatment, not in nonresponders or untreated normal control subjects. Because of BDD's similarities to OCD, it's possible that SRIs may have a similar effect in people with BDD.

It's particularly fascinating to consider that this study demonstrated that the SRI fluoxetine (Prozac) actually makes the brain *normal.* Some people worry that medications will somehow disrupt the functioning of their brains or create artificial changes or an artificial state. But Baxter's findings suggest that the opposite is true. They imply that Prozac and other similar medications correct a "chemical imbalance" in the brain—that they alleviate symptoms by normalizing an abnormal state. Similarly, SRIs aren't "happy pills"—that is, they don't create an artificial state of happiness; rather, they correct abnormal brain functioning.

In a way, these study results aren't surprising, because they reflect patients' experiences with recovery. Those who respond to an SRI feel more "normal." They say that they feel like themselves again, or that they have more control over their mind—the way they used to, or the way other people do. "I have much more control over my thoughts now," one woman said. "I'm no longer obsessed. My thinking and my behavior are more normal now, and that's a big relief."

Improvement with the SRIs

People who respond to an SRI generally experience improvement in a variety of ways. They spend less time obsessing and, if they start thinking about the defect, it's easier to push the thoughts aside and think about other things. The thoughts are less tormenting. Some people think they actually look better than they used to, so the thoughts are less painful for this reason, whereas others think they look the same but they're better able to cope with their appearance problem emotionally. BDD-related behaviors generally improve as well. It's easier to resist the mirror checking, comparing, skin picking, reassurance seeking, and other behaviors. Many people are able to improve their social life. It's much less painful to be around other people, and many find it easier to work or do schoolwork.

There are usually other benefits as well. Anxiety, depression, and suicidal thinking often diminish. Self-consciousness often decreases, and self-esteem and self-confidence get a boost. One of my patients said that she felt "wonderful—like a new person." She had stopped worrying about her nose and hair for the first time in 30 years.

"With Anafranil I can talk to people without feeling they're staring at me," Nathaniel said. "It's easier to resist mirror checking. I spend less time worrying. It comes into my mind less and it's easier to get rid of the thoughts. I can argue with myself that my obsession is irrational—I tell myself, 'just shrug it off!' I'm not so self-conscious around people anymore. It's not a life or death problem for me now."

"I'd say I got 95% better on Prozac," Ned said. He'd had severe BDD for

30 years and had been hospitalized more than 10 times for his symptoms. He had also tried 13 non-SRI medications, without results. "My obsessions mostly went away, and I could stay out of the mirror. I stopped being hospitalized. I was so impressed that I bought stock in the drug company."

I and my colleagues (Dr. Susan McElroy and Drs. James Hudson, Harrison Pope, and Katherine Atala of Harvard Medical School) have treated many people with BDD. Of 61 treatment trials with an SRI in 41 patients, 70% resulted in clinically significant improvement in BDD symptoms.* In reviewing the past treatment history of patients I've seen who were treated by other clinicians, I found that 42% of 65 SRI trials (fluoxetine, clomipramine, paroxetine, sertraline, or fluvoxamine) resulted in clinically significant improvement, in contrast to 8% of 247 trials with a wide variety of other psychiatric medications. I suspect our higher success rate with SRIs (70% versus 42%) is attributable to more vigorous treatment (with higher doses or longer treatment trials or both).

On the basis of these promising results, Dr. McElroy and I decided to take the next step, by conducting what is known as an "open-label" treatment study of BDD. This is a type of study in which both patients and the doctor know that the patient is receiving the medication—in other words, a placebo ("sugar pill") isn't used. In this ongoing 16-week study of fluvoxamine (Luvox), 65% of 26 patients were considered significantly improved after treatment at the time of this writing.† On one of our outcome measures (again using the Clinical Global Impressions Scale), 35% were considered "much improved" and 31% "very much improved."

This study provided better data than that previously obtained because it was obtained prospectively (that is, response was assessed forward over time as opposed to looking back in time). In addition, standard, reliable, and commonly used rating instruments were used, patients were evaluated at regular and planned intervals, and adequate medication doses and length of treatment were used.

Evidence suggesting that the SRIs are effective in BDD—perhaps more effective than other medications—also comes from the work of several other researchers. Dr. Eric Hollander and his colleagues were the first to report this. They found that five patients who had failed to respond to a wide variety of psychiatric medications responded to the SRIs fluoxetine

* Response was assessed with the Clinical Global Impressions Scale, a commonly used global rating scale of treatment response.

† On the Yale-Brown Obsessive Compulsive Scale modified for BDD (BDD-YBOCS). See pages 325–333 in Appendix B for a further description. Significant improvement on this scale consisted of a decrease of 30% or more in total score.

and clomipramine. Drs. Kathleen Brady and Bruce Lydiard of the Medical University of South Carolina subsequently reported that three patients with BDD responded to fluoxetine. In a later retrospective study, Dr. Hollander and his colleagues found that 35 SRI trials resulted in clinically significant improvement in BDD symptoms, whereas trials with non-SRI antidepressants resulted in no overall improvement in BDD symptoms.

Several other studies also suggest that SRIs may be effective for BDD. One is an open-label study of fluvoxamine, similar to the study Dr. McElroy and I did. This study was done by Drs. Guilio Perugi, Daniele Giannotti, Sabrina Di Vaio, Franco Frare, Saettone Marco, and Giovanni Cassano of the University of Pisa in Italy. In this 10-week study, 10 of 15 (67%) patients—and 10 of 12 of those who completed the study—were considered markedly improved.

An ongoing study comparing the SRI clomipramine (Anafranil) to desipramine (a non-SRI antidepressant) is being done by Drs. Eric Hollander, Daphne Simeon, Concetta DeCaria, Bonnie Aronowitz, and Lisa Cohen of Mount Sinai School of Medicine. This is a "cross-over" trial, in which patients are first treated with one of the medications and then with the other. It is a double-blind trial, meaning that neither the patient nor the investigators know when the patient is taking which medication. Preliminary results at the time of this writing indicate that no one has responded to desipramine, whereas nearly half have responded to clomipramine. While preliminary, these findings suggest that SRIs may be preferentially effective for BDD.

Let's take a closer look at what symptoms improve with an SRI. This varies to some extent for different people, with many responding to the medication only partially and others responding completely. Generally, responders experience improvement in a variety of ways.*

Preoccupation   People who respond to an SRI report less preoccupation with their appearance. Those who respond completely may spend only minutes—or no time at all—instead of hours a day obsessing. A partial responder may still be preoccupied, but the time spent decreases—for example, from six hours a day to three. The decrease in preoccupation is usually due to the thoughts' entering the person's mind less frequently and to a better ability to resist and push them away. This change alone can be liberating. Time is freed up to think about more important things. Concentration improves because the distracting thoughts aren't present as often. Feelings of control increase.

* Most responders experience a decrease on all items on the BDD-YBOCS.

Ability to resist and control the obsessional thinking A particularly distressing aspect of BDD is the feeling of not being in control of your own mind. This usually changes with response to an SRI. People who respond usually find it easier to resist and control the distressing thoughts, which results in less time obsessing about the appearance problem. They regain control over their thinking and their mind. They—not the obsessions—are in charge.

Emotional pain The emotional pain and suffering caused by BDD usually diminish as well. The pain may become more tolerable or may vanish. The thoughts are no longer as depressing, anxiety-provoking, or tormenting. This appears to be due in part to their decreased frequency; in addition, when they do occur, they're less emotionally painful. Their power is diminished.

Level of functioning Functioning may also improve. It often becomes easier to go to work or school and to concentrate. It becomes less difficult to be around other people and to leave the house. BDD sufferers may repair wounded relationships, start socializing more, or begin dating. "Our social life improved dramatically every time my wife took Prozac," an engineer told me. "Every time she stopped it, our social life stopped too."

Improvement in functioning may be quite rapid and dramatic. A woman I treated started school again within several weeks of responding to fluvoxamine, a change she'd wanted to make for 10 years but which her symptoms had made impossible. But others change more slowly, and the changes are smaller. Habits can become very ingrained; it isn't always easy to effect major changes. But most people who respond to an SRI do make some progress toward functioning the way they would like.*

BDD-related behaviors Behaviors associated with BDD usually improve as well. Less time is spent checking mirrors, skin picking, hair cutting, reassurance seeking, and performing other BDD behaviors. They're easier to resist and control, and the anxiety that can be caused by doing them, or not doing them, diminishes. "The main thing Prozac did for me was help me stay out of the mirror," one person told me. "I go into the bathroom, and my heart races, but I have the fortitude not to look. It's a very important change. The mirror no longer controls me."

---

* It's fascinating to consider that animal research shows that enhancement of serotonin with medications like Prozac leads to more "social" behavior—decreased avoidance, vigilance, and social solitude. Animals with extreme depletion of serotonin show significantly less "social" interaction than other animals.

Table 10   BDD–YBOCS Scores Among Responders Before and After Treatment with an SRI

BDD–YBOCS Item	*Average Score Before Treatment with an SRI*	*Average Score After Response to an SRI*
BDD PREOCCUPATIONS		
Preoccupation due to thoughts	3.2 (between severe [3–8 hrs/day] and extreme [more than 8 hrs/day])	1.2 (between mild [less than 1 hr/day] and moderate [1–3 hrs/day])
Interference due to thoughts (social, occupational/academic, other)	2.3 (between moderate and severe)	0.4 (between none and mild)
Distress due to thoughts	2.8 (between moderate and severe)	1.0 (mIld)
Resistance of thoughts	2.6 (between some effort and little effort)	0.7 (between always makes an effort and makes an effort most of the time)
Ability to control thoughts	3.3 (between little control and no control)	1.0 (much control)
BDD BEHAVIORS		
Time spent on behaviors	2.5 (between moderate [1–3 hrs/day] and severe [3–8 hrs/day])	1.0 (mild [less than 1 hr/day])
Interference due to behaviors (social, occupational/academic, other)	2.0 (moderate)	0.4 (between none and mild)
Distress if behavior prevented	2.5 (between moderate and severe)	0.9 (between none and mild)

continued

Table 10   BDD–YBOCS Scores Among Responders Before and After Treatment with an SRI *(continued)*

BDD–YBOCS Item	*Average Score Before Treatment with an SRI*	*Average Score After Response to an SRI*
Resistance of behaviors	2.9 (between some effort and little effort)	0.8 (between always makes an effort and makes an effort most of the time)
Ability to control behaviors	3.1 (between little control and no control)	0.9 (between complete control and much control)
INSIGHT	2.3 (between fair and poor)	1.4 (between good and fair)
AVOIDANCE		
(due to thoughts or behaviors—e.g., other people, work/school, going places, doing things)	2.2 (between moderate and severe)	0.6 (between none and mild)
TOTAL SCORE	31.7	10.3

Avoidance   In keeping with improved functioning, avoidance usually lessens. It's easier to do things, go places, and be around others. People become more active—their life becomes more colorful and interesting. Spending less time obsessing or checking the mirror frees you to do other things. It's also easier to do things and be around others when the thoughts and compulsions are less painful and powerful. In addition, self-consciousness and fear around other people may diminish, making it easier to socialize.

Table 10 presents changes in the preceding areas among the responders in our fluvoxamine study and patients from my clinical practice for whom I had BDD-YBOCS scores from before and after treatment. Keep in mind that these are *average* scores—some responders had less of a response to an SRI and others had more. Each item is rated on a five-point scale (0–4), with higher scores reflecting more severe symptoms.

While the items listed in Table 10 are the standard symptoms assessed by BDD researchers, other symptoms may also improve with an SRI.

Depression and anxiety   Symptoms of depression and anxiety often improve with SRI treatment of BDD. Depressive symptoms that improve include depressed or irritable mood, lack of interest and motivation, low energy level, poor concentration, low self-esteem, problems with sleep and appetite, and suicidal thinking. Anxiety symptoms, such as worrying, being on edge, and tension, usually diminish as well. In the fluvoxamine (Luvox) study, two standard measures of depression* revealed significant improvement in depression in a majority of patients.

Body image   A question I find especially interesting is whether body image changes with SRI treatment. This aspect of treatment response has been less well studied than the others I've discussed so far. My clinical experience suggests that some, although not all, SRI responders experience improvement in body image. The medication seems to have the potential to correct a faulty view of one's body.

In the fluvoxamine (Luvox) study, I systematically asked study participants whether their defect had changed since the beginning of the study. More than half of the responders said it had improved. The changes appeared to fall into two categories:

1. Some said the defect visually looked the same, but *it wasn't as distressing or anxiety provoking* as it used to be. They no longer judged themselves as harshly; that is, the cognitive and emotional response to it changed. People said things like, "It still looks the same, but I can live with it. It doesn't upset me as much. It's more of a normal dislike." Or "I'm not overreacting the way I used to. I can live with it now. It's no longer consuming me and ruining my life."

2. A higher percentage said the defect actually *looked different visually.* As I discussed in Chapter 11, some people seem to experience a change in their visual perception, the defect improving or disappearing with the medication and reappearing when it's discontinued. They say such things as "The marks on my face are gone. I don't *see* them anymore." Or "My face used to look blotchy and red. Now it looks fine. I must have been misperceiving." One

* The 24-item Hamilton Rating Scale for Depression and the Montgomery-Asberg Depression Rating Scale.

woman told me, "My features seem to have fallen into place. I look more attractive." She reported that her appearance had physically and visually changed—it wasn't just that she could cope better with it. Occasionally, SRI responders not only don't despise the defect any more—now they really *like* their body! About half reported that both kinds of changes occurred—a more purely cognitive as well as a visual change.

This raises the fascinating question of whether the SRIs can actually improve visual perception and change what may be, in at least some cases, a visual illusion. As I noted previously, serotonin appears to play an important role in vision in animals and may do the same in humans. The drug LSD, which causes visual illusions, affects serotonin in the brain. The SRIs may correct a chemical imbalance involving serotonin that leads to faulty perception or faulty interpretation of visual images.

"I look much better now," said one woman who'd responded to fluvoxamine (Luvox). "I look completely different, like a different person. My skin looks clearer, and my face is more proportionate. I don't notice the rashiness or blemishes anymore. I look normal, but I didn't used to. I like it! . . . I even asked my mother if I looked different and she said no—but I look different to me. . . . It's a nice experience to feel more confident. What I see now is the correct view."

Concern with more noticeable appearance problems   Another fascinating change I've observed is that sometimes the SRIs decrease an obsessional preoccupation with a noticeable aspect of appearance, such as obesity. Some people whose appearance problem wouldn't qualify for BDD (because the defect isn't nonexistent or slight) may nonetheless become less preoccupied with and less upset by these problems when treated with an SRI. For example, some people who are quite overweight become less consumed by their weight obsessions—they're still not happy with their weight, but they're no longer obsessed with it. Both their BDD-related concern and their concern with a more noticeable appearance problem diminish.

In a way, this observation makes sense. It isn't possible for the medication to distinguish between a slight appearance problem (i.e., BDD) and one that's more noticeable. The medication doesn't have eyes! The SRIs probably work by decreasing excessive, obsessional thinking, regardless of what the person actually looks like.

This issue requires more research and goes beyond BDD. It raises the question of whether accident victims or people with congenital deformities who are overly preoccupied with and distressed by very noticeable defects might benefit from SRI treatment. Might they become less consumed by their concern—less preoccupied, less distressed, and better able to function?

Insight   Some SRI responders experience improved insight, becoming more aware that their view of the defect was distorted. In some cases this seems due to resolution of a likely visual illusion. In the fluvoxamine (Luvox) study, we found that, on the whole, responders experienced significantly improved insight.* As one woman said, "I used to be 97% convinced that I looked horrible. Now I'm 97% convinced that I don't. I realize I was distorting." Improved insight occurred in 75% of the patients with nondelusional BDD and in 80% of those with delusional BDD; that is, people who were delusional before treatment were no longer delusional after treatment.

One of my more interesting research findings is that people with delusional BDD appear as likely as those with nondelusional BDD to respond to an SRI; that is, people who are *completely* convinced that their view of the defect is accurate, and who can't be talked out of this belief, have a high rate of response to an SRI. As I discussed in Chapter 12, people with delusional BDD would actually qualify for a diagnosis of delusional disorder. While the treatment of delusional disorder is an understudied area, medications known as neuroleptics are commonly used to treat such patients. My research findings, however, suggest that the BDD type of delusional disorder may actually respond to SRIs. At this time, I first treat patients with delusional BDD with an SRI. If they don't respond adequately, I may then add a neuroleptic (antipsychotic) medication to the SRI. But if a patient with delusional BDD is severely ill (e.g., hospitalized), I sometimes begin treatment with an SRI and a neuroleptic simultaneously.

This is an aspect of BDD that I'm further studying. In an ongoing study of fluoxetine (Prozac), I'm taking a more methodologically rigorous look at the question of whether delusional BDD—the preoccupation, behaviors, and insight—responds as well to an SRI as nondelusional BDD does.

These findings have implication for other psychiatric disorders. Do other types of delusional disorder also respond to SRIs? Do patients with delusional jealousy, who are falsely convinced that their partner has been unfaithful, respond to SRIs? My clinical experience suggests that the answer

---

* Insight was assessed with the Brown Assessment of Beliefs Scale (BABS), a scale developed by Dr. Jane Eisen of Brown University School of Medicine, myself, and Drs. Doug Beer, Katherine Atala, Steven Rasmussen, and Lee Baer. This scale has been shown to be a reliable and valid measure of insight (degree of delusionality).

may be yes. Does delusional OCD, in which people are absolutely convinced that a feared event may occur, respond to SRIs? Again, the answer appears to be yes. These are important, virtually unstudied questions that I hope we'll have answers to in upcoming years.

Commonly Asked Questions about SRIs in the Treatment of BDD

How likely am I to improve with an SRI? In our fluvoxamine (Luvox) study, 65% of the patients we've treated thus far have improved to a clinically significant degree. Dr. Perugi obtained the same result in his fluvoxamine study. In my clinical practice, in which I've used a variety of SRIs, 70% of 61 treatment trials have been successful.* Most responders appear to respond partially.† But even partial improvement may be an immense relief and make a real difference in the lives of BDD sufferers.

How many people who've failed to respond to one SRI respond to another? I found that of 37 patients who had no response, or only a minimal response, to an SRI, about a third responded to another SRI. This percentage is encouraging and suggests that we shouldn't give up trying these medications. In addition, I've found that response to an SRI can be enhanced by adding certain other medications, which I'll discuss later in this chapter.

To determine the response rate to SRIs with greater certainty, larger and more methodologically sophisticated studies of BDD need to be done. I and other researchers are conducting such studies, which will provide more data to answer this question.

---

* These improvement rates are based on a score of "much improved" or "very much improved" on The Clinical Global Impressions Scale or at least a 30% improvement on the BDD–YBOCS Scale. While a 30% decrease in symptom severity may seem relatively small, this degree of improvement correlates highly with both clinicians' and patients' ratings of "much improvement." In addition, 25% to 35% improvement on the Y-BOCS is the standard used by OCD researchers to indicate significant improvement in OCD, which has many similarities to BDD.

† On The Clinical Global Impressions Scale, 50% of the patients I've treated in my clinical practice have been considered "much improved," and 20% have been considered "very much improved." The rest (30%) were considered nonresponders—they were only minimally improved or unimproved. The mean change on this scale was 1.8, where 1 = very much improved and 2 = much improved. Dr. Eric Hollander has reported a similar degree of improvement in his patients (a change of 1.9 in one study). On the BDD–YBOCS scale, I've found that scores decrease an average of about 50%.

How long does the medication take to work? In our fluvoxamine (Luvox) study, it took an average of 6 weeks for BDD symptoms to decrease to a clinically significant degree.* The majority (68%) of responders improved to this extent between weeks 2 and 10. The earliest that anyone in the study responded was 2 weeks, the latest 14 weeks. Sixteen of 17 responders responded within 12 weeks. In my clinical practice, it took an average of 7 to 8 weeks for patients to respond, perhaps reflecting a slower rate of increase in medication dose than in the fluvoxamine study. In the Perugi study, patients responded within 6 to 10 weeks.

Because improvement usually occurs gradually, symptoms generally start to improve even before this. It isn't uncommon for a difference to be noticed within a few weeks of beginning medication. Rarely, improvement, which is often transient, occurs after taking only several doses of an SRI. While this very early improvement might be what's known as a placebo response—that is, not really due to the medication—in some cases it may be a medication effect. My experience suggests that this is a positive sign that may predict a later and more sustained response.

But a very early response is the exception rather than the rule. My advice is not to get discouraged, even if the medication hasn't begun to work after several months. Sometimes it takes longer than that. I recommend staying on the medication for three months, or even a little longer, before concluding that it isn't going to work. Patience and persistence are needed.

Occasionally, the medication begins to work in a dramatic fashion. Sometimes people can pinpoint the day, or even the hour, that it starts working. But typically the onset of effectiveness is gradual. People say things like "I felt a little better three days ago and today, but not for very long, so I don't know if it's really working." Don't get discouraged if this happens, because it's to be expected. These ups and downs—what I call a "sawtooth pattern" of improvement—gradually give way to more sustained periods of feeling better. Good hours gradually turn into good days, and good days transform into good weeks.

Some patients continue to improve further with time. After achieving a significant degree of improvement, with continued treatment symptoms may further respond over the following months.

What dose do I need? What's required to answer this question is a study that directly compares different doses of medication, which hasn't yet been done. In the meantime, we can look at the available data. In the

---

* By at least 30% on the BDD-YBOCS.

fluvoxamine (Luvox) study, patients responded to an average dose of 230 mg/day, and in Perugi's fluvoxamine study, an average dose of 208 mg/day was needed. In my clinical practice, patients responded to an average dose of 50 mg/day of fluoxetine (Prozac) and 175 mg/day of clomipramine (Anafranil). The range of doses to which patients respond is quite broad. Whereas some need a relatively low dose, it isn't uncommon to require the maximum recommended dose.

For patients with very severe symptoms, I tend to raise the dose relatively quickly, as it's tolerated. After a response occurs, the dose can always be gradually decreased to find the lowest effective dose.

If a lower dose of the medication hasn't worked, the dose should be raised, reaching the maximum recommended dose if necessary. As long as you're taking the medication, you might as well find out if a higher dose is more effective. If it isn't, the dose can always be lowered again. It's a mistake to keep the dose too low and to then conclude the medicine isn't working.

Does improvement last?   We also need long-term studies to learn what percentage of patients maintain their response to medication. In my clinical experience, the vast majority of people who respond to an SRI continue to feel well over months and even years while taking medication. Some patients I've treated who responded to medication five years ago are still taking it and doing well.

How long should I stay on the medication?   Studies of the relapse rate when people discontinue medication at different points in time are also needed. My clinical experience suggests that symptoms do recur in the majority of people who stop their medication. But some people remain relatively symptom free after stopping their SRI.

Until we have further scientific data on this question, I generally advise responders to stay on the SRI for at least a year after recovery—or longer if their BDD has been very severe. After all, they need a break. A year of decreased symptoms can allow them to get back to work or do their job more effectively, socialize more, and start enjoying their lives. At the end of this period, my patients and I discuss their options. Some people decide they'd like to try to stop the medication to see what happens. If their symptoms recur, they can always start it again, and in my experience the symptoms usually improve again when this is done. But since it appears that many people—if not the majority—relapse after discontinuing medication, some people opt to stay on it. They don't want to risk a recurrence of their symptoms. For people with very severe BDD, especially those who've attempted suicide because of their symptoms, this is probably the wisest choice. I was recently referred a man with severe BDD after his fluoxetine

(Prozac) dose had been decreased from 80 to 60 mg a day; as a result of this decrease, his BDD symptoms returned, which led to a serious suicide attempt that caused permanent lung damage.

If you decide to stop the medication, I recommend a very slow and gradual tapering, over months. This way, if the symptoms recur and the decision is made to increase the dose again, some medication is already "on board," which might decrease the time to response. In addition, a slow tapering can allow the lowest effective dose to be found; that is, the lowest dose that keeps the symptoms at a tolerable level can be identified, which is useful information. My clinical experience also suggests that reemerging symptoms may be less severe if the medication is gradually tapered rather than abruptly discontinued.

Are there any side effects?   In general, the SRIs are well tolerated. Reviewing lists of all these medications' possible side effects can lead to unrealistic worry; like all medications, the SRIs have the potential to cause side effects, but they're often quite minimal and may improve or disappear with time. Most people have no side effects or fairly minimal and tolerable ones. The SRIs, like other antidepressants, aren't habit forming or addicting. As a class, they've been prescribed safely for decades and are one of the most commonly prescribed classes of medication. They've been taken by many millions of people, often for many years and in some cases for decades.

Nonetheless, side effects can occur. Some of the more common ones are nausea, insomnia, feeling jittery, fatigue, decreased sex drive and sexual functioning, sweating, and decreased appetite. Anafranil can cause side effects such as dry mouth and constipation. These side effects are problematic in a relatively small percentage of people, and they do go away after stopping the medication. None of the SRIs have been documented to have any life-threatening side effects. In my experience, people with BDD who experience side effects are often willing to tolerate them because they so appreciate the relief they obtain from their symptoms.

When side effects do occur, they can often be diminished. Approaches include increasing the dose more slowly (if the dose is being raised), slowly decreasing the dose (while watching carefully for the reemergence of symptoms), or adding other medications to counteract side effects. Often, such strategies are helpful. If they aren't, another medication can be tried. One SRI may be better tolerated than another.

Patience is extremely helpful! I say this because side effects, if they occur, often appear before the medication has had time to work. This can be very frustrating. Keep in mind that some side effects get better, or even disappear, as treatment is continued. And the longer medication is continued (up to a point), the more likely it is to start working.

Is one SRI better than another? Which one should I try? The SRIs
haven't been directly compared to one another in the treatment of BDD, so
this question can't be answered with certainty. In my clinical experience,
they are all effective, although most of my experience has been with fluoxetine (Prozac), fluroxamine (Luvox), and clomipramine (Anafranil). Many
people respond to many, or all, of the SRIs, although some respond better
to one than another. At this time there's no way to predict which SRI will
most benefit an individual. The only way to know whether you'll respond
is to try one. Patients should discuss their options with their doctor and
determine whether one is preferred over another.

What If an SRI Doesn't Work?

What if an SRI doesn't work or works only partially? This is an important
question that clinicians and patients sometimes face. Some people are
pleased enough with a partial response that they don't want to pursue additional treatment, whereas others are interested in trying to further improve
their symptoms. While there are very little research data to answer this
question, my clinical experience suggests that a number of approaches may
be effective.

Maximize the SRI trial   While it isn't yet clear what an adequate SRI
trial for BDD consists of, my approach is to try to reach the highest dose
recommended by the manufacturer (if tolerated) if lower doses aren't effective. I also recommend extending the treatment trial to three months.
Sometimes, increasing the dose and extending the length of treatment lead
to improvement.

Add another medication to the SRI   If maximizing the SRI trial doesn't
work or isn't possible, another medication can be added to the SRI in an
attempt to enhance its effect. This approach, known as *augmentation,* is
commonly used in other disorders, such as OCD and depression. This strategy is particularly appealing if the SRI alone has been partially effective;
continuing the SRI and adding another medication (augmentation) allows
the partial response to the SRI to be maintained, whereas stopping the SRI
risks losing the partial response.

Buspirone (Buspar)   I've had some success by adding buspirone (Buspar)
to an SRI. Buspirone is an antianxiety medication with effects on serotonin
that is sometimes used to treat depression and OCD, often as an augmenting
agent. Unlike other antianxiety medications, buspirone is generally not sedat-
ing and has no potential for causing physical dependence or addiction.

I used this approach with 13 patients with BDD who had no response, or only a partial response, to an SRI. All had received the highest SRI dose recommended or tolerated for at least 10 weeks before buspirone was added. Six of 13 patients (46%) improved with buspirone augmentation. When three of the responders decreased or discontinued buspirone, their BDD symptoms worsened again, and when one then resumed her previous buspirone dose, she improved again; these findings suggest, although do not prove, that the medication was responsible for the change in BDD symptoms.

It's interesting that people who had had a partial response to an SRI (as opposed to no response) were more likely to respond to the addition of buspirone: 56% of those with a partial response to the SRI responded to buspirone, in contrast to only 25% of those who had not responded to the SRI. This pattern of response is similar to that seen in OCD.

Patients responded to buspirone, on average, in about six weeks, and the average effective buspirone dose was 48 mg a day. I recommend trying this approach for at least eight weeks and raising the dose to 60 mg a day if lower doses aren't effective. A few people I've treated further improved when the dose was cautiously raised above the commonly used maximum dose of 60 mg a day. The medication combination was generally well tolerated.

I've also treated a small number of patients with buspirone alone who preferred not to take an antidepressant medication. Several experienced some improvement in BDD symptoms, although none had the robust response that can occur with an SRI.

While these data are limited by the very small number of patients treated and by the open nature of the study, they suggest that buspirone augmentation of SRIs may be a useful alternative for people who fail to respond or respond only partially to an SRI. Like the other promising treatments described, this one warrants further study in a controlled study (in which the medication is compared to placebo).

Pimozide (Orap) Pimozide is a neuroleptic (antipsychotic) medication that's often used to treat delusional disorder and other disorders, such as Tourette's disorder (characterized by repetitive, uncontrollable verbal utterances or physical movements known as tics, which are similar to the compulsive behaviors of OCD).

There are several reasons to think that pimozide may be useful for BDD. Many years ago, a Canadian researcher, Dr. Alistair Munro of the University of Halifax, reported that pimozide was effective in a large percentage of patients with the somatic type of delusional disorder, including the delusional form of BDD. This study was open (uncontrolled) and involved only a small number of patients; nonetheless, the results were promising and led to pimozide's use for delusional BDD in clinical settings.

In addition, pimozide has been shown to be effective in OCD when added to an SRI, especially for patients with coexisting Tourette's disorder. Dr. Wayne Goodman and his colleagues at Yale University found that adding pimozide to fluvoxamine (Luvox) led to further and significant improvement in OCD symptoms than had been attained with fluvoxamine alone. Because of BDD's similarities to OCD, these results also have promising implications for BDD. Furthermore, Dr. Hollander and I have had some success in decreasing referential thinking associated with BDD by adding pimozide and similar medications to an SRI. One of my patients, for example, found it much easier to ride public transportation again, because he no longer thought that people were staring at him and making fun of him on the bus.

These three lines of evidence suggest that pimozide may be useful for BDD. My data, while very limited, suggest that pimozide alone generally isn't effective (with 0 of 10 trials successful), but I think that pimozide has promise when added to an SRI. I am currently studying this approach in a study funded by the National Alliance for Research on Schizophrenia and Depression (NARSAD). Those patients who fail to respond to fluoxetine (Prozac) and who have limited insight will be treated with placebo or pimozide. (People assigned to placebo will subsequently receive free treatment with pimozide.) Until these results are available, my advice is to use an SRI, and not pimozide alone, for BDD (including delusional BDD), but for those with delusional or poor-insight BDD who don't respond adequately to an SRI, adding pimozide is a reasonable and promising approach. And when treating severely symptomatic patients with delusional BDD, I sometimes simultaneously begin treatment with an SRI and pimozide in the hope that the combination might be more effective than either medication alone. Pimozide shouldn't be combined with clomipramine (Anafranil), but may be safely combined with fluvoxamine (Luvox), fluoxetine (Prozac), paroxetine (Paxil), and sertraline (Zoloft).*

Combine SRIs   I sometimes combine the SRI clomipramine (Anafranil) with one of the selective SRIs (fluvoxamine [Luvox], fluoxetine [Prozac], paroxetine [Paxil], or sertraline [Zoloft]) if response to an adequate trial of one of them isn't sufficient. A number of patients I've treated have done better on the combination than on either medication alone. This option may be particularly appealing if a partial response has been attained on one of these medications; rather than risking losing the partial response, the

---

* EKGs should be done periodically when using pimozide.

other medication can be added. Because the selective SRIs have the potential to increase clomipramine blood levels, a lower dose of clomipramine may be required than is usually used. I recommend checking a clomipramine level when this medication is combined with a selective SRI to ascertain that it isn't too high.

Switch to another SRI   Some people who fail an adequate trial of one SRI may respond to another. My approach is, if necessary, to try one SRI after another, in the hope that one will be more effective than others. In some cases, several SRI trials must be undertaken before an effective medication is found. As I've already discussed, various augmentation and combination strategies can be used before switching to another SRI.

Venlafaxine (Effexor) and nefazodone (Serzone) are newer antidepressant medications that have significant effects on serotonin and which may have promise in treating BDD. Venlafaxine seems particularly promising. Although I've treated too few patients with these medications at this time to comment on their efficacy, it's possible that they will be shown to be useful for BDD.

While I consider the above strategies to be first-line approaches for dealing with treatment-resistant BDD, other approaches are sometimes helpful for certain individuals. I've added lithium to an SRI in a number of patients, and although only one responded, the addition of lithium was very helpful, significantly decreasing both her BDD and depression.

Combining a benzodiazepine (commonly used medications for anxiety and insomnia) with an SRI can very helpful for some people with BDD, especially those with severe anxiety that isn't adequately decreased by an SRI. Temporary use of benzodiazepines can be very valuable for severely anxious, agitated, suicidal, or sleep-deprived patients in the early weeks of treatment, while waiting for an SRI to work.

If adding pimozide to an SRI isn't effective, I sometimes try adding another neuroleptic (antipsychotic) to an SRI for people with BDD who are delusional or have prominent referential thinking. Occasional patients have done well with neuroleptics such as trifluoperazine in combination with an SRI. Risperidone (Risperdal) and clozapine (Clozaril), which are newer neuroleptics, also appear promising; several people I've treated have done well when these medications were added to an SRI. One woman experienced a notable decrease in all aspects of her BDD symptoms, and several others experienced decreased referential thinking.

MAO inhibitors, another class of antidepressants with effects on serotonin, should also be considered if the SRIs don't work. Although the response rate doesn't appear to be as high as with the SRIs, it seems higher than with other medications. You may recall that Jane, whom I described in Chapter 3, had a very good response to an MAO inhibitor. Although we need more definitive data on their effectiveness, at this time I consider them a valuable alternative for people who haven't responded to a number of SRIs. (MAO inhibitors should never be combined with an SRI.)

In addition, cognitive-behavioral treatment, which I'll discuss in the next chapter, may be helpful in combination with medication. While this combined approach hasn't been adequately studied, clinical experience suggests that it may be useful.

Each person with BDD requires an individualized assessment of BDD and other symptoms. If other disorders are present along with the BDD, this may influence the medication selected. I recommend a comprehensive evaluation by a psychiatrist and development of an individualized treatment plan. Creativity and expertise in psychopharmacology are needed in more treatment-resistant cases. So is persistence. With enough tries, in my experience most patients eventually improve with medication.

Other Medications and Somatic Treatments

Over the years, reports have been published in the psychiatric literature of one person, or several people, with BDD responding to a particular medication. Most of these positive reports have been counterbalanced by negative ones. For example, response of BDD symptoms to imipramine (a non-SRI antidepressant) was reported for one patient, but in four other reports, BDD symptoms didn't improve with this medication. On balance, most of these reports suggest that non-SRI medications are generally ineffective for BDD.

My research findings support these case reports. Based on my treatment of patients and on information I've obtained on their prior treatment, I've found that only 8% of treatment trials with medications other than SRIs resulted in clinically significant improvement of BDD symptoms. With a class of antidepressants known as tricyclics (excluding the SRI clomipramine [Anafranil], which is a tricyclic), 15% of 48 trials resulted in improvement. Response rates to other non-SRI antidepressants (e.g., bupropion) appear similar. In my experience, these medications sometimes improve depression but usually not accompanying BDD symptoms. Amy, for example, experienced complete relief from her depressive symptoms on desipramine but no improvement whatsoever in her severe BDD symptoms. Both her BDD and depression subsequently resolved with an SRI. Occasionally, however, BDD symptoms do seem to improve with a tricyclic antidepressant.

MAO inhibitors (e.g., tranylcypromine [Parnate] and phenelzine [Nardil]), are antidepressants with significant effects on serotonin. My data (which are mostly retrospective) suggest that approximately 30% of people with BDD respond to these medications. While lower than with the SRIs, this rate is higher than that obtained with other medications.

Only 2% of neuroleptic (antipsychotic) trials, and 6% of trials with a variety of other psychiatric medications, such as benzodiazepines, resulted in improvement in BDD. Neuroleptics appear to be ineffective even for people with delusional BDD, a group they might be expected to help. It's worth emphasizing, however, that most of my data on neuroleptics are retrospective; in addition, it appears that neuroleptics may be helpful in combination with SRIs for some people with BDD. And benzodiazepines can be very effective in decreasing severe anxiety, although they generally don't appear to significantly decrease the BDD obsessions or compulsive behaviors themselves.

In published case reports, ECT, or shock therapy, was reported to be effective for BDD in two of eight patients. My data suggest a similarly low response rate, with 0 of 8 people responding. These findings, while limited by the very small number of patients, suggest that this treatment isn't effective for BDD. Nonetheless, ECT, which is the most effective treatment available for depression, may be worth considering for someone with BDD who is also severely depressed. Sometimes, when depressive symptoms become very severe, BDD symptoms can become less severe and even fade away. In such cases, ECT can be useful for the depression. Because ECT is a very effective treatment for depression and has the potential to be lifesaving, it should remain an option for someone with BDD who is very depressed and suicidal.

While brain surgery might seem like a drastic measure, some people are so tormented by their symptoms that they seriously consider it or have it done. I'm aware of three cases in which this approach was used for BDD. A published case reported improvement in BDD symptoms with a procedure known as a modified leucotomy. A colleague of mine told me of a young woman with debilitating and intractable BDD who had an excellent response to a similar procedure (bilateral anterior cingulotomy and subcaudate tractotomy). Another colleague described a woman with BDD who responded to a procedure known as a capsulotomy, a treatment being investigated for people with severe OCD who don't respond to standard treatments. These data are extremely limited, and I don't at this time recommend brain surgery for BDD, especially if many other treatment options haven't been tried or haven't been adequate. But it will be important to see whether future studies demonstrate that certain types of brain surgery offer hope for severely ill people with BDD who don't respond to other treatments.

Needed Studies

More studies of SRIs and other medications in BDD are greatly needed. The greatest current limitation is that, with the exception of studies that are still in progress, available data and studies are either retrospective or "open," which are potentially subject to bias. A good response to medication in these types of studies could result from spontaneous improvement or to a desire to please oneself or the doctor (a placebo response). A number of factors, however, suggest that placebo response in BDD is uncommon. For one thing, BDD is usually a chronic illness, so spontaneous remission isn't to be expected. In addition, many patients experience reemergence of their symptoms when stopping their SRI and remission when restarting it. Furthermore, some of my patients who've responded to medication have, out of curiosity, tried to bring their obsessions back, but couldn't. Another supporting piece of evidence is that non-SRI medications appear to be rarely effective for BDD.

Nonetheless, to prove that the SRIs really work, we need studies known as controlled studies. I am currently doing the first placebo-controlled study in BDD, comparing fluoxetine (Prozac) to placebo, which is funded by the National Institute of Mental Health (NIMH). (Patients who are assigned to placebo will subsequently receive free treatment with fluoxetine.)* Dr. Hollander's "cross-over" study, in which the same patient is sequentially treated with clomipramine (Anafranil) and desipramine, a non-SRI antidepressant, is also in progress.† If significantly more patients improve on clomipramine than on desipramine, this, too, is strong evidence that the SRIs are effective for BDD, and in fact more effective than another type of antidepressant. While findings from studies like these are necessary to prove the effectiveness of the SRIs, clinical experience and the available data are very promising.

* To obtain information about participating in this study, write to Katharine Phillips, M.D., Butler Hospital, 345 Blackstone Blvd., Providence, RI 02906.

† To obtain information about participating in this study, write to Eric Hollander, M.D., Box 1230, Mount Sinai School of Medicine, One Gustave Levy Place, New York, NY 10029-6574.

·· *fourteen* ··

Cognitive-Behavioral Therapy and Other Treatments

Cognitive-Behavioral Therapy

Cognitive-behavioral therapy is another promising treatment for BDD. Alan responded partially to this approach, and David found it helpful in combination with an SRI. Our knowledge of its effectiveness is still preliminary, with little published data and no placebo-controlled studies. Nonetheless, I and other researchers and colleagues find it useful for some people with BDD and consider it a promising approach.

Cognitive-behavioral therapy, or CBT, is a broad term encompassing a number of specific therapeutic approaches. It is a practical "here and now" approach that focuses on changing problematic thoughts and behaviors. When used by trained therapists, CBT has been shown to be effective for such disorders as depression, phobias, panic disorder, obsessive compulsive disorder, and eating disorders. Not all therapists, however, have been trained in CBT.

The *cognitive* aspect of cognitive-behavioral therapy focuses on cognitions—that is, thoughts. The goal of cognitive therapy is to identify and change distorted and unrealistic ways of thinking. The *behavioral* aspect of cognitive-behavioral therapy focuses on problematic behaviors, such as checking and social avoidance. The aim is to help the person stop such behaviors and substitute healthier behaviors. Often, cognitive and behavioral approaches are combined—hence, the commonly used term "cognitive-behavioral therapy," or CBT.

Available data and clinical experience suggest that a specific type of behavioral therapy known as *exposure and response prevention* may be particularly effective for BDD. *Exposure* consists of exposing the defect in feared and avoided situations—for example, social situations or work. With enough exposure, anxiety in these situations may gradually diminish, as may avoidance. *Response prevention* is not performing compulsive behaviors. Mirrors aren't checked, comparing isn't done, and reassurance isn't asked for or provided. With time, the behaviors may decrease in frequency. Exposure and response prevention are probably more effective than other behavioral approaches for BDD, although this hasn't yet been studied. While cognitive approaches may also be helpful, at this time I consider exposure and response prevention the most effective aspects of CBT for BDD (although cognitive approaches are often usefully combined with exposure and response prevention). Exposure and response prevention has been shown to be very effective for OCD—more effective than other behavioral strategies—and is currently considered the cornerstone of nonmedication therapy for OCD.

The first stage of cognitive-behavioral treatment for BDD involves education about BDD and its treatment. The patient is also asked to monitor BDD-related thoughts and behaviors, ideally recording them in a diary. Detailed descriptions of situations that trigger BDD thoughts and behaviors, the frequency of their occurrence, and the anxiety level produced by the situation should also be recorded. These initial steps alone can help people see how excessive their BDD behaviors are and how often they make them feel worse rather than better. This realization can set the stage for resisting such behaviors—that is, for response prevention.

This first stage is followed by the use of exposure and response prevention techniques, which I'll now describe in more detail.

Exposure

Exposure involves confronting feared and avoided situations, such as social situations, that trigger obsessive thoughts. The goal is to confront or enter such situations repeatedly, exposing the perceived defect until anxiety diminishes. Ritualistic behaviors intended to decrease anxiety in these situation, such as reassurance seeking, are not done. With enough exposure of the defect, anxiety and fear may gradually decrease. Learning theory would predict that avoidance of social situations is reinforcing (because anxiety may stay at a more manageable level in the short run) and prevents a person from habituating to his or her fear. It's better not to avoid.

Exposure can be done in several ways. It can be done by imagining oneself with the defect exposed in the anxiety-provoking situation (imaginal exposure) or by actually putting oneself in the feared situation (in vivo exposure). In vivo exposure is probably more effective, but if it's too anxiety provoking, doing imaginal exposure first may make in vivo exposure possible. The two approaches can be effectively combined.

The groundwork for exposure therapy involves constructing an anxiety hierarchy. The patient, with the therapist's assistance, develops a list of situations that cause BDD-related anxiety. For many people with BDD, these are social situations. Using the Subjective Units of Distress Scale (SUDS), the patient rates the amount of anxiety experienced in each situation. The numbers 0 to 100 are used, with 0 representing no anxiety and 100 representing a state of panic. The number assigned often reflects such factors as the number of people in the situation in which the defect is exposed, the familiarity of these people, and the distance of the exposed body part from others.

Sandra's anxiety hierarchy is shown in Table 11. She rated going out to the mailbox at night 5 on a scale of 0 to 100. Going to the mailbox during the day was rated 10, because the slight scar on her face was more visible in daylight. She gave shopping a higher rating, because this involved being around more people, who might notice her scar. Talking to a classmate or a stranger face-to-face from several feet away was rated 60, whereas talking with them from less than a foot away was a 70 because the scar would be more visible. The list of feared situations and the numbers assigned will differ for each person and should be individualized.

After constructing a hierarchy, the next step is to expose yourself, and the perceived defect, to a feared situation with a relatively low number. The key is to identify a situation that produces some anxiety but not too much. Sandra started with jogging around the neighborhood with the scar exposed. Initially, she was very anxious, but the more she did this, the less anxious she became. She then moved up her hierarchy, frequently going to the grocery store and doing other kinds of shopping. At first, she felt very anxious because she feared others would notice her scar, but the more she

Table 11   Sample Anxiety Hierarchy for Exposure Therapy

Feared Situation	Anxiety Rating
Getting the mail at night	5
Getting the mail during the day	10
Jogging around the neighborhood	20
Going shopping—for example, grocery shopping	30
Asking a store clerk about an item	40
Going to class and sitting near classmates	50
Talking to a classmate or stranger face-to-face from several feet away for at least 5 minutes	60
Talking to a classmate or stranger face-to-face from less than a foot away for at least 5 minutes	70
Speaking up in class	80
Talking with a man at a party	90
Going out on a date	100

went, the better she felt. She then continued moving up the hierarchy. She forced herself to go to night school again, first three times a week and then five times. Gradually, over several months, she put herself in increasingly anxiety-provoking situations, eventually talking with a man at a party. Eventually, her fear and avoidance diminished.

It's important to stop using camouflage in the exposure situations, unless it allows entry into the avoided situation early in treatment. Stop wearing covering makeup, a hat or wig, bulky clothing, and sunglasses. Shave off your mustache or beard if it's hiding a defect, and avoid covering the defect with hands or hair. Some therapists have patients actually magnify the defect, for example, messing up their hair or combing it straight back to expose a slightly receding hairline.

It's also important to refrain from doing other things that might be a distraction from the anxiety caused by exposure. Avoidance behaviors shouldn't be engaged in; nor should ritualistic behaviors, such as reassurance seeking, that could decrease anxiety. It's important to experience some anxiety during the exposure, which should gradually diminish with time.

To increase chances of success, it's also important to remain in the feared and avoided situation with the defect exposed long enough for anxiety to diminish. When first entering the situation, anxiety usually increases (and it should for exposure to work), but after a long enough time it actually falls again, to a level that may be even lower than the original anxiety level. The exposure shouldn't be discontinued until anxiety falls again. Therapists use the term *habituation* to refer to this phenomenon. If a situation is left prematurely, when anxiety is still very high, it will be that much harder to go back to the situation the next time. Exposure also needs to be done frequently enough—usually many times a week—so habituation may occur. With repeated exposure, anxiety should eventually decrease.

After developing her anxiety hierarchy, Barbara, who thought her hair didn't "look right" and spent hours a day styling it, was told to limit her styling and grooming to one hour, then 30 minutes, and then 10 minutes a day. Later, she was asked to no longer blow dry or style her hair at all and to mess it up while talking to staff in the therapist's office. In subsequent sessions she was exposed to people in stores and was instructed to talk with them for longer and longer periods of time without having styled her hair.

Exposure may be conducted in the therapist's office, but it's better if the therapist accompanies the patient into the feared situation, such as a store, modeling and prompting exposure and other adaptive behavior. Homework that includes self-administered exposure assignments is essential because consistent exposure makes habituation occur more readily. Family members or friends may be taught to assist in homework as co-therapists. Progress may be slow at first and then increase. It's helpful to keep a daily diary of the progress that's made—which situations are engaged in and the amount of anxiety experienced.

The approach I've been describing is known as *graded exposure*; that is, the exposure is done in a gradual, step-by-step fashion, beginning with the least frightening situation and gradually working up to more frightening situations. An alternative approach is *flooding*, a nongradual approach in which the person quickly confronts their most feared situation and remains in the situation until anxiety dissipates. Removal of camouflage can also be done with either graded exposure or flooding. With a graded approach, a hat might be inched back a little further each time, gradually exposing more of the hairline, or less and less makeup is used. With a flooding technique, the hat or makeup are simply removed and the defect exposed to others.

In my and my colleagues' experience, the graded approach is often successful and better tolerated than flooding, which is often too anxiety provoking. We've even had patients become suicidal when flooding was tried. I therefore recommend graded exposure, rather than flooding, especially for patients who are very depressed or suicidal. The effectiveness of flooding versus graded exposure needs to be further studied and directly compared.

An unresolved and important question is whether mirror exposure is useful. Sometimes, instead of being instructed to avoid mirrors, patients are told to expose themselves to the mirror and look at their defect until their iety diminishes. Others are instructed not to focus on the defect but on themselves as a whole. Or they may be told to expose themselves to the mirror for a certain amount of time each day—for example, an hour—and to avoid mirrors at other times. But some patients find mirror exposure unhelpful because they become far too anxious, and their anxiety never abates. I don't recommend doing this kind of exposure without a therapists' guidance until it's determined whether it's useful for a given individual.

My colleagues who specialize in CBT (Leslie Shapiro, MSW, of Butler Hospital in Providence, RI, and Dr. Robin Goldstein of McLean Hospital in Belmont, MA) sometimes use this approach. For example, a young woman who picked her skin was instructed to look in the mirror for an hour a day without picking. She was also instructed to avoid mirrors at other times. This approach was somewhat helpful. Another patient was instructed to look in the mirror for 20 minutes a day without specifically focusing on the "defect" in order to see himself more realistically. He, too, was instructed to avoid mirrors at other times. This approach was helpful for this patient because he realized that his view of the defect was distorted, and looking in the mirror confirmed that he actually looked okay. It was tried only after other approaches had failed, however, and his therapist made sure that the mirror exposure didn't substitute for mirror checking, which, fortunately, didn't occur.

If exposure therapy is too anxiety provoking, a lower-rated activity on the hierarchy should be tried. If this, too, is too anxiety provoking, the hierarchy may need to be modified, so less anxiety-provoking situations are included. Sometimes the SUDS levels need to be reevaluated and modified because patients can underestimate the actual anxiety level they experience in the situation. Here, too, medications can be extremely helpful. Partial response to an SRI may diminish symptoms, including anxiety, to the point where exposure therapy can be used. Anti-anxiety medications can also make exposure therapy possible by decreasing anxiety to a tolerable level.

Response Prevention

Response prevention is stopping the performance of compulsive behaviors. The patient is instructed to stop checking mirrors, asking for reassurance, picking their skin, comparing themselves with others, measuring, or engaging in any other repetitive BDD-related behaviors. The ritual should be avoided to the greatest extent possible.

The rationale for this approach is that these behaviors sometimes decrease anxiety and thus are done again and again, in the hope that this will be one of those times. But relief of anxiety is usually only temporary, if it occurs at all. In addition, the behaviors can actually maintain the fear and prevent disconfirmation of beliefs about the perceived defect. For example, if a scar is always covered by makeup, the person never has the opportunity to see that people won't shun him if it's uncovered.

Stop checking the mirror Avoiding mirrors is a commonsense approach that patients sometimes figure out themselves. For the many people whose obsessions are triggered or worsened by mirrors, the less often a glimpse of the defect is obtained, the better. Similarly, checking defects without a mirror should be stopped. Mirrors should be taken down and thrown away or covered with something (e.g., a towel) that's difficult to remove. Pocket mirrors should be discarded. Covering or removing other reflecting surfaces from the environment may also be necessary. One man kept his shiny toaster locked in the trunk of his car and removed it only when needed to make toast. Following this approach only halfway—for example, putting the mirror under the bed—isn't as helpful, since it's fairly easy to retrieve and check when the urge occurs.

It may be hard to believe that it's possible to live without mirrors, but patients tell me it is. They shave, put on makeup, and comb their hair without one. Some substitute a small mirror that's used only to briefly groom each morning, not to check the defect. While it may be difficult for family members or roommates to remove or cover mirrors, my advice is to get rid of as many as possible. Mirrors generally aren't needed in the living room or hallways, for example.

Stop asking for and providing reassurance Providing reassurance may decrease anxiety temporarily, but soon the anxiety returns, as does the urge to ask again. Quite often, a reassuring reply isn't believed, so anxiety doesn't diminish even temporarily. No response or a different response should be given instead—for example, "We've agreed that it isn't useful for me to reassure you; this is a BDD ritual that I don't want to reinforce." With time, if reassurance isn't provided, the behavior and the need for reassurance may eventually become less frequent or even stop.

Limit grooming time   Time spent on grooming activities, such as applying makeup, shaving, or styling hair, should be limited to a reasonable amount, for example, 15 minutes a day. Time, rather than how the person feels, should be used to determine when the behavior should stop, because people with BDD typically never feel really satisfied with how they look.

Stop other compulsive BDD-related behaviors   Avoid looking at fashion magazines if pictures of models trigger increased obsessions and anxiety. Stop comparing yourself with others; try, for example, to focus on aspects of other people's appearance unrelated to the defect. Stop measuring, weighing, clothes changing, skin picking, and seeking frequent surgical or dermatologic consultations. Telling yourself that these are BDD rituals— not things you *have* to do—can be helpful.

Using a step-wise approach to response prevention may be valuable. Because it can be very difficult to simply stop the behaviors, an initial goal could be to delay the behavior or decrease its frequency. For example, time spent in the mirror could first be decreased from four hours a day to three. The time could then be further decreased, in a gradual fashion, to 30 minutes.

Recording the time spent doing these behaviors facilitates success. A diary should be kept of situations that seem to trigger or worsen the checking behavior. This can help patients anticipate difficult situations, devise techniques for dealing with them, and monitor progress.

Keeping busy may also be useful. I advise patients to develop a list of enjoyable activities, which they can refer to and do instead of ritualizing when the urge to ritualize occurs. Some find it helpful to put this list on the refrigerator, where they can easily find it. Reminding yourself to go for a walk, pick up a crossword puzzle, listen to your favorite music, or go jogging instead of checking the mirror are just some examples of activities to substitute for BDD thoughts and behaviors. Keeping busy can decrease the obsessions and behaviors to some extent by shifting attention away from them, although it isn't, by itself, adequate treatment for BDD.

Some people find response prevention too difficult because the urge is too strong. A therapist may be able to devise ways to make resisting them easier. In addition, medications are a powerful ally, decreasing the urge to perform behaviors and increasing control over them. SRIs work hand-in-hand with response prevention and often increase success with this approach.

Systematic Desensitization
and Other Behavioral Techniques

Systematic desensitization, which is no longer widely used but which has similarities to exposure therapy, was reported by Dr. Dennis Munjack of LAC-USC Medical Center in Los Angeles to be effective in one patient. This method incorporated elements of imaginal exposure and used relaxation training. The patient, who was preoccupied with his "overly red" complexion, learned relaxation techniques and then constructed an anxiety hierarchy, which he called his "criticism about red face hierarchy." This included such things as being at a meeting at work without having to say anything, being at a meeting but having to speak (which might cause anxiety and increase facial redness), worrying that someone would say his face matched his shirt, and being teased about the color of his face (e.g., being called "beetface"). The patient also developed a "scrutiny hierarchy," which included similar items. He then imagined these anxiety-evoking scenes, starting with the least distressing, while remaining relaxed using his relaxation techniques. After 11 sessions, he was no longer bothered or preoccupied by his concerns with facial redness.

Other behavioral techniques may be helpful when combined with exposure and response prevention. For example, relaxation techniques may make exposure more tolerable, although I don't recommend them alone as treatment for BDD. Other patients may benefit from social skills training, in which adaptive social behaviors are learned. These approaches are optional rather than core behavioral treatments for BDD.

Cognitive Therapy

While exposure and response prevention focuses on changing problematic *behaviors,* cognitive therapy focuses on identifying and changing cognitions—that is, the negative *thoughts and beliefs* that underlie and fuel problematic behaviors. Cognitive therapy aims to help people overcome negative attitudes about themselves, and may also make it easier to do exposure and response prevention. Cognitive therapy is usually combined with exposure and response prevention.

Cognitive therapy was started by a psychiatrist, Aaron Beck, and has been developed by many others over the past several decades for the treatment of depression and anxiety disorders. This type of therapy is based on the premise that our internal world can be divided into thoughts, feelings, and behaviors, which interact in a complex way with the environment, as illustrated in the figure below.

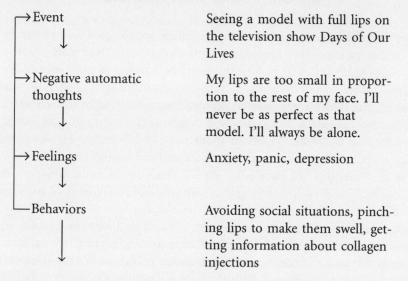

→Event	Seeing a model with full lips on the television show Days of Our Lives
→Negative automatic thoughts	My lips are too small in proportion to the rest of my face. I'll never be as perfect as that model. I'll always be alone.
→Feelings	Anxiety, panic, depression
Behaviors	Avoiding social situations, pinching lips to make them swell, getting information about collagen injections

Figure 1   An Example of BDD-Related Thoughts, Feelings, and Behaviors and How They Interact with the Environment

Cognitive therapy involves overcoming negative thoughts and feelings such as these, which should in turn change problematic behaviors. It typically involves the following steps, which take place over a number of therapy sessions:

1. Identifying the *unrealistic and negative automatic thoughts* that trigger upsetting feelings and behaviors (for example, "My lips are too small in proportion to the rest of my face"). Triggering situations for the thoughts may also be identified (e.g., seeing a model on TV).
2. Identifying the *unrealistic core beliefs, attitudes, and rules* that *underlie* the negative thoughts and drive the BDD symptoms (e.g., "If I don't look right, I'll always be alone").
3. Challenging the unrealistic beliefs and seeking *alternative, more realistic beliefs and attitudes* to replace the unrealistic beliefs (e.g., "Appearance isn't everything; I have many positive traits").
4. *Practicing* the alternative, realistic beliefs.

5. After the underlying beliefs have been at least partly modified, challenging the negative automatic thoughts and *developing more realistic alternative thoughts* to replace them with (e.g., "My lips look fine; I don't need to worry about them).

6. *Practicing* all of the above in a state of *emotional arousal* (e.g., anxiety). Homework assignments should include monitoring for any negative and distorted thoughts, challenging them, and substituting more realistic alternative thoughts.

The patient in the example above was helped to identify the automatic negative thoughts about her small lips as well as the painful feelings (such as anxiety and panic) and problematic behaviors (such as avoidance) the thoughts triggered. Her underlying beliefs about the importance of appearance were identified and challenged, and new beliefs and thoughts replaced the old problematic ones. For change to occur, steps 5 and 6 need to be combined with exposure and response prevention.

Cognitive therapy has been adapted for use in BDD by, among others, Dr. David Veale and his colleagues at Grovelands Priory Hospital in London. Dr. Veale and his colleagues first put a lot of effort into engaging the person in therapy and developing a psychological model for how negative thinking and behavior may maintain BDD symptoms. Aesthetic judgments about the appearance of the perceived defect are generally not directly challenged. Negative automatic thoughts are identified, but before attempting to modify them, Dr. Veale first has the patient examine the *core beliefs* that underlie the negative thoughts. These beliefs consist of assumptions or rules the person has about his or her appearance. Such assumptions or rules might include beliefs such as the following:

1. I have to look perfect.
2. My worth as a person depends on whether I look good.
3. If I don't look right, I'll always be rejected and alone.
4. I must always be approved of by everyone.
5. When people notice me, it must be because they're thinking how ugly I am.
6. If I don't get asked out, it must be because I'm ugly.
7. Life would be fine if it weren't for this ugly feature.

Cognitive therapy involves identifying and chipping away at negative attitudes and beliefs such as these which drive the BDD symptoms. The therapist works with the patient to develop alternative beliefs. The process of attitude change is assisted by collecting information in an "alternative data log" and reviewing it at regular intervals. The information collected is data the patient usually discounts or distorts.

Another technique used by Dr. Veale and Professor Isaac Marks is role play, with the therapist pretending to be the patient and playing "devil's advocate." The therapist argues in support of the patient's beliefs as if he or she were a prosecuting lawyer in court—for example, "I put it to you that you are ugly and will remain unloved for the rest of your life!" The patient is asked to play the lawyer for the defense and to refute the prosecution's case. In other words, the patient argues the case for an alternative belief— for example, that beauty is subjective and appearance is just one aspect of a person. This method helps patients look for evidence that doesn't fit with their beliefs and practice new ways of thinking.

After chipping away at the underlying core beliefs with methods such as these, it may then be helpful to question and challenge the negative automatic thoughts that spring from these beliefs. In Dr. Veale's experience, challenging the automatic thoughts early in therapy (or challenging them without first modifying the underlying beliefs) often doesn't work in BDD because most patients don't really believe the alternative thoughts. The underlying beliefs about being defective are often held too rigidly and may not be very susceptible to evidence or logic. Patients often dismiss or distort positive or neutral information that doesn't fit with their way of seeing the world (their underlying beliefs). For example, pointing out that the patient's spouse finds him attractive may be dismissed with "she only stays with me so she doesn't hurt me." This is similar to how a racist person might react after being helped by someone of another race; he processes the information by ignoring or distorting it—e.g., by thinking the helpful person was only trying to get something from him.

Patients are taught to be scientists, to treat their automatic thoughts as hypotheses and test them in experiments. For example, when a person with BDD sees a friend walking by who appears to ignore him, he might automatically have the negative thought, "I look terrible today—no wonder she's ignoring me." This thought triggers anxiety and feelings of depression. He feels worse about himself and withdraws more from others, creating a vicious cycle (as was shown in the Figure). A cognitive therapist helps the patient question his negative thinking and look for alternative explanations for being ignored (e.g., his friend was daydreaming). The patient also tests various alternative explanations, for example by calling his friend and asking her about the incident.

Taking this process a step further, some therapists find it useful to think of underlying beliefs and automatic thoughts as types of cognitive (thinking) errors (i.e., errors in reasoning) and to have patients identify these errors. Such errors include the following:

All-or-nothing (dichotomous) thinking: This involves seeing the world in extremes—good versus bad, or black versus white. The subtle shades of gray get lost. A BDD-related example: "With hair like this, I'll always look *totally* ugly," or "All that matters is my appearance. My other qualities don't count."

Overgeneralization: This involves making far-reaching, global conclusions on the basis of a single interaction or event. BDD-related examples: "I didn't get asked out this weekend—no one in the whole world likes me!"

Arbitrary inference: This involves drawing a mistaken conclusion from an experience, which is very common in BDD. Many people with BDD wrongly assume that if someone looks at them it's because there's something wrong with how they look. A BDD-related example: "When Jim looked at me he must have been thinking how bad my breasts looked."

Personalization: This involves not only drawing a mistaken conclusion, but also misinterpreting events in personal terms. Events that have nothing to do with the person are considered to be related to them. People with BDD often assume that a negative event, such as a look of disgust on someone's face, is directed toward them and a reaction to their appearance.

Exaggerating/catastrophizing: This involves exaggerating the negative aspects of an event and viewing negative events as catastrophic. BDD-related example: "This haircut is such a disaster that life's not worth living anymore."

Mind reading: This type of cognitive distortion involves assuming that other people are thinking the same negative thoughts you think about yourself—for example, "I know that person is thinking my nose looks funny."

The following examples illustrate what I've just discussed—identification of negative automatic thoughts, the cognitive errors being made, and underlying core attitudes and beliefs, as well as more realistic alternative beliefs and thoughts to replace them with.

Here are some examples of questions the therapist can ask the patient,

Table 12   Examples of Replacements for BDD-Related Negative Thoughts and Underlying Beliefs

Negative Automatic Thought	Cognitive Error	Underlying Belief/Attitude	Alternative Belief	Alternative Thought about the Event
This haircut is a *total disaster*. I won't be able to go out tonight."	Exaggerating/ catastrophizing	People won't want to be with me if I don't look right.	My friends like me for who I am, not because of how I look.	This haircut isn't perfect, but it isn't the end of the world. I may not like it, but I can live with it and go out tonight.
"That woman must be looking at me because my jaw's so wimpy."	Arbitrary inference Mind reading	Everyone views me only in terms of my appearance. Appearance is the only thing that matters.	Appearance isn't all that matters. It isn't the only thing that people notice.	Her looking at me probably has nothing to do with my jaw. She could be thinking that I'm attractive or that I seem like a nice person.

or the patient can ask himself or herself, to identify each of the categories in Table 12:

- *Negative automatic thoughts:* "What went through my mind when I was most upset?"

- *Cognitive error:* "What thinking error did I make?"

- *Underlying belief/attitude:* "What does this mean about me or the situation I'm in?"

- *Alternative belief:* "After considering the evidence, what alternative meanings are there?"

- *Alternative thought about the event:* What would be an alternative way of viewing the situation?"

For cognitive therapy to be effective, some emotional arousal should be experienced while doing it—otherwise, the therapy process may simply be an intellectual discussion, which is unlikely to lead to change. One way to accomplish this is to practice the alternative beliefs in an exposure situation. Some patients find it helpful, for example, to practice in front of a mirror or with the therapist looking at the perceived defect with a magnifying glass. Many patients, however, find this far too anxiety provoking and over-whelming and first need to discuss the beliefs and thoughts in a more intellectual way, or as if they were talking about somebody else, not them-selves. Whatever the method used, it needs to be repeatedly practiced. The patient should keep a diary to review with the therapist, recording informa-tion like that in Table 12. The ultimate aim is for patients to practice over and over again and eventually learn to be their own therapist. This should help prevent recurrence of symptoms in the future.

Another cognitive approach is having patients make positive self-state-ments that reframe their negative thoughts as a symptom of BDD. At times, Eva realized that her view of her thighs wasn't accurate. But at other times she lost sight of this and thought they looked really bad; at times like these it helped to replay in her mind statements like, "This is my BDD; my thighs look larger to me than they do to other people. I'm seeing myself in a distorted way." This approach appears more successful with people who already have some insight into the fact that their view of the defect is distorted and exaggerated.

Yet another approach used by some therapists involves instructing pa-tients to carry their negative and distorted thoughts to an extreme, for example, "As people drive by me, they're laughing at me because I'm the hairiest person in the world," or "Even people overhead in airplanes are noticing how ugly I am." As the thoughts become paradoxically absurd, they may become less upsetting and even humorous. This approach should be used only with the guidance of a qualified cognitive-behavioral therapist and, in my view, only with selected patients.

Some Commonly Asked Questions About Cognitive-Behavioral Therapy for BDD

How likely is it to work?   CBT has been studied in only a small number of patients, so we don't have a definitive answer to this question. Nonetheless, available data are encouraging. Drs. Fugen Neziroglu of Hofstra University and Jose Yaryura-Tobias of the Institute for Bio-Behavioral Therapy and Research in New York reported success with 4 of 5 patients using exposure and response prevention in combination with cognitive therapy. They found that most patients continued to feel ugly, but less than before treatment. They were also less distressed by their appearance and could more easily expose themselves to and tolerate the scrutiny of others. Professor Isaac Marks and Dr. Joseph Mishan also reported decreased avoidance, improved functioning, and improved insight with exposure and response prevention in three patients (although two were also taking medication, so it's unclear which treatment caused the improvement). In a retrospective chart-review study of 30 patients with BDD, Drs. Juan Gomez-Perez, Isaac Marks, and Juan Gutierrez-Fisac reported improvement in about half of the 21 patients who completed CBT treatment.

Dr. James Rosen found that exposure and response prevention plus cognitive techniques were effective in 77% of 27 patients who received this treatment in eight weekly two-hour sessions in a group format. BDD symptoms were significantly decreased, and self-esteem also improved. A strength of the study is that it was controlled to an extent—that is, subjects were randomly assigned to CBT or no treatment. However, because the control subjects didn't receive any treatment, it's possible that it wasn't specifically CBT that was effective but some nonspecific aspect of treatment such as the attention subjects received. It's also worth noting that the study didn't include men, many subjects appeared to fall in the diagnostic gray zone between BDD and eating disorders (most had concerns about weight or body shape), and the study follow-up period was brief. In addition, many subjects appeared to have mild BDD, and severely depressed or suicidal people were not included. Nonetheless, the results are very encouraging.

Dr. David Veale has also reported a successful outcome using CBT in a study in which 19 nondelusional patients were randomly allocated to either CBT or a wait list control group over 12 weeks. Those in the control group did not improve, whereas those who received CBT had significant improvement in BDD and depressive symptoms.

While these success rates are promising, most of the cognitive-behavioral therapists I've spoken with have the impression that it's harder to treat BDD than OCD with CBT. In addition, the improvement rates are likely to be biased because most patients who agree to participate in and complete CBT are highly motivated; those who aren't motivated to tolerate the anxiety and face the challenges posed by this treatment are unlikely to agree to participate in the first place (although some patients prefer trying CBT rather than medication). Some patients begin treatment but drop out because the anxiety is too great to tolerate. Others cheat, rendering the treatment ineffectual. Some hide mirrors under their bed, others don't do their homework. For CBT to work, persistence and commitment are needed. Dr. Veale's experience suggests that cognitive therapy may make it easier to comply with exposure and response prevention.

In my and my colleagues' experience, cognitive approaches often fail in people with delusional BDD. By definition, delusional thinking involves complete certainty that can't be changed by rational argument or discussion. Professor Marks, however, reported that several patients with delusional BDD did well with the role play technique in which the therapist presents exaggerated views of the defect, while the patient defends their appearance as normal, in a debate-like format. The question of whether certain cognitive techniques are effective for the delusional form of BDD needs to be researched.

In my experience, SRIs are more often effective than CBT for BDD. This statement reflects my opinion; we don't know for a fact which form of treatment is more effective, as they haven't been compared. My view may reflect the fact that we need to learn more about what specific CBT techniques are most effective for BDD. It could also reflect the fact that most of my patients have had moderate or severe (as opposed to mild) BDD, and that medications may be more effective for more severe symptoms. At this time, I would recommend against using CBT without an SRI in patients with intolerable anxiety, severe depression, or suicidal thinking. Partial response to an SRI, and temporary use of low to moderate doses of an anti-anxiety medication (benzodiazepine), can make participation in CBT possible and increase its chance of success. In addition, CBT is probably less effective for people who are delusional or who have no BDD-related behaviors—that is, for those with preoccupations alone.

The likelihood of success depends on the training, skill, and creativity of the therapist, who should be well trained in CBT. In some cases, standard approaches don't work, and ingenuity and persistence are required for devising successful techniques.

What is the recommended number of sessions?   It appears that fairly intensive and frequent treatment is needed. In their report, Drs. Neziroglu and Yaryura-Tobias used 90-minute sessions 5 days per week for 4 weeks or 12 weeks, or weekly 90-minute sessions for 12 weeks. They noted that sessions more frequent than once a week may be necessary. If the exposure sessions are too brief or infrequent, anxiety may not decrease, and may even increase, because there isn't enough time for habituation to occur—that is, for anxiety to decrease during exposure. Homework between sessions increases the intensity of treatment, which probably increases the chance of success. Patients with more severe BDD and more difficulties in functioning will probably require more days of treatment per week and longer treatment. Many experts consider an adequate trial for OCD to consist of a total of at least 15 to 20 hours of treatment. It isn't known whether this guideline is appropriate for BDD.

Can I stop my medication if I start behavioral therapy?   It hasn't been established that CBT is an effective substitute for medication. I recommend continuing the medication for a minimum of one year after recovery—and longer if that's the person's preference or if the BDD has been very severe—whether or not CBT has been received. It isn't known whether successful participation in CBT increases the chance of remaining symptom free after stopping medication. This is an important question to be studied. Until we have scientific data, I wouldn't assume that CBT protects against relapse. I know of patients who received high-quality CBT for BDD who relapsed after their medication was discontinued.

Can I combine cognitive-behavioral therapy and medication?   Yes! These two treatments work hand-in-hand. It appears that CBT may further improve response to medication; conversely, if BDD symptoms are severe, partial response to an SRI may make participation in CBT possible. The SRI may decrease BDD symptoms, depression, or anxiety, or may increase insight to the point where the person is willing and able to try CBT. If necessary, an antianxiety medication may also facilitate participation in CBT. For severe BDD, or BDD with severe depression or suicidal thinking, I consider medication essential.

Needed Studies

Much larger and more methodologically rigorous studies of CBT are needed, especially controlled treatment trials, in which CBT is compared to a placebo treatment and to other active treatments such as medication. Some additional questions that require investigation are the following: Is CBT more effective for mild than severe BDD, or for nondelusional than delusional BDD? Is medication plus CBT better than medication or CBT alone? Is improvement maintained over the longer term? What is the optimal frequency and length of treatment? These are just some of the many important questions that I hope are studied and answered in upcoming years.

Treatments That May Be Useful
When Combined with Core Treatments

The following treatments appear useful for some people when combined with the "core" treatments just described; they do not, however, appear to be effective for BDD when used alone. This impression is based on information I've systematically obtained from study subjects about their past treatment response as well as my clinical experience. At this time, these strategies haven't been adequately studied, so definitive judgments about their effectiveness can't be made. Five, ten, and twenty years from now, it will be possible to make more definitive statements about their efficacy.

Group Therapy

The potential usefulness of group therapy for BDD is intriguing. In the previous section, I described the good outcome reported by James Rosen, who used cognitive-behavioral approaches in a group setting. In addition, I and Leslie Shapiro have run several groups for people with BDD, most of whom found the group helpful.

Each group consisted of six to ten patients, all of whom were also in individual treatment and had moderate to severe BDD. The groups met once a week for 90 minutes for a total of 12 to 16 weeks. The format focused on (1) education about BDD, (2) support, and (3) learning cognitive-behavioral techniques for BDD.

The education portion of the groups consisted of brief presentations about BDD and patients' discussion of their own experience with the disorder. They also learned cognitive-behavioral strategies and did homework, as described in the preceding section. The group strategized together, helping one another devise cognitive-behavioral approaches to deal with their symptoms. Group members also provided one another with much-valued support. It was an amazing experience for some of them to meet other people with BDD—to interact with others who truly understood their own experience.

While patients found the group treatment generally helpful, BDD symptoms per se didn't greatly improve with group treatment. The better outcome reported by Dr. Rosen might reflect the specific techniques he used, which may have been more effective, although we used similar treatment strategies. Another possible explanaiton is that his patients may have had less severe BDD. I think it's likely that group treatment alone is more likely to be effective for mild BDD and that it is important that patients with more severe BDD also receive medication and/or individual cognitive-behavioral treatment. At this time, I require all my group patients to be in individual treatment as well.

Although the available data on group treatment are preliminary, they're promising. I would hypothesize that group treatment based on cognitive-behavioral approaches is more likely to be effective than other types of group treatment. I also think it's likely that groups focused on BDD are more likely to be effective than groups in which the treatment focus isn't on BDD. Many people with BDD have great difficulty participating in non-BDD-focused groups and may drop out because they're so embarrassed by their appearance and their symptoms. They're often reluctant to divulge their concerns, and they may simply spend the group time comparing themselves with others and thinking that everyone else is noticing how ugly they are. Such an approach appears very unlikely to be effective for BDD when used as the only form of treatment.

Insight-Oriented Psychotherapy

Insight-oriented psychotherapy, also known as psychodynamic or exploratory psychotherapy, is a type of individual "talking therapy." This approach focuses on increasing self-awareness and bringing about behavioral change (e.g., improving relationships with others) through exploration of one's perceptions and interactions with others. Better awareness of one's inner life and motivations, and improvement of one's problems, should result.

Available evidence, although very limited, suggests that this type of treatment alone—as well as psychoanalysis alone—is generally ineffective for BDD. I've seen countless patients who have been in insight-oriented psychotherapy for months or years, as the only treatment for their BDD, only to end up unimproved and frustrated over their lack of improvement. They never figured out the "reason" for their BDD; even if they thought they did, their symptoms generally didn't improve as a result. Most of the psychoanalysts I've queried have said that in their experience psychoanalysis alone is generally ineffective for BDD.

Having said this, insight-oriented psychotherapy or psychoanalysis may be useful for some patients as an adjunct—that is, in addition—to the core BDD treatments. Psychologically minded people may benefit from an insight-oriented therapy that explores BDD-related themes—for example, low self-esteem, sensitivity to rejection, or relationship problems. This type of therapy may also be very helpful—if not essential—for certain problems unrelated to BDD. At this time, however, I do not recommend using it without the concomitant use of medication, as it appears unlikely to effectively diminish BDD preoccupations or behaviors when used alone. The effectiveness of this treatment is harder to study than that of medication or cognitive-behavioral treatment; nonetheless, I hope such studies will be done.

Supportive Psychotherapy

Supportive psychotherapy is another type of talking therapy that focuses on the creation of emotional support and a stable, caring relationship with patients. The therapist concentrates more on providing support than on increasing patients' understanding of themselves. Advice, learning new social skills, and assistance in problem solving are often components of this approach. The goal is to help patients attain the highest possible level of functioning. This approach is often usefully combined with other therapeutic approaches, such as medication treatment or cognitive-behavioral therapy.

For patients with BDD, this therapeutic approach offers understanding and support for their struggles with the disorder. It can help the BDD sufferer cope better with life—for example, the effects of BDD on friendships, intimate relationships, school, or work. For some patients, the provision of support by a psychiatrist who is prescribing medications, or support offered in the course of cognitive-behavioral therapy, may suffice. Some patients do, however, benefit from additional supportive psychotherapy, and for some it's essential.

While supportive psychotherapy can be a very helpful addition to the core BDD treatments, I don't recommend it as the only treatment for BDD because it appears unlikely by itself to effectively diminish BDD preoccupations or behaviors. Like insight-oriented psychotherapy, the role of supportive psychotherapy in the treatment of BDD needs further study.

Family Therapy

Family meetings or family therapy may be another helpful adjunctive approach. Such meetings may include spouses, parents, or other family members. I often meet with family members, at least once, to get to know them and hear their view of the problem. They often find it helpful to learn about BDD—what it is and what the treatment options are. If family members participate in BDD-related rituals, we discuss ways in which they can avoid being part of these behaviors.

More extended family meetings or formal family therapy may be helpful for selected individuals, particularly families of children and adolescents. This approach may increase understanding of BDD's effect on the patient and the family, provide a forum for devising coping strategies, and teach family members how to assist in behavioral treatment. Other family problems, if present, can also be addressed.

Vocational Rehabilitation

While medication and CBT may improve work or school functioning, some patients—particularly those who've been underemployed or unemployed for a long time— also benefit from a formal vocational program. Response to medication may get these individuals to the point where they can usefully participate in such a program. For someone who hasn't been working, the first step may be a volunteer job, with gradually increasing hours, then a paying job, perhaps first on a part-time basis. Other people with BDD won't need to take this stepwise approach.

Individuals with BDD who abuse drugs or alcohol should also be in a treatment program that focuses on their drug or alcohol problem.

Self-Help Groups

I'm sometimes asked whether self-help groups are helpful. My answer is that it depends on the group, and that self-help groups alone are unlikely to effectively treat BDD. I do recommend certain self-help groups, but in addition to the core treatments I've described.

There are as yet no self-help groups designed specifically for BDD, although some are getting started. But some people with BDD find that other types of support groups are helpful. Some benefit from participation in the Obsessive Compulsive Foundation (OCF), because of the many similarities between BDD and obsessive compulsive disorder.* Others benefit from participating in such organizations as the National Alliance for the Mentally Ill (NAMI), Freedom From Fear, or, especially if they have accompanying depression or manic-depressive illness, the Manic Depressive and Depressive Association (MDDA). These are national organizations with local chapters that offer education and support groups for people with psychiatric problems. I recommend groups like Alcoholics Anonymous and Narcotics Anonymous for people with a coexisting alcohol or drug problem.

Other types of self-help groups that don't educate members about psychiatric illness or don't support psychiatric treatment are unlikely to be helpful and may be harmful. My hope is that in the near future groups will form that are specifically geared to people with BDD.

Combining Treatments

All the treatments I've described can be combined, sometimes with a better outcome than with any one treatment alone. While some patients, like Christina, experience remission of their symptoms with medication alone, others derive greater benefit from a combination of medication and cognitive-behavioral treatment. Others do best with a combination of medi-

---

* Obsessive Compulsive Foundation, P.O. Box 70, Milford, CT 06460-0070; tel: 203-878-5669. The OCF can also provide information on support groups for BDD that are getting started.

National Alliance for the Mentally Ill (NAMI), 2101 Wilson Boulevard, Suite 302, Arlington, VA 22201; tel: 703-524-7600.

Freedom From Fear, 308 Seaview Avenue, Staten Island, NY, 10305; tel: 718-351-1717.

Manic-Depressive and Depressive Association (MDDA), 730 N. Franklin Street, Chicago, IL 60610; tel: 312-939-2442.

The Dean Foundation for Health, Research, and Education (8000 Excelsior Drive, Suite 302, Madison, WI 53717-1914; tel: 608-836-8070) can provide information on BDD.

cation, supportive psychotherapy, and a group. As I've previously emphasized, I advise everyone with BDD to take medication or be in cognitive-
behavioral treatment.

How do you know which combination, if any, should be used? It depends on the individual. The treatment plan for any given person should
be tailored to their individual needs and life situation. In general, the treatment plan should be based on (1) the severity of BDD symptoms, (2)
whether other disorders or problems are present, (3) the patient's preference, and (4) the availability of therapists trained in CBT.

If a person has severe BDD and is very depressed or suicidal, treatment
with medication is critical, and a supportive therapy (which may be part of
medication visits) is also desirable. In such cases, family meetings can be
very helpful. Patients who fit this description may be too ill to meaningfully
engage in CBT. Participating may be too stressful until the symptoms are
at least partially alleviated by medication.

People who have significant problems in addition to BDD may benefit
from therapeutic approaches in addition to medication and cognitive-
behavioral treatment. They may, for example, benefit from an insight-
oriented therapy or couples' therapy aimed at resolving relationship difficulties, self-esteem problems, or sensitivity to rejection, problems that don't
always adequately resolve with medication or CBT. Or they may benefit
from vocational rehabilitation or a partial hospital program in addition to
medication. Coexisting disorders may require additional medications. The
advice of a psychiatrist or other mental health professional should be obtained to make this determination.

Patient preference should also influence the treatments selected. Some
people strongly prefer trying medication only, whereas others prefer CBT.
Others benefit by obtaining a better understanding of their inner life and
are helped by an insight-oriented psychotherapy in addition to medication.
Others benefit from the support of a group. Another factor to consider is
that relatively few therapists are well trained in CBT.*

I suggest that patients seriously consider the recommendations of a mental health professional who has thoroughly evaluated their difficulties and
that medication (especially for patients with moderate or severe BDD and
those with severe depression or suicidal thinking) or cognitive-behavior
therapy be part of the treatment plan.

---

* Information on therapists trained in CBT can be obtained from the Obsessive
Compulsive Foundation and from the American Association for Advancement of Behavior Therapy (for addresses and telephone numbers see pages 314 and 315).

Surgery, Dermatologic Treatment, and Other Nonpsychiatric Medical Treatments

Sophie's experience with surgery was like that of many people with BDD. She was initially happy with her nose surgery but after several months became increasingly dissatisfied and had another operation. This time, she thought the surgeon ruined her nose. She even considered suing him, even though other people told her how nice her nose looked.

"I don't care what other people say," she said. "He made me look like an idiot!" A third nose operation was also unsuccessful. "People still look at my nose and think it's ugly," she said. "They're thinking I look like a dog." Sophie believed this even though she'd often been asked to work as a model. Her explanation for these requests was, "They've asked me to model because they feel sorry for me because of my atrocious appearance."

Jack estimated that he'd seen 10 to 15 dermatologists and plastic surgeons for the scars on his face. The problem had begun during childhood, when he had chicken pox. "My father forced me to go to school, even when I still had some scars, and I freaked out because people could see the scars. I picked to get rid of them, which made them even worse." For many years, Jack had worn his hair long so it covered much of his face. Most of the surgeons and dermatologists told Jack he looked fine—that his scarring was minimal—and didn't provide treatment. "They thought it wasn't really a problem," Jack explained. But recently he'd found a dermatologist who'd agreed to do dermabrasion. "I was so happy with having it done that I cut my hair short," he said. "Then I took the bandages off, and I realized the scars were still there." Jack was so upset over this that he quit his job as a cashier.

Kate saved up her money and spent thousands of dollars on skin remedies. She'd seen many dermatologists and plastic surgeons as well as countless cosmetologists and aesthetisists, and she'd tried numerous acne medications, cosmetics, and facials. She'd even managed to buy liquid nitrogen through a mail-order catalog to remove a few freckles from her face. "I felt desperate for treatment—I'd try anything. I knew I'd have no peace until I could solve the freckle problem. I constantly called the doctor when the treatment didn't seem to be working. I was an obnoxious patient."

A majority (72%) of the people I've seen have sought nonpsychiatric medical or surgical treatment, and 61% actually received such treatment. Some people finally received treatment after being turned down by other physicians. The most common reason such treatment wasn't received is that the physician thought it wasn't necessary and didn't provide it. The defect wasn't present or was minimal enough so that surgery or other forms of medical treatment weren't worth the risk.

Dermatologists are most often seen, with 49% of those in my study having seen, and 38% having been treated by, a dermatologist. This isn't surprising, since skin and hair concerns are so common. People with BDD who pick their skin are particularly likely to seek such treatment. When dermatologic treatment wasn't received, it was usually because the doctor thought it wasn't warranted.

Surgery was sought by 33%, about a third of whom didn't receive it, usually because they weren't able to find a surgeon who would agree to operate. Seventy-one percent had surgery on their nose, 14% on their ears, 11% on their eyes or eyelids, and 11% on their breasts or chest. Lip, chin, jaw, or skin surgery had each been received by 7%, and cheekbone, eyebrow, or penis surgery had each been received by 4%. Those who received surgery had an average of two surgeries and as many as six; 61% had more than one operation. Most patients who had more than one operation had at least one repeat operation on the same body part, usually because they were dissatisfied with the previous results.

A recent study by Dr. Christopher Thomas, a psychiatrist in England, compared 20 individuals with BDD to 20 patients awaiting rhinoplasty (a nose job) and 20 normal controls. Compared to the other two groups, those with BDD were more dissatisfied with their facial appearance and were more "neurotic," introverted, anxious, and depressed.

Eleven percent of the patients in my study had seen other medical doctors, 6% had seen dentists, and 13% had sought or received nonmedical treatment such as electrolysis. Most people sought or received treatment from more than one of these categories—for example, they'd seen both a dermatologist and a surgeon. As health plans increasingly require patients to see primary-care doctors before they see a specialist, primary-care doctors will increasingly see people with BDD.

Some patients have surgery on a body part that looks acceptable to them to make it even more attractive and thereby "distract" attention from the "defective" body part. One handsome man was planning a total facial reconstruction, even though his face looked fine to him because, if it looked even better, people might not notice his supposedly thinning hair. A beautiful young woman had a cheekbone implant so people would look at her cheekbones instead of her "ugly" lips.

Although studies show that most people are pleased with the results of cosmetic surgery, this doesn't appear to be the case for people with BDD. Two-thirds of those who had surgery or nonpsychiatric medical treatments reported no change or even a worsening of their concerns. They were just as, or even more, preoccupied, distressed, or impaired by their concern with their perceived defect. One man thought that orthodontia had pulled his ears down. Another man became more preoccupied after trying minoxidil for his supposedly thinning hair. "I was much more obsessed," he said. "I kept wondering, 'Was it growing?' I spent even more time in the mirror."

"I hated the results of my surgery," Nicole said. "Too much bone was taken off one side of my nose. Now you can see a shadow on the smooth side and a bump on the other side. It was the biggest mistake of my life. It took all of my looks away." Jeff, who had multiple surgeries, told me, "Overall, surgery made my appearance worse. I wouldn't do it if I could do it over." Some people feel temporarily better, but the improvement doesn't last. "My nose looked better for a while after I had surgery," a 35-year-old salesclerk told me. "But then it seemed to grow back after six months, and I wasn't happy with it anymore."

Many people with BDD seem to have very high and unrealistic expectations for surgery, expecting the surgical outcome to be perfect. Scott was an example of this: "The surgeries I had were somewhat helpful, but they weren't good enough. I'm a perfectionist." Surgery after surgery may be obtained in pursuit of this elusive perfection.

Others with BDD have a very particular idea of how they should look after surgery, which may not conform to conventional views of beauty. They may expect an outcome that to others would be undesirable. As the husband of a woman with BDD said, "The surgeons always focus on something different than my wife wants them to." One man was so desperate over his nose that he asked to have it completely removed!

In other cases, people with BDD may not have conveyed their desire to the surgeon or may feel that their directives weren't followed; some requests are vague. Or they may not have anticipated how they'd actually look after the desired change was accomplished. A 30-year-old man told me, "I wanted my nose shorter, but the surgeon changed the whole shape because he thought it would look better that way. He took my whole nose off. I didn't want him to do those things. I feel I lost my identity, and I'm sorry I ever had it done." Another person, whose nose had been changed exactly as he'd wanted, was nonetheless disappointed because he hadn't anticipated how his new nose would look in relation to the rest of his face, and he was angry at the surgeon for not telling him how he'd look.

Even when the treatment outcome is good by objective standards, which is usually the case, some people blame the surgeon for ruining their looks. This can fuel a desire for even more surgery, leading to procedure after procedure. "I first saw a plastic surgeon who refused to operate because he said nothing was wrong," Claire said. But she subsequently did have surgery, first liposuction of her neck as well as chin and cheekbone implants. "Overall I felt somewhat better, but my chin was still off center. I needed another operation to center the chin and build up the right jaw." After another surgery, Claire still thought that her chin wasn't centered. "After my third surgery, I was happy with the chin centering but not my jaw." She was planning a fourth surgery to fill out her jaw and make it look symmetrical, even though her savings were nearly depleted.

Some people repeatedly visit the surgeon after surgery, asking for reassurance about the "faulty" operation. Others sue. Still others get extremely depressed and even suicidal after having surgical or medical treatment that they believe has ruined their looks. A woman lawyer, who had many unsuccessful surgical procedures, told me that she thought she might ultimately kill herself over the results of future surgery. I've worked with many patients who were suicidal over their belief that a powerful acne medication caused irreversible damage, such as dry and flaky skin, or a change in their skin color. "In using the Accutane, I threw gasoline onto the fire," one patient told me. "I've caused irreparable damage to myself. The tragic mistake I made is always on my mind. . . . Because of this, I prefer not to live."

"My life has never been the same since my surgery," Walter said. "I went to have my nose done, and the surgeon volunteered that I could use an implant in my chin, even though my chin had never bothered me. It ruined my life. I was horrified by the surgery. My nose was ruined—I have awful scar tissue there. I was very angry and upset. I got suicidal because of it. I also got swallowing and saliva problems because of the chin implant. I had to go to the emergency room because I was so upset."

Educating patients about BDD and their distorted view of their appearance, or their unrealistic expectations for surgery, is sometimes helpful in decreasing their anger and motivating them to obtain psychiatric treatment.

One-third of the people I've seen reported improvement in their concern with the treated body part, but in most of these cases (about three-quarters), the BDD didn't improve. What often happened is they subsequently obsessed more about something else. Some worried more about a previous concern; others started obsessing about a new body part. As a 50-year-old business executive said, "My obsession stayed regardless of my appearance. After surgery, it just moved on to something else."

After dermatologic treatment, Ellen became more sensitive to smaller imperfections in her skin. And another woman told me, "I've seen six dermatologists, and I think they made my skin look better, but I don't worry any less because I worry just as much about small pimples as big ones. And now I'm hypervigilant. I worry my skin will get bad again."

This type of outcome isn't surprising, considering that the problem in

BDD isn't physical—it's obsessional. Fixing the perceived defect generally doesn't cure the tendency to worry and obsess. As G. A. Ladee wrote in the 1960s, BDD is "the self-detested body image . . . which no mirror and no surgeon can correct." What's needed is psychiatric treatment that gets at the root of the body-image problem by treating the tendency to obsess.

It can be difficult, though, to turn down requests for surgical or other medical treatment. Some people with BDD suffer so greatly that it can be very hard to deny them the treatment they so desperately seek. "The doctors and my friends and family tried to talk me out of surgery," Andrew told me. "But they couldn't turn me down because I was so miserable." Another man said, "I can't believe the doctor did liposuction because now I know I look fine. But I was so unhappy back then that he gave in and did it."

No one can predict with certainty how someone with BDD will respond to surgery or other medical treatment, but it appears that most don't improve, and some are devastated by the results. Psychiatric treatment is more likely to be helpful and is a much more conservative route to take. The results aren't irreversible, as they may be with surgery. There's nothing to lose by trying it.

Having said this, there is a group of people with BDD who may benefit from a combination of psychiatric and dermatologic treatment. These are people who pick their skin, some of whom damage it, creating infections or other skin problems. But while some require and may benefit from dermatologic treatment, this treatment generally doesn't decrease the BDD symptoms—the preoccupation and picking behavior—that caused the skin damage in the first place. Psychiatric treatment is needed to break the picking cycle and prevent further skin problems. I found that 85% of 20 people with BDD who picked experienced no decrease in their skin obsessions or skin picking with dermatologic treatment but that 75% subsequently improved with a serotonin-reuptake inhibitor.

BDD has been virtually unstudied in dermatologic, surgical, and other medical settings. Yet these patients have been described in the professional medical literature. In the dermatology literature, BDD has been referred to as "dermatologic hypochondriasis," "hypochondriacal preoccupation with trivial lesions," and "dermatological non-disease." Skin picking associated with BDD is subsumed by the term "neurotic excoriations." In some reports the term "monosymptomatic hypochondriacal psychosis" is used, which refers to delusional BDD.

BDD is less precisely identified in the surgery scientific literature. Some studies done in surgical settings may have included some people with BDD, but how many and which patients had BDD is unclear because the disorder wasn't clearly identified. Surgery studies that included patients with "minimal deformities," "perceived defects," or "psychological problems" can't be assumed to pertain to BDD because it isn't clear which patients in these studies, if any, had BDD. Although people with BDD have no deformity, a minimal deformity, or a perceived deformity, the criteria also require preoccupation and clinically significant distress or impairment in functioning as a result of the concern.

One study from Japan was an exception in that the patients were identified as having BDD. This was a study of 274 patients with BDD who went to a surgery clinic requesting cosmetic surgery. A review of the patients' charts indicated that many were dissatisfied with the results of surgery. The researchers concluded that surgery in people with BDD is risky because they often have unrealistic expectations, are often unhappy with the outcome, and may be angry with the surgeon about the results. These surgeons therefore tended to avoid operating on people with BDD. Similarly, a review of BDD in a German surgery journal concluded that such patients should not be treated with surgery.

It's been estimated, on the basis of several studies, that approximately 2% of people seeking cosmetic surgery have BDD, although a number of authors and some surgical colleagues of mine suspect the actual number is higher. Preliminary data from a general medical outpatient setting, which I've obtained in collaboration with Dr. Mark Zimmerman of Brown University School of Medicine, suggest that the prevalence of BDD may be relatively high in this group. We found that of 316 patients who were seen in this setting, 4.4% appeared to have BDD. While this finding requires confirmation, it's surprisingly high and suggests that BDD may be relatively common in this setting.

While my results suggest that few people with BDD are pleased with surgery or dermatologic treatment, it could be argued that they're biased, because people who improve with such treatment might not subsequently see a psychiatrist. The results of the Japanese study I just mentioned, however, suggest that my findings of a generally unsatisfactory outcome with surgical treatment may not be biased and may also apply to a surgical setting.

What is needed are prospective studies, in which patients are followed over time and carefully assessed before and after surgery to see whether their BDD improves, is unchanged, or worsens. Patients should be clearly identified as having BDD, and their outcome with surgery should be assessed over a long period of time.

Although available evidence indicates that many people with BDD improve with psychiatric treatment, people who initially consult surgeons or other nonpsychiatric physicians may be reluctant to see a psychiatrist. They may be more willing to do so when they understand that they may be unhappy with the results of surgery or dermatologic treatment. And they may be more likely to accept psychiatric treatment when they realize that they worry too much and that such treatment can decrease the preoccupation and emotional pain, improve their depression, help them get their life back on track, and aid them in coping more successfully with the problem. It helps put the problem in perspective and diminishes the power of the obsessions.

Ineffective Treatments for BDD

There are a number of other treatment approaches and coping strategies that are sometimes used for BDD but that appear ineffective.

- *Diet*   I recently saw a magazine article on my research that blazoned the headline: "Feeling ugly? Eat a banana." It was accompanied by a photograph of an attractive woman with half her face covered by a mask. After noting that I had found that boosting serotonin levels may lessen appearance preoccupations, the author went on to recommend that BDD sufferers eat chicken, avocado, corn, and bananas to cope with their symptoms. While certain foods do contain precursors of serotonin, there is no evidence whatsoever that foods affect serotonin levels enough to diminish BDD symptoms. I don't recommend diet alone to treat BDD.

- *Natural remedies*   A number of people I've seen have tried various other "natural remedies," such as homeopathic approaches and megavitamins. There is no evidence that such approaches are effective for BDD.

- *Uncovering a presumed trauma*   There is no evidence that BDD is caused by childhood trauma. While some people with BDD have experienced trauma, it's a mistake to assume that everyone with BDD has undergone serious trauma, that the presumed trauma is necessarily related to the development of BDD, or that uncovering a presumed trauma will cure the disorder. Some patients who clearly have experienced trauma may find it helpful to deal with this issue in psychotherapy, but this doesn't constitute treatment for BDD.

- *Reassurance*   BDD does not respond to reassurance alone. Trying to talk a person with BDD out of their worries doesn't cure the disorder and generally leads to frustration among everyone involved.

- *Hypnosis*   Some of my patients have tried hypnosis for their BDD, but many were too anxious, tense, and preoccupied to be successfully hypnotized. One person improved with hypnosis but only temporarily. Similarly, while relaxation techniques may be a useful part of cognitive-behavioral therapy, they don't appear to be effective when used alone.

- *Trying harder*   Many people try this approach alone, thinking it will be enough. But trying harder, by itself, won't treat BDD. Nor does it help for others to tell the BDD sufferer to "pull themselves up by their bootstraps." They're usually trying as hard as they can. The problem with this approach is that, in addition to not diminishing BDD symptoms, the BDD sufferer may feel even worse about themselves—not only because they think they look bad, but also because they can't talk themselves out of being so concerned about it.

But making an effort and having a healthy attitude are important components of getting better. The right attitude needs to be combined with treatments that at this time appear effective for BDD. It's important, for example, to try hard by:

- Making a commitment to psychiatric treatment.

- Complying with behavior therapy, which can be challenging and difficult; forcing oneself to resist rituals and do anxiety-provoking exposures.

- Trying medications; staying with them even if experiencing side effects, in the hope that they'll prove tolerable or will pass; waiting for medications to begin working, which can take time; and trying another medication if previous ones haven't worked. A healthy attitude and medications work hand in hand—they are powerful allies.

- Maintaining hope and not giving up. Most people do get better with psychiatric treatment.

In upcoming years and decades, more treatment studies of BDD will be done. Our knowledge about BDD, and hope for BDD sufferers, will grow.

·· fifteen ··

BDD and the Family

"At least one can be patient, understanding, and loving, and prevent them from feeling isolated."   **A mother**

"The Selfish Disease": A Husband's Perspective

"There aren't enough days on a calendar to tell you how many times I've wanted to leave my wife," Sam told me. "I'm a very loyal person, and I love her. But at times it gets to be too much. She's late when we go out, and sometimes she won't go at all. She can get so wrapped up in her obsessions that she ignores me completely. She doesn't give the children the attention they need. BDD is the selfish disease."

Sam sometimes accompanied his wife, Beth, to her sessions and told me about how he tried to cope with her illness. "My wife has had this problem for decades," he said. "No one knew what it was." I heard about Beth's fixation on her nose and the many unsuccessful surgeries she'd had. Her preoccupation had made it difficult for her to raise her children. Later, after they'd grown, she'd found it difficult to focus on a job; despite her desire to work, she'd been largely unemployed.

"This is a problem that affects family members, too," Sam told me. "I know how much pain this problem has caused my wife—I don't want to downplay how hard it's been for her. But it's also had a major impact on me. I hope this doesn't sound too selfish, but sometimes I think I've suffered as much as my wife has!"

Sam and Beth had been married for ten years. Beth's previous husband had left her because of her symptoms. "You might be skeptical that that was the reason, that it was because of my nose obsession," she told me. "Some people think it's an excuse—that he really left me for some other reason. But it was mostly because of the BDD. I hounded him all day long. I'd plead with him to help me find another surgeon, and I'd constantly talk about how surgery would solve my appearance problem. We hardly had a social life. When we went out, I'd be late a lot of the time. I'd be in the mirror putting on makeup and styling and restyling my hair to make my nose look smaller. Sometimes I wouldn't go to social events at all because I thought I looked so bad. That really drove him crazy.

"I did manage to raise my children and actually did a pretty good job, I think, but it was very hard. I don't know how I did it. I was so focused on my nose. I couldn't stop thinking about it. It was really hard for my husband, because he ended up working two jobs and doing a lot of the child care too. I don't want you to think I was a *total* basket case—I wasn't—but life was a lot harder with my problem. My husband finally got fed up, and he left me."

Like Beth's first husband, Sam had also gotten very involved in her disorder. At her insistence, Sam held mirrors and lights so she could get a better look at her nose, a ritual that could take more than an hour a day. Beth also often talked to him about her nose, saying she wanted surgery or asking if her nose looked okay. "The questioning is especially hard," Sam told me. "No matter what I say, she doesn't really believe me. She just asks me again and again! I don't know what to say." They'd missed family get-togethers and had few friends because his wife often felt too ugly to be around other people. A few times Sam even drove her to an emergency room because she'd looked in the mirror and felt she couldn't go on living.

"There's no worse illness on earth than BDD," Sam told me many times. "People who haven't lived with it probably wouldn't understand, but this is the most devastating thing in the world. I've seen death. I've seen murder. This is as bad. . . . Maybe it's harder for me than my wife because I'm more helpless than her. I can't do anything about it."

One of the most difficult aspects for Sam had been the isolation. "I've felt very alone because friends and family don't understand. I've mostly dealt with this on my own. I took a risk and told a few relatives, but they don't understand it; they think it's strange. But it's the most devastating illness there is."

Like Beth's first husband, Sam had thoughts of leaving his wife. Nonetheless, he resolved to stand by her. Beth did eventually get much better with sertraline (Zoloft), and the strain on their marriage diminished.

Sam's story isn't unusual. I've met many husbands, wives, girlfriends, boyfriends, parents, and friends who've experienced BDD. They've been deeply affected by the disorder and have struggled to find ways to cope.

I never met Craig's wife because she'd left him years ago. "She left me because of my skin obsession," he told me. "I was totally obsessed. Sometimes it wasn't so bad, but when it got really bad, I'd miss work and I wouldn't go out. I'd even spend entire weekends in bed. I'd feel that life wasn't worth living and I totally ignored my wife. I was completely wrapped up in the obsession.

"We couldn't agree about whether to have children. My wife wanted to, but I was afraid that with my symptoms I wouldn't be able to take responsibility for a child. I had a hard enough time taking care of myself. My wife stuck it out with me for a couple of years. But eventually she couldn't take it anymore, and she left me. If I didn't have the disorder, I think we'd still be together today."

While divorce as a result of BDD isn't the norm, it isn't rare. It's an extreme and striking indication of how painful this disorder can be for those who are close to BDD sufferers. I've heard similar stories from many people. Some are dramatic, many are not. But every story reflects the myriad ways in which BDD can interrupt lives and cause needless suffering. Husbands, wives, girlfriends, boyfriends, sons, daughters, close friends, and acquaintances may all experience the disorder. Sometimes they don't know the cause of the difficulties they experience—they don't know that BDD is the root of their loved one's problems because the symptoms are kept secret—but they experience its effects nonetheless.

You may recall the people I described earlier in the book who were affected by BDD. Some of their experiences were dramatic. Dwayne's girlfriend pulled a knife on him and threatened to harm him if he didn't stop talking about getting surgery. Jonathan's symptoms were so severe that his wife left him. I've heard many stories about missing important ceremonies and events—not showing up for graduations or weddings, or not seeing a close friend before death.

Other examples are less dramatic but no less painful. Ted's wife pleaded with her husband to try medication that might decrease his symptoms; he preferred to try "natural remedies" instead, which hadn't worked for 15 years. As a result, their marriage suffered. Ivan's girlfriend tried to get him to go to parties with her, telling him that he looked fine—that he was very handsome—and that no one would be focusing on his hair except him. She often ended up going alone. Teachers may experience the frustration of trying to get a student with BDD to work harder, not understanding why their grades are dropping. A boss may try to understand why his employee is sometimes late for work and takes too many sick days. They are all affected by BDD.

The "selfish disease"—the phrase used by Sam to describe BDD—reflects the experience of many family members. The person with BDD can be so wrapped up in their obsession that family members are ignored. The BDD sufferer seems to put his or her needs first—missing the social engagement, forgoing a wedding, spending too much money on beauty products, talking about their appearance rather than showing interest in others. Even if the BDD sufferer does none of these things, he or she may seem distant, preoccupied, and self-absorbed, rather than focused on the people around them.

But, as I've emphasized throughout this book, people with BDD have little control over their obsessions. If they could take their mind off the preoccupation, they would. BDD may seem selfish to those who are affected by it, but BDD isn't a problem of selfishness. Effective treatment often puts an end to the "selfishness"—what appeared to be selfish behavior turns out to have been symptoms of BDD.

"I Knew Something Was Wrong with My Daughter": A Parent's Perspective

"I knew something was wrong with my daughter when she'd be in the bathroom for an hour and was upset when she came out." This mother had tried very hard to help her daughter cope with her BDD. Although some of the approaches she tried—such as reassuring her—weren't successful, others were. Her daughter finally agreed to see a psychiatrist and responded well to paroxetine (Paxil).

Parents may suffer greatly as a result of BDD. They may have to cope with their 14-year-old daughter's dropping grades and avoidance of friends and activities. They may care for a 35-year-old son who is unable to support himself or live on his own. They may finally, in desperation, take their handsome adolescent son for a chin implant because they can no longer tolerate his relentless pleas for cosmetic surgery, only to find that he's even more unhappy after the surgery.

Jennifer's mother worried endlessly about her daughter—how to get her back into school, how to help her find a job, how to get her to *stop worrying* so much about how she looked. Other parents do too. "We tell our daughter that she looks fine and to stop worrying so much," Molly's parents told me. "We hate seeing her so unhappy." "I know I drive them crazy, asking them if I look okay and telling them I'm ugly," Molly replied. "But it makes me mad when they say I'm attractive. They love me and want to reassure me, so they tell me I look fine. But I don't."

Coping with BDD may be particularly difficult for parents because they may feel responsible for their child's difficulties. Did they cause the problem? Did they overemphasize the importance of appearance? Should they have raised their child differently? Blaming themselves only compounds their suffering.

One mother felt helpless when it came to helping her son cope with his hair, and she blamed herself. "He's so upset over his hair that he can't function because of it. We try not to reassure him, but he's so desperate, we have to. He's having temper tantrums because he thinks his hair is getting worse. We don't know what to do!"

Her son, too, told me how his appearance concern caused his family to suffer. "I can't enjoy being with them, because I'm so upset over how I look," he said. "I can't even have a good Christmas with them. I have to ask them 'Does my hair look okay? Does it look thin?' And they say to me, 'Don't ruin the day.' But I do. And I feel bad about how much unhappiness I've caused them. I've put them through hell."

I heard from the mother of a boy who had killed himself because of his supposed ugliness. He'd seen many doctors, but BDD hadn't been diagnosed. "For many years I lost patience with my son for always staring in the mirror and saying he was ugly when he was a quite handsome boy," she wrote. "He used to say to me, 'What's this thing that's taking me over, mom?' The night before he died, he said I didn't understand him, which was true, and that there was no hope for him.

"I know that it's almost impossible to sway the mind of someone with body dysmorphic disorder, but at least one can be patient, understanding, and loving, and prevent them from feeling isolated. . . . My tragedy will always be that I didn't know and couldn't tell him that it wasn't his fault."

Common Problems and Coping Strategies for Family Members and Friends

What follows is a description of some of the problems commonly encountered by family members and friends of people with BDD, as well as some approaches to dealing with them. Because of the varied ways in which BDD expresses itself—because each individual's and each family member's experience with BDD is in some ways unique—this advice may not address certain problems that are encountered. But I hope it will cover many of them and that the coping strategies offered are helpful.

All the coping strategies I'll discuss are easier to describe than implement. It can in fact be very frustrating and difficult to do some of them. Yet all are worth trying. It can be helpful to keep in mind that they're more likely to be effective when at least a partial response to medication and/or cognitive-behavioral therapy has been attained.

Most of the approaches discussed here won't actually treat the disorder. That's what serotonin-reuptake inhibitors and cognitive-behavioral treatment appear to do. The coping strategies I'll discuss are additional approaches that may enhance effective treatments for BDD and make the disorder somewhat easier to live with. At the very least, they should prevent worsening of symptoms, which sometimes results from well-intentioned responses and interventions by family members and friends. They should also help counteract feelings of helplessness. Although family members and friends might feel powerless in dealing with BDD, there are many things they can do to help.

Participation in BDD Rituals and Behaviors

BDD can be especially difficult because family members and friends may themselves be drawn into rituals and behaviors that seem senseless and even strange. They may be asked to facilitate these behaviors, making it easier or possible for them to be performed. While many BDD behaviors are typically done silently, in private, without involving other people, virtually any of them can involve others. Other people may be asked to hold mirrors to allow multiple views of the defect or to shine lights on the defect while it's inspected. Or the bathroom may be unavailable for hours each morning while checking and grooming rituals are performed.

Friends and family may be asked to measure a body part or to confirm that a certain measurement was obtained or is normal. They may be asked to cut, groom, or style hair. They may be asked to confirm that a certain outfit is flattering or pay for expensive items, such as wigs, clothing, beauty products, or surgery. They may be asked to vacation in a cold location, where concealing clothes can be worn. Some people with BDD compulsively pick the skin of family members and friends. When family members try to prevent this, the BDD sufferer can get very upset. As one woman said, "Usually they just give in and let me do it," she said. "It's the easiest thing for them to do."

Coping strategy: Don't participate in BDD rituals   Family members and friends should avoid participating in BDD behaviors and rituals. Participation helps keep them going and may even make them possible. The behaviors and rituals may in turn feed the appearance preoccupations. Participation also drains the time and energy of everyone involved.

Family members often participate in the hope that they're helping the BDD sufferer. After all, they're responding to a request from someone they care about, who is often extremely distressed. They participate in the hope that something good will result—that once the view in the mirror is obtained, the worry will finally end. They hope this time it will be different. But participating in BDD-related behaviors never has and never will cure the disorder. It can even make it worse by reinforcing those behaviors.

Don't hold special lights to allow a better view. Cover or take down mirrors. Don't groom or style hair. Don't give reassurance about clothing. Don't pay for yet another outfit, or for surgery after surgery. Don't allow your skin to be picked. Consistency is crucial so the sufferer learns that the behaviors aren't acceptable or helpful.

Not participating in rituals isn't easy. The BDD sufferer may insist that others participate and may become very distraught or even angry if they're turned down. It's important to first discuss with the BDD sufferer that you'll no longer participate in their rituals because it isn't in their best interest to do so. Explain that you know they're in pain but that participating in the behaviors can actually increase preoccupations and fears. Even if anxiety is relieved, the relief is only temporary. Resisting the compulsive behaviors is better in the long run. All family members need to agree on this. Fortunately, treatment with medication or CBT often diminishes the rituals as well as requests that others participate in them.

Questioning and Reassurance Seeking

This BDD behavior is one of the most frustrating for family members. It always involves others; asking for reassurance, or trying to convince others of the defect's ugliness, requires a listening ear.

If the questioning is infrequent, it may not be particularly problematic for others. Some people refrain from reassurance seeking because they realize how bothersome it can be. But others simply can't—the urge is irresistible. Parents of a 20-year-old woman with BDD told me, "We don't know how to cope. No matter what we say, the questioning persists. We love our daughter and want to reassure her that she looks fine. She thinks we're lying but we're not. We don't know what to do."

Coping strategy: Avoid providing reassurance   The typical—and understandable—response is to provide the reassurance the BDD sufferer seeks. After all, the person with BDD looks fine, so the natural tendency is to say so. Common responses include "You look fine!" "I can't see it at all," "It's hardly visible," or "It's not as bad as you think—it's hardly noticeable!" The problem with these responses is that although they're true, they don't stop the questioning for long, if at all. Furthermore, reassurance doesn't put an end to the appearance concerns.

Paradoxically, responding to questioning with a reassuring reply can actually perpetuate the reassurance-seeking behavior. If the response does temporarily decrease the BDD sufferer's anxiety, this transient relief fuels the attempt to obtain more relief by asking the question again. While it might seem cruel to refuse to respond to requests for reassurance, it isn't. Refraining from providing reassurance may actually stop this time- and energy-consuming behavior.

When possible, I meet with family members, along with the person with BDD, to discuss BDD more generally and this behavior in particular. We all agree that providing reassurance isn't helpful and benefits no one. The individual with BDD can generally acknowledge that they aren't reassured very much by the responses they get, and family members can readily acknowledge that no matter what they say, it really doesn't seem to help. We then agree that, for the benefit of the BDD sufferer, family members will no longer respond to the questioning. Instead, if necessary, they will remind the questioner that the questioning is a ritual—part of their disorder—and that it isn't helpful for them to respond. They may also remind the questioner that they agreed as a group not to respond as part of treatment.

Different families come up with their own response. "I'm sorry; I know you're suffering, but I'm not going to respond to your question," "We agreed it isn't helpful for me to reassure you," or "I know you're anxious, but my reassuring you won't help" may work quite well. The main point is to avoid commenting on the person's appearance as part of the response. It's also important to avoid giving reassurance to the greatest extent possible. Providing reassurance only occasionally—for example, only 20% of the time—may seem like very little, but it may be frequent enough to reinforce and maintain the behavior.

Having said this, there are times when I've given reassurance to my patients. I give it only once, and I give it only when they are in extreme and intolerable distress. But I do it with reluctance, and I convey my concern that I may be reinforcing their ritual by responding. I also do it very rarely. These occasions bring home to me how difficult it can be for family members to refrain from providing reassurance. At times, their loved one may be in such distress that reassurance seems like the only solution. Ideally, these occasions will be relatively rare.

I also recommend that family members not take the BDD sufferer to the surgeon, dermatologist, or other medical professional to obtain reassurance about the defect's appearance or after receiving surgical or other medical treatment they're dissatisfied with.

Occasionally, in great frustration, family members may say that the defect looks terrible. They don't actually believe this, but they say it in anger, or because giving reassurance has been fruitless. I also recommend avoiding this response because it can cause the BDD sufferer great pain and may strengthen the BDD preoccupation.

Reasoning About the Defect

Some family members and friends make a considerable effort to talk the person with BDD out of their belief. This approach, too, is understandable. The person with BDD looks okay, so why not just explain this to them? Why not just reason with them? After all, they're reasonable in other ways. Maybe all that's needed is a compelling argument or a heartfelt attempt to convince them of this.

This approach is highly unlikely to effectively treat BDD. More often, it results in frustration over the failed attempts. In my experience, this approach almost always fails with someone with delusional BDD—that is, who is completely convinced that their view of the defect is accurate. You may recall Steven's statement: "I'm as convinced of what I see as you are that the box on this table is rectangular, not round." Try arguing with conviction of this strength!

Coping strategy: "Reality checks" may be helpful for certain individuals with BDD, but trying to talk someone out of complete conviction is unlikely to succeed   People with some insight—who realize that their view of the defect is distorted or that their belief is due to a psychiatric disorder—may benefit from reminders that their view is exaggerated and is due to BDD. Reminding them of this—that others don't see them the way they do—can help put things in perspective.

One patient of mine found that comments such as "You view your chest that way, but other people don't" or "This is your BDD flaring up" helped keep his obsession in check. Reminders, or "reality checks," like this were especially useful when his symptoms increased and his beliefs intensified.

Indeed, this approach may be usefully incorporated into cognitive-behavioral therapy for BDD. I recommend that family members consult with a professional to determine whether and how they should use this approach.

It's also helpful to keep in mind that as medication or cognitive-behavioral treatment start to work, insight may improve; that is, the person's view of the defect may become more realistic. At this point, it may be helpful to remind them that their view isn't entirely accurate—that they have "foggy glasses on their brain" that prevent them from seeing themselves as others do.

Angry Outbursts

Angry outbursts, or what some of my patients refer to as temper tantrums, can disrupt the family. Although they aren't a common aspect of BDD, they're a particularly difficult one. The outbursts usually reflect frustration and anger over the psychological pain, isolation, and interference with functioning that the symptoms can cause.

Sometimes the outbursts are precipitated by a painful event, such as the perception of being mocked. Some of my patients routinely become very angry after receiving a "bad" haircut. Unfortunately, family members may be the recipients of their anger and frustration.

Coping strategy: Understand that this behavior is related to BDD In many cases, people with BDD don't intend to express their anger toward their family; their family members or friends happen to be present when they're feeling frustrated. Identifying precipitants of outbursts and trying to avoid them in the future may be useful. Setting limits on destructive behavior and urging the person to talk about how they feel, rather than expressing their feelings in angry behavior or attacking words, may also be helpful. As BDD symptoms respond to treatment, the frustration and anger usually diminish as well.

It may be helpful for family members and the BDD sufferer to meet with the treating psychiatrist or therapist to discuss the outbursts and their effect on the family. Family discussions or family therapy may yield helpful strategies for dealing with anger that are tailored to the particular family. Such meetings are unlikely to effectively treat the BDD itself, but may make it easier to cope with the disorder.

Difficulty Functioning

This consequence of BDD often affects family members, especially parents of children or adolescents. It's the family who may be in the position of urging the BDD sufferer to be on time for work or school, get a job or go to school, go out with friends, or leave the house. In some cases, the person with BDD lives with and is supported by family members long after the time has come to live independently.

In my experience, family members often give this kind of support quite willingly, yet providing it may be a significant strain on their resources, financial and emotional. And they may question whether it's the right thing. Are they doing the BDD sufferer a disservice by having them live with them or be financially dependent on them? Should they instead require independent functioning? Are they "enabling" the disorder in some way?

Alexandra's parents expressed this dilemma. "Our daughter is 33 years old. She should be on her own by now. But we're afraid that if we ask her to leave she won't be able to support herself. We've tried it before, and it didn't work. But we wonder if we're doing the right thing by having her continue to live with us."

Coping strategy: Encourage better functioning but recognize the person's limitations   Unfortunately, there aren't simple solutions to this problem. Each family, with the help of a mental health professional, will need to determine what approach works best for them. In general, I advise patients and families to encourage improved functioning and, if the patient is an adult, the goal is eventual self-support. I also advise family members to encourage the person with BDD to get out of the house and socialize. Adequate psychiatric treatment with medication and behavior therapy can be critical to success.

Family members can also help by encouraging the BDD sufferer to keep busy. This won't cure the disorder, but idleness can worsen preoccupations. Family members can suggest activities or participate in creating lists of activities that the person can refer to when idle or preoccupied. A job can decrease preoccupations because it acts as a distraction.

For some people, the most effective approach to improved functioning is a stepwise one, especially for those who've been ill for a long time. Moving from a volunteer job to part-time and then full-time work can be an effective strategy. The support and encouragement of family members can be extremely helpful as the person with BDD negotiates these changes and challenges. Improvement in functioning can take time; it's better to measure progress over longer periods than day-to-day. Give positive feedback and praise for even small improvements.

Many patients improve their functioning with adequate treatment as well as family encouragement and support. But this isn't always possible. Their symptoms may be too severe for meaningful progress to be made. In such cases, insistence that the person function better is likely to be fruitless. But it's crucial that such a person be in psychiatric treatment (in an outpatient or partial hospital setting) and taking medication. In my view, it's a mistake for family members to observe someone who is this impaired without insisting that they obtain adequate treatment. When patients do respond to such treatment, their functioning may markedly improve; they may be able to go to school or work, and able to support themselves. For patients who require the assistance and support of a therapist or vocational rehabilitation counselor in transitioning to independent living, it can be helpful for the family to meet with these professionals to discuss ways in which they can facilitate this transition.

Avoidance of Family Events

Avoidance of family events may be especially difficult for families. It isn't uncommon for people with BDD to avoid family get-togethers or important events such as graduations, weddings, or funerals. They may anticipate these events with great trepidation and avoid them because of having to face others, fearing they'll be judged negatively because of how they look. "I'm petrified about my brother's wedding," one man told me. "If my hair doesn't start growing back by then, I'm not going. My family will be incredibly upset, but I refuse to go."

Coping strategy: Encourage participation in family events My advice here is similar to that in the preceding section. Encourage the BDD sufferer to attend family events. Remind them that the focus won't be on them; at a wedding, it will be on the bride and bridegroom. People with BDD should be encouraged to face their fears by being around other people. If they do this enough, their fears will eventually diminish. They may even feel better afterward because they didn't miss the event. Avoiding social situations only reinforces BDD symptoms.

But, as I've previously noted, this is easier said than done. It can be extremely difficult for BDD sufferers to be around others. A cognitive-behavioral therapist can be very helpful in facilitating exposure to social situations and can help patients tolerate the specific social events they would like to avoid.

Suicidal Thinking

Nothing is more likely to precipitate a family crisis than suicidal thinking or behavior, which isn't uncommon. When it does, family members may be able to help.

Coping strategy: Obtain psychiatric treatment Family members shouldn't deal with suicidal thinking or behavior on their own. It's crucial to get psychiatric help. Suicidal thinking and behavior are serious warning signs that the person is suffering greatly; furthermore, they may culminate in actual suicide.

A common response is to deny or minimize suicidal thinking in a loved one. It's a very difficult situation to face, and it may be ignored in the hope that it will simply go away. But it's a serious mistake to ignore these warning signs or assume they will pass. They may not, and they may worsen if untreated. If a person with BDD appears severely depressed, it's even advisable for family members or friends to ask if they've had thoughts that life isn't worth living, thoughts of causing self harm, or a plan to end their life.

Usually, suicidal thinking is associated with an underlying psychiatric disorder, such as BDD or depression, which is amenable to psychiatric treatment. Family members and friends should insist that their loved one obtain psychiatric treatment, including medication, which often effectively treats BDD symptoms as well as associated depression, anxiety, and suicidal thinking.

Reluctance to Get Treatment

Family members, relatives, or friends may need to deal with the BDD sufferer's reluctance to enter treatment. This can be very difficult. There are treatments that appear to help, yet the person who is suffering the most may be reluctant, or may refuse, to try them. This can cause family members to feel intensely frustrated, sad, and helpless.

Coping strategy: Provide information about BDD and emphasize that treatment may diminish pain and lack of control. As with the other problems described in this chapter, the solutions to this one aren't simple or straightforward. It may be helpful to provide the BDD sufferer with information about the disorder, to convey that it's a recognized problem that other people have and that it often responds to psychiatric treatment. Effective treatment is worth *trying*. Giving it a try doesn't necessarily lead to treatment for life. In addition, the medications that appear effective are generally well tolerated. Consulting a mental health professional about how to get the person to try psychiatric treatment is sometimes helpful as well. Periodically remind the sufferer that you are willing to help and that people with BDD can get better.

It can be helpful to convey to sufferers that they're *overly* preoccupied, that they worry *too much,* and that they're *suffering too much* as a result of their appearance concerns. Their preoccupation has too much power over them. It's interfering with their functioning and their relationships. It has far too strong a hold. They may not like how they look, but this shouldn't control their life or cause them so much anguish.

Effective treatment is the means to regaining control. *They,* not the appearance preoccupation, should be in charge. They should be able to think about whatever they want to think about. They should be able to interact with other people, free of gnawing, painful thoughts that keep them a prisoner. Tell them what some of my patients have said after they've responded to psychiatric treatment. Cassandra described herself as a caged animal— her obsessional thinking had locked her in a place where she had no freedom or pleasure. Effective treatment freed her; it allowed her to regain control of her life.

Another patient said, "The treatment I got was very freeing—it's lifted an amazing burden. I regret that I put it off for so many years." This patient hadn't been interested in psychiatric treatment. He preferred holistic approaches, which he'd tried for 20 years. He finally got tired of trying to treat himself; his approaches weren't working, and he was worn out and not living the life he'd hoped for. He decided he had nothing left to lose.

Feelings of Isolation

Family members may feel isolated in dealing with BDD. It's still an underrecognized problem, and some people feel a sense of stigma because a loved one has a psychiatric problem. If family members do confide in others, they may be met with disbelief. Others may find the concerns hard to understand. Reactions like these may intensify feelings of isolation.

Coping strategy: Realize that you're not alone Remember that BDD isn't a rare disorder. Millions of family members are trying to make sense of it and cope with it. I encourage family members to share their struggles with someone they trust; the support can be quite helpful. Educating supportive people about BDD may help them better understand the problem.

I hope that BDD will continue to be increasingly recognized and that local and national support groups will develop. This has occurred for other psychiatric disorders, such as depression, manic depressive illness, and OCD. Many family members and friends find these groups helpful sources of information and support. Until such groups are developed for BDD, some of the existing groups for other mental illnesses may be of help.

In the meantime, remember that you're not alone—you may *think* you don't know anyone else who is coping with BDD, but you probably do. BDD affects millions.

More Advice for Family Members and Friends

Take the disorder seriously As I've conveyed throughout this book, BDD is a serious psychiatric disorder. It isn't simply vanity. Nor is it something that will necessarily be "grown out of" or disappear by simply trying harder. Identifying and confronting the problem are the necessary first steps to a successful outcome.

Talk openly about BDD BDD sufferers may be reluctant to talk about their concern because of embarrassment or for other reasons. If your family member has any of the signs of BDD discussed in Chapter 4, ask if he or she has troubling appearance concerns. Avoid reassuring them that they look okay; instead encourage them to talk openly about their worries. Share information about BDD with them.

Encourage and support psychiatric treatment Psychiatric care could be considered a coping strategy for all the dilemmas I've just discussed. Family members and friends can make a big difference in this regard. Sometimes it's only because of their concern and assistance that people with BDD obtain effective treatment.

Trying harder isn't, by itself, adequate treatment for diabetes, heart disease, or cancer. Nor is it adequate treatment for BDD. BDD is no different. As I discussed in the treatment chapter, making an effort is important. But it doesn't constitute sufficient treatment.

Family members can be extremely helpful in encouraging compliance with psychiatric treatment. While many people with BDD welcome psychiatric treatment because it offers them hope of relief, others are reluctant. Family support can make a crucial difference. It can be helpful to remind the person taking medication that side effects may not occur; when they do, they may be relatively mild and transient. Waiting it out for a while may allow side effects to pass and the medication to begin working. If they're more problematic, another medication can be tried. Cognitive-behavioral treatment is challenging and difficult at times. Encourage the sufferer to remember that this is to be expected—that treatment isn't likely to work if it isn't challenging. In addition, family members can participate in exposure activities once they learn how to do this. They can move the avoidant person further along with their interest and support.

Support psychiatric rather than surgical treatment   Supporting psychiatric rather than surgical treatment is sometimes difficult. People with BDD may be desperate to get surgery, and may beg and plead with family members to give them financial or moral support for it. As I discussed in the last chapter, scientifically rigorous studies of surgical outcome in individuals with BDD need to be done. However, available data suggest that people with BDD are often unhappy with the results of surgery; they sometimes say that they wish someone—including their family members—had talked them out of getting the procedure.

Based on what we now know about BDD's treatment response, the best advice at this time is to encourage a family member with BDD to avoid surgery. I recommend this especially if the person has already had multiple surgeries, without alleviation of their appearance-related concerns. At the very least, it's prudent to first give psychiatric treatment a good try. Encourage your loved one to try this approach first. The surgery will always be there—why not try psychiatric treatment first? There's no significant downside to a psychiatric approach. In addition, on the basis of available data, the psychiatric treatments I've discussed appear more likely to be effective, and are also less costly and less risky than surgery.

Be patient   Patience is enormously helpful when dealing with a loved one with BDD. It's needed when waiting for a response to medication. While some people respond relatively quickly—within a few weeks—it often takes longer. Any given medication may take up to three months—and occasionally even more time—to work. If the first medicine doesn't work, another should be tried for another three months. Occasionally, it takes many tries to find the right one. Persistence and patience are needed in such cases.

Similarly, the initial CBT strategies tried may not be effective. It can take creativity and a good understanding of the person and their symptoms to come up with the behavioral strategies that will work for them. As with medications, more than one try may be needed.

Patience may also be needed while waiting for functioning to improve. Some people function better nearly immediately—as soon as their symptoms abate. In other cases, much more time is necessary. Recognize also that symptoms may flare during stressful times.

For people who are reluctant to get adequate treatment, keep in mind that time and the family's continued support may make a difference. I've treated many people with BDD who finally, after many years—even many decades—of suffering, decided to give psychiatric treatment a try. In many of these cases, the continued support and patience of family members made a difference.

Don't blame yourself Some family members—parents in particular—wonder if they're responsible for BDD. We don't know its cause, but it's unlikely to result largely from something parents have done wrong. Instead of looking back and blaming yourself, focus on the present and future—do what you can now to help the BDD sufferer overcome their symptoms.

Maintain hope Never give up hope. Most people respond to psychiatric treatment. Symptoms may not entirely disappear, but they often get much better. Sometimes the first treatment tried is helpful; sometimes it's the third, fourth, or fifth. Unusual combinations may be needed, and sometimes they work. Keep in mind that time and patience may be required to find the treatment that works best for any given individual. Although some people with BDD don't respond to available treatments, our knowledge of BDD's treatment response is still in its very early stages. Much more will be learned about effective treatments in the coming years.

Epilogue

I hope I've conveyed what my patients would want you to know about body dysmorphic disorder. BDD affects many lives, it causes great suffering, and certain psychiatric treatments appear very promising and hold out much hope for BDD sufferers.

BDD is a common but underdiagnosed disorder. Sufferers often keep their pain a secret, even from their loved ones. Courage is often needed to tell others about it. Despite the suffering it causes, it's easily trivialized. Many people with this disorder feel isolated and alone.

A woman with BDD contributed this poem to this book. It conveys how many people with BDD feel.

BEAUTY DISEASE

Absorbed solemn silence, she's locked at the glass
Every morning same again
Morning is now after one p.m.
Eyes cropped puffy, hue of spilled dirtied kerosene
    reflect so hunted
There's no use telling her that eyes closed never shine
Long thin oranged burnt threads of hair hanging lower each day
Tugging her hair tangled, brushing till all tangles, each one
    is hidden

Turning with disgust, her many other tangles sting

She draws up to make up her face again, resisting to spit in
each tingling bright Wild Fuschia false promise

Lips so trivial peeling away each day more wasted Romance Rose
Sun Kissed Sienna, Perfect Plum wears transparent

In her mouth now the taste of metal shavings, her fillings
are eroding

She never knows when she has finished dressing, it never hides
scars or shame, ashtray tints or the palette of
a tired carpet

Could the doctor really remove them? Don't try to speak of
pulling them out through her tearducts

Enough tears are already fallen

—AEP

I hope the voices in this book have spoken as strongly and as clearly as the facts. I hope that readers with BDD and their family members will take comfort in knowing they aren't alone.

Have hope! Although we still have a great deal to learn about BDD and how to heal it, the psychiatric treatments I've discussed appear very promising and have already made a difference—in some cases, a tremendous difference—in the lives of many people with BDD.

If you have BDD or know someone who does, it's important to be evaluated by a psychiatrist (a medical doctor with specialized training in psychiatric disorders) who can confirm the diagnosis and prescribe medication. People with more treatment-resistant BDD may benefit from seeing a psychiatrist with particular expertise in psychopharmacology, since experience and creativity in prescribing psychiatric medications may be needed. Because of BDD's many similarities to obsessive compulsive disorder, seeing a psychiatrist with expertise in OCD is a good approach to take.

If you decide to try cognitive-behavioral therapy, seek out a therapist who is not only familiar with BDD but who has training in and experience with cognitive-behavioral therapy—particularly with exposure and response prevention. As is the case for medication treatment, seeing a cognitive-behavioral therapist with expertise in treating OCD is a good approach. The Obsessive Compulsive Foundation* and the Dean Foundation† may be

* Obsessive Compulsive Foundation, P.O. Box 70, Milford, CT 06460-0070; tel: 203-878-5669.

† The Dean Foundation for Health, Research, and Education, 8000 Excelsior Drive, Suite 302, Madison, WI 53717-1914; tel: 608-836-8070.

continued

able to help you find a psychiatrist and a cognitive-behavioral therapist. The American Association for Advancement of Behavior Therapy* may also be able to help you find a therapist with expertise in CBT.

I have no doubt that in the coming years we'll learn a great deal more about BDD. I and other researchers are rapidly learning about it, and more and more researchers are starting to study it. In five, ten, and twenty years, some of what I've written will be out of date. We'll have many more clues about its causes, and we'll certainly know much more about treatment. New treatments should become available as more medications are developed and as we learn more about cognitive-behavioral and perhaps other treatment strategies. What won't be out of date is what BDD sufferers have to say about their experience, just as the Wolf Man's experience, described in 1928, still rings true today.

In the future, BDD should cause less pain as the disorder becomes better known and is more accurately diagnosed, and as more people try psychiatric treatment.

Never give up! The odds are that most people with BDD who try psychiatric treatment will benefit. Remember the words of some of my patients—some of whom were very hesitant to try psychiatric treatment—who were successfully treated with this approach:

Nathaniel: "I can talk to people without feeling they're staring at me. I'm better able to resist mirror checking. I spend less time obsessing. It comes into my mind less and it's easier to get rid of the thoughts. I can argue with myself that my obsession is irrational—I tell myself, 'just shrug it off!' I'm not so self-conscious around people anymore. It's not a life or death problem for me now."

Christina: "I just wasn't seeing myself clearly before. I feel calmer, happier, and more confident. It's hard to believe the medication has made this much of a change, but it has. I feel the way I used to feel, before the BDD ever started. I feel great!"

Sandy: "The medication definitely curbs the obsession. It released a logjam. My life felt like a stream that had thousands of huge boulders and logs in it—the water couldn't flow through smoothly. Now it flows with ease. I feel full of energy and creativity."

Luke: "Suicide is the furthest thing from my mind now. I have a great life. Thank God I got treatment. I owe my life to it."

---

*American Association for Advancement of Behavior Therapy, 305 7th Ave., New York, NY 10001-6008; tel: 212-647-1890.

Appendix A

Brief Descriptions of
Selected Psychiatric Disorders

What follows are brief descriptions of the psychiatric disorders I've referred to in this book. They are based on, and are briefer versions of, definitions in DSM-IV, the official manual of definitions and descriptions of psychiatric disorders.

Mood Disorders

Major Depression A depressive disorder characterized by depressed mood or loss of interest or pleasure as well as other symptoms, such as abnormal sleep or appetite (too much or too little), fatigue, low self-esteem or feelings of worthlessness, guilt, difficulty concentrating, and thoughts that life isn't worth living.

Atypical Subtype A type of major depression in which mood is reactive (that is, it brightens in response to actual or potential positive events) as well as two or more of the following features: significant weight gain or increase in appetite, an increase in sleep, "leaden paralysis" (heavy, leaden feelings in the arms or legs), and sensitivity to rejection by others leading to difficulties in social or occupational functioning.

Bipolar Disorder (Manic Depressive Illness) A type of mood disorder characterized by episodes of depression as well as mania or hypomania (a milder form of mania). Mania consists of a distinct period of abnormal and persistent elation, euphoria, or irritability and is accompanied by some of the following symptoms: decreased need for sleep, excessive talkativeness, increased energy, inflated self-esteem or grandiosity, racing thoughts, distractibility, increased activity or physical agitation, and excessive involvement in pleasurable activities with a high potential for painful consequences (e.g., unrestrained buying sprees or sexual indiscretions).

Dysthymic Disorder   A type of depressive disorder characterized by less severe depressive symptoms that have been present for at least half of the time during the past two years. While depressed, two or more of the following symptoms must be present: poor appetite or overeating, difficulty sleeping or sleeping too much, low energy or fatigue, low self-esteem, poor concentration or difficulty making decisions, and feelings of hopelessness.

Anxiety Disorders

Panic Disorder   Panic disorder consists of recurrent panic attacks that come out of the blue; at least one of the attacks has been followed by one month or more of one (or more) of the following: concern about having more attacks, worry about the consequences of the attacks, or a significant change in behavior related to the attacks. **Panic attacks** consist of a discrete period of intense fear or discomfort that peaks within 10 minutes of onset and is accompanied by a number of physical symptoms, such as heart palpitations, sweating, trembling or shaking, shortness of breath, chest pain or discomfort, feeling dizzy, and fear of dying.

Agoraphobia   Anxiety about being in places or situations from which escape might be difficult or embarrassing, or in which help might not be available, in the event of having a panic attack or panic-like symptoms. Typically, people with agoraphobia feel anxious in or avoid being outside of their home alone, in a crowd, or on a bridge, or traveling in buses, cars, or trains.

Social Phobia (Social Anxiety Disorder)   A marked and persistent fear of one or more social or performance situations in which the person is exposed to unfamiliar people or to possible scrutiny by others. The person fears appearing anxious or doing something humiliating or embarrassing in front of others. The fears may occur in most social situations (generalized type) or in a specific situation (e.g., fear of public speaking).

Specific Phobia   This disorder consists of marked and persistent fear due to the presence or anticipation of a specific object or situation—for example, flying, heights, or spiders.

Obsessive Compulsive Disorder (OCD)   OCD is characterized by obsessions or compulsions (usually both) that cause marked distress, are time consuming (take more than one hour a day), or significantly interfere with functioning. Obsessions are recurrent, persistent, and intrusive thoughts, impulses, or images. Compulsions are repetitive behaviors (e.g., hand washing or checking) or mental acts (e.g., counting) that are performed in response to an obsession and are aimed at preventing or reducing distress or a dreaded event.

Post-Traumatic Stress Disorder (PTSD)   PTSD develops following exposure to a traumatic event. The disorder is characterized by persistent reexperiencing of the traumatic event (e.g., recurrent distressing dreams), persistent avoidance of stimuli associated with the trauma and numbing of general responsiveness, and persistent symptoms of increased arousal (e.g., difficulty falling or staying asleep or an exaggerated startle response).

Generalized Anxiety Disorder   Excessive anxiety and worry about a number of events or activities (such as school or work performance). The worry is difficult to control and is associated with a number of symptoms, such as muscle tension or feeling on edge. The symptoms cause clinically significant distress or impairment in functioning.

Substance-Related Disorders

Substance-related disorders consist of drug abuse or dependence. This includes alcohol and other drugs, such as cocaine, marijuana, opioids (e.g., heroin), and hallucinogens (e.g., LSD).

Somatoform Disorders

Somatization Disorder   This disorder consists of many physical complaints that aren't fully explained by a medical condition. They begin before the age of 30, occur over several years, and result in seeking treatment or significant impairment in functioning. Symptoms consist of pain, gastrointestinal (stomach or intestinal) symptoms, sexual symptoms, and neurological symptoms.

Pain Disorder   This disorder is characterized by pain that is the primary reason for seeking treatment and that causes significant distress or impairment in functioning. Psychological factors are judged to play an important role in the onset, severity, exacerbation, or maintenance of the pain.

Hypochondriasis   Preoccupation with fears of having, or the idea that one has, a serious disease based on a misinterpretation of bodily symptoms. The preoccupation persists despite appropriate medical evaluation and reassurance, and it causes clinically significant distress or impairment in functioning.

Eating Disorders

Anorexia Nervosa   Anorexia nervosa consists of a refusal to maintain body weight in the normal range and an intense fear of gaining weight or becoming fat despite being underweight. It also involves body-image disturbance—a disturbance in the way one's body weight or shape is experienced, undue influence of body weight or shape on self-evaluation, or denial of the seriousness of the low body weight. Amenorrhea (the absence of at least three consecutive menstrual cycles) also occurs.

Bulimia Nervosa   This disorder is characterized by recurrent episodes of binge eating, recurrent compensatory behaviors to prevent weight gain (e.g., self-induced vomiting), and a disturbance in body image (self-evaluation is unduly influenced by body weight and shape).

Binge Eating Disorder   Recurrent episodes of binge eating, which are associated with such things as eating much more rapidly than normal, eating large amounts of food when not feeling hungry, and eating until feeling uncomfortably full. Marked distress over the behavior is also present. (This disorder has been proposed for inclusion in DSM and is being researched but isn't yet an official diagnosis.)

Psychotic Disorders

Delusional Disorder This disorder consists of nonbizarre delusions (i.e., involving situations that occur in real life) of at least one month's duration. The criteria for schizophrenia have never been met.

Olfactory Reference Syndrome (ORS) The erroneous belief that one emits a foul or unpleasant body odor (a type of delusional disorder).

Schizophrenia Schizophrenia consists of symptoms such as delusions, hallucinations, disorganized speech, behavior that is grossly disorganized or abnormal (e.g., purposeless agitation), and symptoms such as lack of emotion or motivation. The symptoms cause impairment in functioning.

Other Psychotic Disorders These include other disorders characterized by symptoms such as hallucinations or delusions. They include schizoaffective disorder.

Other Disorders

Koro Koro occurs primarily in Southeast Asia and consists of a preoccupation that one's penis is shrinking and will disappear into the abdomen, resulting in death.

Trichotillomania Recurrent pulling out of one's hair, resulting in noticeable hair loss as well as clinically significant distress or impairment in functioning.

Tourette's Disorder A disorder characterized by the persistent presence of motor (movement) and vocal tics. A *tic* is a sudden, rapid, recurrent, nonrhythmic, stereotyped movement (e.g., blinking or shrugging) or vocalization (e.g., shouting or coughing).

Personality Disorders A personality disorder is an enduring pattern of inner experience and behavior that deviates markedly from the expectations of the individual's culture, is pervasive and inflexible, and leads to distress or impairment. Personality disorders usually begin in adolescence or early adulthood and are stable over time.

Appendix B

Instruments for Assessing BDD

The BDD Diagnostic Module:
A Clinician-Administered Instrument
to Diagnose BDD

When making a psychiatric diagnosis, clinical judgment, based on years of professional training and experience, is indispensable. However, tools that aid in making a diagnosis can be very helpful. Such tools—generally referred to as diagnostic instruments—ascertain that the diagnosis is being made according to accepted guidelines and criteria. Such instruments usually consist of questions that the clinician asks the patient or self-report forms that the patient fills out. These instruments specify that certain questions are asked when determining whether a psychiatric disorder is present. They are useful in a clinical setting because they help clinicians ascertain that their diagnosis is correct, and they're useful to researchers since they assure that different researchers ask similar questions to make the diagnosis.

The most widely used instrument for the diagnosis of a broad range of psychiatric disorders is the Structured Clinical Interview for DSM-IV, or SCID. Its predecessor, the Structured Clinical Interview for DSM-III-R, was used prior to the DSM-IV version. These instruments were developed by Drs. Robert Spitzer, Janet Williams, Miriam Gibbon, and Michael First of Columbia University. The SCID is intended for use by a clinician, who asks specified questions to determine whether diagnostic criteria for a particular disorder are met.

Because the SCID is the standard diagnostic instrument in psychiatry, I developed a SCID-like diagnostic module for BDD, which is presented on the next page. This instrument follows the SCID format, which provides DSM criteria for the disorder on the right-hand side; the questions the clinician asks to ascertain the presence or absence of each criterion are on the left-hand side, opposite each criterion. If the person answers "yes" to the questions on the left, which in turn indicates that they meet the opposite criterion for the disorder, the next question is asked. More "yes" answers leads to progression through the subsequent questions. If one of the disorder's criteria aren't met, the subsequent questions aren't asked. A disorder is diagnosed if all the diagnostic criteria for that disorder are met (all the questions are answered "yes").

Following this format, the DSM-IV diagnostic criteria for BDD (which I discussed in Chapter 3) are listed on the right-hand side of the BDD module. The questions to assess the presence or absence of these criteria are on the left-hand side. These questions, or probes, must be asked as written, but further questions can also be asked if necessary to clarify whether the criterion is met. Examples of impairment, for example, should be given to ascertain whether impairment is present and how severe it is. The additional questions that may be asked are determined by the interviewer and based on clinical judgment.

To briefly review the Diagnostic Module's questions, those opposite criterion A are straightforward ways of asking about preoccupation with appearance. An alternative question is "Some people are very bothered by the way they look. Is this a problem for you? Tell me about it." This can then be followed by "How often do you think about it? (For example, at least an hour a day?)"

The concern must relate to appearance and that the body part is unattractive, defective, or "not right" in terms of how it looks. As the module indicates, it's worth giving some examples of commonly disliked body parts by asking "What about the appearance of your face, skin, hair, nose, or the shape or size or other aspect of any other part of your body," because some people are too shy or embarrassed about their concerns to volunteer all of them. If the person can't identify a particular part, but indicates dislike of their entire face, or their overall appearance, this response is compatible with the diagnosis of BDD.

Finally, to meet criterion A, the questions about preoccupation should be asked. The question in parentheses about whether others have said the person is too concerned is optional. Some people with BDD will answer no

---

Body Dysmorphic Disorder Diagnostic Module

Have you ever been very worried about your appearance in any way?
If yes: What was your concern? Did you think (body part) was especially unattractive?

What about the appearance of your face, skin, hair, nose, or the shape/size/other aspect of any other part of your body?

Did this concern preoccupy you? That is, you thought about it a lot and wished you could worry about it less? (Did others say that you were more concerned about _____ than you should have been?)

What effect has this preoccupation had on your life? Has it caused you a lot of distress?

Has your concern had any effect on your family or friends?

(If concern is completely attributable to Anorexia Nervosa, do not diagnose BDD)

A. Preoccupation with an imagined defect in appearance. If a slight physical anomaly is present, the person's concern is markedly excessive

Note: *Give some examples even if person answers no to these questions.*
Examples include: skin concerns (e.g., acne, scars, wrinkles, paleness), hair concerns (e.g., thinning), or the shape or size of the nose, jaw, lips, etc. Also consider perceived defects of hands, genitals, or any other body part.

B. Preoccupation causes clinically significant distress **or** impairment in social, occupational, or other important areas of functioning.

Note: *If slight physical defect is present, concern is clearly excessive*

C. The preoccupation is not better accounted for by another mental disorder (e.g., dissatisfaction with body shape and size in Anorexia Nervosa).

---

to this question because they've never told anyone about their concern. Such a response should not be counted against the diagnosis.

The questions used to determine whether distress or impairment are present (criterion B) usually need to be followed up by additional questions created by the questioner. Asking the person to say more about their distress, to get a better sense for how severe it is, and asking for examples of impairment, are useful.

Criterion C doesn't have any questions accompanying it, because the interviewer is expected to be familiar with anorexia nervosa and its diagnostic criteria, which are provided in DSM-IV. A brief description of anorexia nervosa is given in Appendix A. Criterion C, as previously discussed, ascertains that people who have anorexia nervosa, without any other body image concerns, are not diagnosed with BDD. However, it's possible for a person to have both BDD and anorexia nervosa—for example, a significantly underweight person who thinks she's too fat (as a symptom of anorexia) can also have BDD preoccupations, such as thinking she has a huge and ugly mole.

Criterion C also applies to disorders such as bulimia nervosa; that is, body-image concerns that are better accounted for by bulimia nervosa are not diagnosed as BDD. But, as with anorexia, an individual can have both BDD and bulimia. While criterion C is usually easy to assess, it's occasionally difficult. As discussed in Chapter 12, differentiating BDD from anorexia nervosa and bulimia nervosa is occasionally a complicated clinical judgment.

A person who—on the basis of the questions in the Diagnostic Module, as well as additional questions determined by the interviewer—meets BDD criteria A, B, and C is considered to have BDD.

Available data indicate that the BDD Diagnostic Module has excellent interrater reliability (kappa = 96). That is, two clinicians who assess individuals in separate interviews with the Diagnostic Module are able agree on whether the diagnosis is present in a high percentage of cases.

A fair amount of clinical judgment may be necessary to determine whether the criteria for BDD are met; in particular, determining whether distress or impairment are severe enough to qualify for a psychiatric diagnosis requires clinical judgment. Indeed, criterion B specifies that distress or impairment must be "clinically significant." Such judgment is also needed to ascertain whether particular body-image concerns are a feature of an eating disorder or BDD. The more severe and classic the BDD symptoms are, the more obvious it is that BDD is the correct diagnosis. But clinical judgment is particularly important when assessing less classic cases, cases with features of both BDD and an eating disorder, and milder BDD, which must be differentiated from normal concern. Thus, in general, the ratings should depend on the patient's report, but the final rating is based on the interviewer's clinical judgment.

I've also developed a longer version of the BDD Diagnostic Module, which additionally assesses insight, whether the disorder is currently present (i.e., present during the past month) or present only in the past, what percentage of the past five years the symptoms have been present, and at what age the disorder began.

The BDDQ:
A Self-Report Screening Instrument
for BDD

The BDDQ, or Body Dysmorphic Disorder Questionnaire, is a self-report screening instrument for BDD that is filled out by the patient, as was shown in Chapter 4. A person who appears to have BDD according to this instrument should ideally be seen by a clinician to confirm the diagnosis—to determine that the defect is actually nonexistent or minimal, and whether distress or impairment are clinically significant.

Available data suggest that there is excellent agreement between the BDDQ and a clinician's judgment of whether BDD is present (as assessed with the BDD Diagnostic Module). I and my colleagues, Drs. Katherine Atala and Harrison Pope of Harvard Medical School, found that the BDDQ had a sensitivity of 100% and a specificity of 89% among 66 individuals with a psychiatric diagnosis. What this means is that in a group of individuals who are judged by a clinician to really have BDD, the BDDQ will accurately ascertain that BDD is present in 100% of the cases. And in a group of individuals whom a clinician judges really don't have BDD, the BDDQ will accurately determine that BDD is *not* present in 89% of the cases. These data were obtained in a psychiatric setting; whether the BDDQ agrees as well with the Diagnostic Module in other settings, such as a surgical setting, has yet to be determined.

An advantage of the BDDQ over the clinician-administered BDD Diagnostic Module is that the possible presence of BDD can be assessed when a clinician isn't available to use the Diagnostic Module. Because the BDDQ is a brief self-report instrument, larger numbers of people can be easily assessed. In addition, some people might feel less self-conscious when filling out a self-report form and more willing to reveal their concerns.

The BDD-YBOCS:
A Measure of Severity

There are several methods for assessing the severity of BDD. These include the Yale-Brown Obsessive Compulsive Scale Modified for BDD (BDD–Y-BOCS), the Clinical Global Impression Scale, and the NIMH Obsessive Compulsive Scale Modified for BDD.

The Yale-Brown Obsessive Compulsive Scale (Y-BOCS) modified for BDD (the BDD-YBOCS) is a particularly useful instrument for assessing the severity of BDD. The BDD–YBOCS is based on the Y-BOCS, which was developed in the 1980s to assess the severity of obsessive compulsive disorder (OCD). The Y-BOCS is the standard rating scale to assess severity of OCD. It was developed by researchers at Yale University School of Medicine and Brown University School of Medicine (Drs. Wayne Goodman, Lawrence Price, Steven Rasmussen, Carolyn Mazure, Pedro Delgado, Roberta Fleischmann, Candy Hill, George Heninger, and Dennis Charney). Because of the many similarities between BDD and OCD, the Y-BOCS was slightly modified by Eric Hollander and myself to assess the current severity of BDD. Other researchers involved in its development are Bonnie Aronowitz, Concetta DeCaria, Steven Rasmussen, and Wayne Goodman.

The BDD–YBOCS rates the severity of BDD symptoms during the past week. The first five items rate BDD-related *thoughts,* and the second five items rate BDD-related *behaviors.* The BDD–YBOCS also includes two additional items: item 11 (insight) and item 12 (avoidance).

This rating scale, like the BDD Diagnostic Module, is intended for use as a semi-structured interview, meaning that the interviewer should assess the items in the listed order and use the questions provided. However, additional questions can be asked to clarify responses. In general, the ratings should depend on the patient's report, but the final rating is based on the interviewer's clinical judgment.

If the person being assessed volunteers information at any time during the interview, that information should be considered. Ratings should be based primarily on reports and observations gained during the interview. Each item is rated for the time period *during the past week* up until and including the time of the interview. Scores should reflect the average occurrence of each item for the entire week. For questions 1 through 5 (which rate BDD-related thoughts), the *total* (composite) effect of *all* body parts of concern are rated. For items 6 though 10 (which rate BDD-related behaviors), the *total* (composite) effect of *all* behaviors is also rated.

Before proceeding with questions 1 to 5, the rater must first determine that the person has BDD and must identify the body parts the person is excessively concerned with. The previously described BDD Diagnostic Module can be used for this purpose.

Associated behaviors, which are inquired about with questions 6 through 10, must also be identified before proceeding with the BDD–YBOCS. They can be identified by asking the person whether they engage in any behaviors in association with the appearance concern. The behaviors on page 329 should be specifically asked about to determine whether they are present.

Body Dysmorphic Disorder Modification of the Y–BOCS (BDD–YBOCS)

For each item, circle the number identifying the response that best characterizes the patient during the **past week**.

1. **Time occupied by thoughts about body defect**

   How much of your time is occupied by **THOUGHTS** (*not* including associated behaviors) about a defect or flaw in your appearance (such as your face, nose, hair, skin, breasts, genitals, hands?)

   0 = None
   1 = Mild (less than 1 hr/day)
   2 = Moderate (1–3 hrs/day)
   3 = Severe (greater than 3 and up to 8 hrs/day)
   4 = Extreme (greater than 8 hrs/day)

2. **Interference due to thoughts about body defect**

   How much do your **THOUGHTS** about your body defect(s) interfere with your social or work (role) functioning? Is there anything you aren't doing or can't do because of them?

   0 = None
   1 = Mild, slight interference with social or occupational activities, but overall performance not impaired.
   2 = Moderate, definite interference with social or occupational performance, but still manageable.
   3 = Severe, causes substantial impairment in social or occupational performance.
   4 = Extreme, incapacitating.

3. **Distress associated with thoughts about body defect**

   How much distress do your **THOUGHTS** about your body defect(s) cause you? (Rate "disturbing" feelings or anxiety that seem to be triggered by these thoughts, *not* general anxiety or anxiety associated with other symptoms.)

   0 = None.
   1 = Mild, and not too disturbing.
   2 = Moderate and disturbing but still manageable.
   3 = Severe and very disturbing.
   4 = Extreme and disabling distress.

continued

BDD Modification of the Y–BOCS (continued)

4. **Resistance against thoughts of body defect**

   How much of an effort do you make to resist these **THOUGHTS?** How often do you try to disregard them or turn your attention away from these thoughts as they enter your mind? (Only rate effort made to resist, NOT success or failure in actually controlling the thoughts. How much patient resists may or may not correlate with ability to control them.)

   0 = Makes an effort to always resist, or symptoms so minimal doesn't need to actively resist.
   1 = Tries to resist most of time.
   2 = Makes some effort to resist.
   3 = Yields to all such thoughts without attempting to control them but yields with some reluctance.
   4 = Completely and willingly yields to all such thoughts.

5. **Degree of control over thoughts about body defect**

   How much control do you have over your **THOUGHTS** about your body defect(s)? How successful are you in stopping or diverting these thoughts?

   0 = Complete control, or no need for control because thoughts are so minimal.
   1 = Much control, usually able to stop or divert these thoughts with some effort and concentration.
   2 = Moderate control, sometimes able to stop or divert these thoughts.
   3 = Little control, rarely successful in stopping thoughts, can only divert attention with difficulty.
   4 = No control, experienced as completely involuntary, rarely able to even momentarily divert attention.

6. **Time spent in activities related to body defect**

   How much time do you spend in **ACTIVITIES** related to your concern over your appearance or a body defect, (such as, but not limited to, mirror checking, trying to conceal the defect, or

   0 = None
   1 = Mild (spends less than 1 hr/day)
   2 = Moderate (1–3 hrs/day)
   3 = Severe (spends more than 3 and up to 8 hrs/day)
   4 = Extreme (spends more than 8 hrs/day in these activities)

continued

BDD Modification of the Y–BOCS (continued)

consulting plastic surgeons or dermatologists or undergoing surgical procedures to correct the defect)?

Read list of activities (check all that apply)

__ Checking mirrors/other surfaces

__ Rearranging/selecting clothing

__ Grooming activities

__ Applying makeup

__ Camouflaging with clothing and other things

__ Scrutinizing others' appearance/comparing

__ Questioning others about your appearance

__ Skin picking

__ Touching

__ Other_____

7. *Interference* due to activities related to the body defect

   How much do the above **ACTIVITIES** interfere with your social or work (role) functioning? Is there anything you don't do because of them?

   0 = None
   1 = Mild, slight interference with social or occupational activities, but overall performance not impaired.
   2 = Moderate, definite interference with social or occupational performance, but still manageable.
   3 = Severe, causes substantial impairment in social or occupational performance.
   4 = Extreme, incapacitating.

8. *Distress* associated with behaviors related to body defect

   How would you feel if prevented from performing these **ACTIVITIES**? [Pause] How anxious would you become?

   0 = None
   1 = Mild, only slightly anxious if behavior prevented, or only slight anxiety during the behavior.
   2 = Moderate, reports that anxiety would mount but remain manageable if behavior is prevented or

continued

BDD Modification of the Y–BOCS (continued)

that anxiety increases but remains manageable during such behavior.

3 = Severe, prominent and very disturbing increase in anxiety if behavior is interrupted, or prominent and very disturbing increase in anxiety during the behavior.

4 = Extreme, incapacitating anxiety from any intervention aimed at modifying activity, or incapacitating anxiety develops during behavior related to body defect.

9. *Resistance* against compulsions

How much of an effort do you make to resist these **ACTIVITIES**? (How much the patient resists these behaviors may not correlate with his/her ability to control them.)

0 = Makes an effort to always resist, or symptoms so minimal doesn't need to actively resist.

1 = Tries to resist most of the time.

2 = Makes some effort to resist.

3 = Yields to almost all of these behaviors without attempting to control them, but does so with some reluctance.

4 = Completely and willingly yields to all behaviors related to body defect.

10. *Degree of control* over compulsive behaviors

How strong is the drive to perform the behaviors? [Pause] How much control do you have over them?

0 = Complete control, or control is unnecessary because symptoms are mild.

1 = Much control, experiences pressure to perform the behavior, but usually able to exercise voluntary control over it.

2 = Moderate control, strong

continued

BDD Modification of the Y–BOCS (continued)

pressure to perform behavior, can control it only with difficulty.

3 = Little control, very strong drive to perform behavior, must be carried to completion, can delay only with difficulty.

4 = No control, drive to perform behavior experienced as completely involuntary and overpowering, rarely able to even momentarily delay activity.

11. *Insight*

Is it possible that your defect might be less noticeable or less ugly than you think it is?

How convinced are you that (body part) is as unattractive as you think it is?

Can anyone convince you that it doesn't look so bad?

0 = Excellent insight, fully rational.

1 = Good insight. Readily acknowledges absurdity or unreasonableness of thoughts or behaviors but does not seem completely convinced that there isn't something besides anxiety to be concerned about.

2 = Fair insight. Reluctantly admits that thoughts or behavior seem unreasonable but wavers. May have some unrealistic fears, but no fixed convictions.

3 = Poor insight. Maintains that thoughts or behaviors are not unreasonable.

4 = Lacks insight, delusional. Definitely convinced that concerns and behavior are reasonable, unresponsive to contrary evidence.

continued

BDD Modification of the Y–BOCS (continued)

---

12. *Avoidance*

Have you been avoiding
doing anything, going any
place, or being with anyone
because of your thoughts or
behaviors related to your
body defect? (If YES, then
ask: How much do you
avoid? Rate degree to which
patient deliberately tries to
avoid things.)

0 = No deliberate avoidance.
1 = Mild, minimal avoidance.
2 = Moderate, some avoidance
    clearly present.
3 = Severe, much avoidance;
    avoidance prominant.
4 = Extreme, very extensive
    avoidance; patient avoids
    almost all activities.

- Checking mirrors or other reflecting surfaces (or checking directly without a mirror)
- Seeking reassurance about the appearance of the body part
- Asking others to look at or verify the existence of the "deformity"
- Requesting surgery, dermatologic treatment, or other treatment
- Comparing with others
- Touching the body part
- Grooming behaviors (e.g., hair combing, hair styling, or shaving)
- Skin picking
- Applying makeup
- Camouflaging (e.g., with makeup or with hats or other clothing)
- Rearranging or selecting clothing to hide the "defect"
- Other BDD-related behaviors (e.g., measuring, reading, dieting, weight lifting)

On repeated assessment, the body parts of concern and associated behaviors should be reviewed and, if necessary, revised to reflect currently active symptoms. This instrument can be used over time to assess improvement or worsening in the individual's symptoms.

I've assessed approximately 125 individuals with BDD with this instrument and have found an average score of 23.9 on the first 10 items (with a standard deviation of 6.6), which is similar to the average score found in patients with OCD. On the 12-item version, the average score was 28.5

(with a standard deviation of 7.8). This instrument has been found to have acceptable psychometric properties, with adequate interrater and test-retest reliability, frequency of item endorsement, internal consistency, and validity. It is also sensitive to improvement in symptoms with treatment. Psychometric properties of the 10-item and 12-item versions of the scale are comparable.

The CGI and NIMH OC Scale: Other Severity Measures

Several other scales are useful in assessing the severity of BDD. These scales differ from the BDD–YBOCS in that they rate severity of the disorder globally, with a single rating—for example, "moderately ill." They don't have separate items, nor do they provide questions to be asked by a clinician. The Clinical Global Impressions Scale (CGI) is a 7-point scale that is used in research of many psychiatric disorders; it measures current global severity of the disorder and can also be used to rate improvement or worsening in symptoms with treatment. The NIMH (National Institute of Mental Health) Global Obsessive-Compulsive Scale is a 15-point global rating scale that was developed for OCD and can be easily adapted to assess BDD.

Appendix C

Co-occurrence of BDD
and Other Disorders

Table 13 on the next page shows the rate of BDD among individuals with other psychiatric disorders. These rates were obtained by the researchers indicated in the table's footnotes.

Table 14 shows the converse: the rates of other psychiatric disorders among the approximately 200 individuals with BDD whom I, Dr. Susan McElroy, and Dr. Katherine Atala have assessed. The presence of these coexisting disorders were determined with the Structured Clinical Interview for DSM-III-R (the SCID), previously discussed in Appendix B. A disorder is considered to be current if criteria have been fulfilled during the past month. The lifetime percentage indicates whether the disorder has *ever* been present, either currently or in the past.

While most of the people we saw had at least one other psychiatric disorder, this might reflect a bias. People who see a clinician may be more likely to have multiple disorders than those who don't—the greater number of symptoms may impel them to seek help. The rate of these other disorders is probably lower in nonclinical populations.

While the severity of depression varies, in people with BDD it's often fairly severe. On the Beck Depression Inventory, a self-report measure of depression severity, I found that people with BDD had an average score of 23.3, which is in the moderate to severe range. A majority of those who filled out the scale scored in the extremely severe range. This finding is consistent with several published studies that suggest an association between BDD and depression. A study of dermatology patients by Hardy and Cotterill, for example, found that five of 12 patients with BDD were moderately or severely depressed, compared with none of the comparison subjects

Table 13   Percentage of Individuals with Other Disorders Who Have BDD

Psychiatric Disorder	Percent
MAJOR DEPRESSION	
Typical major depression	5% (8 of 156)
Atypical major depression	14% (12 of 87)
Total	8% (20/243)[a]
SOCIAL PHOBIA	11% (6 of 53)[b]
OBSESSIVE COMPULSIVE DISORDER	37% (25 of 68)[c]
	24% (158 of 646)[d]
	15% (9 of 62)[e]
	12% (51 of 442)[f]
	8% (4 of 53)[b]
TRICHOTILLOMANIA	26% (6 of 23)[g,j]
PANIC DISORDER	2% (1 of 47)[b]
GENERALIZED ANXIETY DISORDER	0% (0 of 32)[b]
POST-TRAUMATIC STRESS DISORDER	20% (11 of 55)[h]
PSYCHIATRIC OUTPATIENTS WITH VARIOUS DISORDERS	12% (60 of 500)[i,j]

[a] Nierenberg AA, Uebelacker LA, Alpert JE, Worthington JJ, Tedlow JR, Phillips KA, Rosenbaum JF, Fava M
[b] Brawman-Mintzer O, Lydiard RB, Phillips KA, Morton A, Czepowicz V, Emmanuel N, Villareal G, Johnson M, Ballenger JC
[c] Simeon D, Hollander E, Stein DJ, Cohen L, Aronowitz B
[d] Hantouche EG, Bourgeois ML, Bouhassira M, Lancrenon S (the 646 subjects had definite or probable OCD or an OCD-spectrum disorder [e.g., trichotillomania])
[e] Phillips KA, Gunderson CG, McElroy SL, Mallya G, Carter W
[f] Simeon D, Hollander E, Stein DJ, Cohen L, Aronowitz B
[g] Soriano JL, O'Sullivan RL, Baer L, Phillips KA, McNally RJ, Jenike MA
[h] Zlotnick C, Phillips KA, Pearlstein T
[i] Zimmerman M, Mattia J, Phillips KA
[j] In these studies, a screening instrument (the BDDQ) was used, which may overestimate to some extent the rate of BDD

(who were healthy or had psoriasis), and that the BDD patients scored significantly higher as a group than the comparison subjects on the Beck Depression Inventory.

Table 14   Percentage of Individuals with BDD Who Have Another Disorder

Psychiatric Disorder	Current	Lifetime
MOOD DISORDERS		
Major depression	57%	83%
Bipolar disorder	8%	11%
Dysthymic disorder[a]	7%	
Total[b]	68%	93%
ANXIETY DISORDERS		
Panic disorder	4%	11%
Agoraphobia	1%	1%
Social phobia[c]	26%	36%
Specific phobia	4%	7%
Obsessive compulsive disorder	24%	29%
Total[b]	49%	62%
PSYCHOTIC DISORDERS[d]		
Schizophrenia	0%	0%
Schizoaffective disorder	1%	1%
Total	1%	1%
SUBSTANCE-RELATED DISORDERS		
Alcohol	6%	31%
Other drug	6%	25%
Total[b]	12%	41%
SOMATOFORM DISORDERS[a]		
Somatization disorder	1%	
Pain disorder	3%	
Hypochondriasis	3%	
Total[b]	6%	
EATING DISORDERS		
Anorexia nervosa	1%	4%
Bulimia nervosa	2%	7%
Total[b]	3%	10%

[a] The lifetime columns are blank because the SCID assesses only the current presence of these disorders.

[b] Because some individuals had more than one disorder in a given category, the total for that category may be smaller than the sum of the individual disorders in the category. For example, 4% of individuals had lifetime anorexia nervosa, 7% had lifetime bulimia, but 1% had both anorexia and bulimia, so the total lifetime percent for the eating disorder category is 10%, not 11%.

[c] This rate applies only to "primary" social phobia—that is, social phobia that doesn't appear to be largely due to BDD. If social phobia due to BDD were included, the percentages would be much higher.

[d] Excluding delusional BDD.

Appendix D

Family History

Table 15   Family History[a,b]

Psychiatric Disorder	Percent (%) of Relatives Affected
MOOD DISORDERS	
Major depression	17
Bipolar disorder	3
ANXIETY DISORDERS	
Panic disorder and/or agoraphobia	4
Obsessive compulsive disorder	4
PSYCHOTIC DISORDERS	
Schizophrenia	0
Schizoaffective disorder	0
SUBSTANCE-RELATED DISORDERS	
Alcohol	17
Other drug	7
EATING DISORDERS	
Anorexia nervosa	1
Bulimia nervosa	3
BODY DYSMORPHIC DISORDER	11

[a]Information was obtained for 219 first-degree relatives (parents, brothers, sisters, or children of the BDD sufferer) who are age 16 or older.
[b]Family history was obtained by the family history method—that is, by asking people with BDD whether their family members had any psychiatric disorders. Because relatives weren't interviewed directly, some of the percentages in the table may be underestimates, especially for disorders that can be kept secret from family members (such as obsessive compulsive disorder, bulimia, and drug abuse).

Information on what psychiatric disorders tend to run in families of BDD sufferers, and how commonly they do, is currently limited. While the data presented in table 15, which is from my own work, provides us with some clues, much larger family studies are needed to provide more definitive information about this. I hope that in the future twin studies will also be done, as they will shed light on the relative contribution of genetic and environmental factors in BDD.

Glossary

Antidepressant A class of medications effective in the treatment of depression as well as a variety of disorders, such as dysthymia, panic disorder, social phobia, eating disorders, obsessive compulsive disorder, hypochondriasis, and others. Certain antidepressants are also used to treat nonpsychiatric disorders, such as headache and pain syndromes. There are many different types of antidepressant medications.

Anxiety hierarchy A tool used in exposure therapy consisting of a list of situations that cause anxiety. The situations are rated according to how much anxiety they produce.

Augmentation The addition of a medication to a "primary" medication to boost its effect. This approach is commonly used for depression and other disorders.

BDD–YBOCS A scale that assesses severity of BDD symptoms during the past week.

Benzodiazepine A type of medication used primarily to treat anxiety and insomnia.

Buspirone (Buspar) A type of antianxiety medication with effects on serotonin.

Clomipramine (Anafranil) A type of serotonin-reuptake inhibitor (a class of antidepressant medications with antiobsessional and anticompulsive properties).

Cognitive-behavioral therapy (CBT) A broad term that encompasses a number of specific therapeutic approaches. The *cognitive* aspect focuses on cognitions—that is, thoughts. The goal of cognitive therapy is to identify and change distorted and unrealistic ways of thinking. The *behavioral* aspect focuses on problematic behaviors, such as excessive checking and social avoidance. The aim is to stop performing such behaviors and substitute healthier behaviors. Often, cognitive and behavioral approaches are combined—hence, the commonly used term "cognitive-behavioral therapy," or CBT. CBT is used to treat depression, phobias, panic disorder, obsessive-compulsive disorder, eating disorders, and other disorders.

Compulsion A repetitive behavior (e.g., hand washing or checking) or mental act (e.g., counting) performed in response to an obsession and aimed at preventing or reducing distress or a dreaded event. May also be referred to as a "ritual." Compulsions are usually difficult to resist or control. They are characteristic of obsessive compulsive disorder and BDD (e.g., mirror checking and reassurance seeking).

Controlled study A type of study in which the treatment being investigated is compared to another type of treatment received by a "control group." The control group may receive a standard and proven treatment, a competing treatment, no treatment (e.g., they may be on a treatment waiting list), or a placebo. A placebo in a medication trial is an inert substance (e.g., a "sugar pill") that physically resembles the treatment under investigation. If treatment is shown in a controlled study to be as effective as a proven treatment, or more effective than placebo, this is strong evidence that the treatment is effective.

Delusion (delusional thinking) A false belief based on incorrect inference about external reality that is firmly sustained despite what almost everyone else believes.

Delusional BDD A form of BDD in which the belief about the defect is held with absolute conviction and certainty. This form of BDD is probably the same disorder as the nondelusional form of BDD, in which the person can acknowledge that their view of the defect may be distorted or inaccurate.

Diagnostic instrument   A questionnaire filled out by patients, or a set of questions asked by clinicians, that is used to make psychiatric diagnoses. Usually, the instrument asks questions that determine whether DSM criteria for a disorder are met.

Dopamine   One of the brain's many neurotransmitters (chemical messengers transmitted between nerve cells). Dopamine plays an important role in certain movement disorders and in many psychiatric disorders, especially those characterized by delusional thinking and hallucinations.

DSM   DSM stands for Diagnostic and Statistical Manual of Mental Disorders. It contains the official classification and nomenclature system for psychiatric disorders used in the U.S. Disorders in DSM are defined by diagnostic criteria that describe their essential features.

   DSM-III-R   The version of DSM in use from 1987 to 1993.

   DSM-IV   The current version of DSM, published in 1994.

Dysmorphophobia   A previous term for BDD. It is sometimes used in a broader sense than BDD, to refer not only to the specific disorder BDD but to any excessive preoccupation with a minimal or nonexistent defect in appearance.

Electroconvulsive therapy (ECT)   Also known as shock therapy, this is a very effective treatment for depression. It is often reserved for more severe depression that hasn't responded to antidepressant medication.

Exposure and response prevention   A type of cognitive-behavioral therapy effective for obsessive compulsive disorder and other disorders. *Exposure* consists of facing feared and avoided situations—for example, social situations or work. Types of exposure consist of "graded exposure," in which exposure is done gradually, and "flooding," in which it is done quickly. Response prevention consists of not engaging in compulsive behaviors.

Fluoxetine (Prozac)   A type of serotonin-reuptake inhibitor (a class of antidepressant medications with antiobsessional and anticompulsive properties).

Fluvoxamine (Luvox)   A type of serotonin-reuptake inhibitor (a class of antidepressant medications with antiobsessional and anticompulsive properties).

Hallucination A sensory perception that seems real but occurs without external stimulation of sensory organs. Hallucinations may be visual (involving sight), auditory (involving hearing), somatic (involving a bodily sensation), tactile (involving the skin), olfactory (involving smell), or gustatory (involving taste).

ICD-10 The current international classification and nomenclature system for medical and psychiatric disorders published by the World Health Organization. Its psychiatric classification system is very similar to that of DSM-IV.

Ideas of reference The belief that casual incidents and events have a special meaning that is specific to the person. This is a type of **referential thinking.**

Illusion A misperception or misinterpretation of a real external stimulus, such as hearing running water as the sound of whispering.

Insight-oriented psychotherapy Also known as psychodynamic or exploratory psychotherapy, this is a type of individual "talking therapy." It focuses on increasing self-awareness and bringing about behavioral change (e.g., improving relationships with others) through exploration of one's perceptions and interactions with others.

Insomnia A subjective complaint of difficulty sleeping.

Magical thinking The erroneous belief that one's thoughts, words, or actions will cause or prevent a specific outcome in a way that defies commonly understood laws of cause and effect.

MAOI (MAO inhibitor) A class of antidepressant medication.

Minoxidil A medication taken to promote hair growth.

Neuroleptic A type of medication used to treat Tourette's disorder, delusional disorder, schizophrenia, and other disorders. Neuroleptics may also be used in combination with other medication to treat obsessive compulsive disorder and certain types of major depression and manic depressive illness. They are also sometimes used to treat physical pain and nausea. Also known as an antipsychotic.

Neurotransmitter   A type of chemical messenger in the brain that transmits messages between neurons (nerve cells). There are many types of neurotransmitters, which include serotonin, norepinephrine, and dopamine. Abnormal functioning of brain neurotransmitters is implicated in many neurological and psychiatric disorders.

Obsession   A recurrent, persistent, and intrusive thought, impulse, or image that is difficult to dismiss despite its disturbing nature. Obsessional thinking is characteristic of obsessive compulsive disorder as well as BDD.

Obsessive compulsive spectrum disorders (OCD spectrum disorders)   A grouping of disorders postulated to be related to obsessive compulsive disorder on the basis of similarities in symptoms and other characteristics. BDD is considered an OCD spectrum disorder because of its many similarities to OCD.

Open study   An uncontrolled study in which both the patient and the doctor know what treatment the patient is receiving.

Overvalued idea   An unreasonable and sustained belief that is held with less than delusional intensity (i.e., the person is able to acknowledge the possibility that the belief may not be true). Synonymous with poor insight.

Paroxetine (Paxil)   A type of serotonin-reuptake inhibitor (a class of antidepressant medications with antiobsessional and anticompulsive properties.)

Pimozide (Orap)   A type of neuroleptic medication.

Placebo   In a medication trial, an inert substance, sometimes called a "sugar pill," that physically resembles the treatment being studied. The patient is unable to discriminate between the placebo pills and active treatment and is unaware of which treatment he or she is receiving. In a "double-blind" trial, the physician is also unaware of whether the patient is receiving placebo or active treatment. This study design guards against bias in assessing treatment outcome. If the treatment being studied is more effective than placebo, this is strong evidence that it is effective.

Prospective study   A study that is done "forward over time." In other words, such studies measure characteristics or events as they occur after the study has started. In contrast, retrospective studies are done "backward over time," in that they collect data about events that have already occurred.

Referential thinking The belief that casual incidents and events have a special meaning that is specific to the person. Includes ideas of reference and delusions of reference.

Response prevention An aspect of behavioral therapy in which behaviors, such as excessive mirror checking, are resisted.

Retrospective study A study done "backward over time"; in other words, data are collected about events that have already occurred. This is in contrast to a prospective study, in which data are collected about events or characteristics at the time they actually occur.

Ritual Another term for a compulsion—that is, a repetitive behavior (e.g., hand washing and checking) or mental act (e.g., counting) performed in response to an obsession and aimed at preventing or reducing distress or a dreaded event.

Selective serotonin-reuptake inhibitor (SSRI) A type of serotonin-reuptake inhibitor (SRI) that has prominent effects on serotonin but little direct effect on other neurotransmitters. The SSRIs are fluoxetine (Prozac), fluvoxamine (Luvox), paroxetine (Paxil), and sertraline (Zoloft). (Clomipramine [Anafranil] also has fairly prominent effects on the neurotransmitter norepinephrine.)

Serotonin One of the many neurotransmitters (chemical messengers) in the brain. Serotonin plays an important role in mood, sleep, appetite, pain, and other bodily functions. Malfunctioning of serotonin is involved in a wide variety of psychiatric disorders, including depression, obsessive compulsive disorder, and eating disorders. It probably plays an important role in BDD.

Serotonin-reuptake inhibitor (SRI) A class of antidepressant medication with prominent effects on serotonin. Unlike other antidepressants, SRIs have anti-obsessional and anti-compulsive properties, and they effectively treat obsessive compulsive disorder. The SRIs currently marketed in the U.S. are clomipramine (Anafranil), fluoxetine (Prozac), fluvoxamine (Luvox), paroxetine (Paxil), and sertraline (Zoloft).

Sertraline (Zoloft) A type of serotonin-reuptake inhibitor (a class of antidepressant medications with antiobsessional and anticompulsive properties).

Supportive psychotherapy   A type of talking therapy that focuses on the creation of emotional support and a stable, caring relationship with patients. The therapist focuses more on providing support than on increasing patients' understanding of themselves. Advice, learning new social skills, and assistance in problem solving are often components of this approach.

Yale-Brown Obsessive Compulsive Scale (Y-BOCS)   A scale developed by Dr. Wayne Goodman and his colleagues which is the most widely used instrument to assess the severity of obsessive compulsive disorder. A slightly modified version has been developed to assess severity of BDD.

Index